EMOTION REGULATION IN PSYCHOTHERAPY

Emotion Regulation in Psychotherapy

Robert L. Leahy
Dennis Tirch
Lisa A. Napolitano

THE GUILFORD PRESS
New York   London

© 2011 Robert L. Leahy, Dennis Tirch, and Lisa A. Napolitano
Published by The Guilford Press
A Division of Guilford Publications, Inc.
72 Spring Street, New York, NY 10012
www.guilford.com

Printed in the United States of America

This book is printed on acid-free paper.

Last digit is print number: 9   8   7   6   5   4   3   2

The authors have checked with sources believed to be reliable in their efforts to provide
information that is complete and generally in accord with the standards of practice that are
accepted at the time of publication. However, in view of the possibility of human error or
changes in behavioral, mental health, or medical sciences, neither the authors, nor the editor and
publisher, nor any other party who has been involved in the preparation or publication of this
work warrants that the information contained herein is in every respect accurate or complete, and
they are not responsible for any errors or omissions or the results obtained from the use of such
information. Readers are encouraged to confirm the information contained in this book with other
sources.

Library of Congress Cataloging-in-Publication Data

Leahy, Robert L.
    Emotion regulation in psychotherapy : a practitioner's guide / by Robert L. Leahy,
Dennis Tirch, and Lisa A. Napolitano.
        p. ; cm.
    Includes bibliographical references and index.
    ISBN 978-1-60918-483-4 (pbk. : alk. paper)
    1. Cognitive therapy.   2. Emotions—Psychological aspects.   3. Psychotherapy.   I. Tirch,
Dennis D., 1968–   II. Napolitano, Lisa A..   III. Title.
    [DNLM: 1. Cognitive Therapy.   2. Adaptation, Psychological.   3. Emotions.
4. Psychotherapy.   5. Stress, Psychological—psychology.   WM 425.5.C6]
    RC489.C63L383 2011
    616.89′1425—dc23
                                                                        2011014843

To Helen
—R. L. L.

To Jaclyn Marie Tirch
—D. T.

To my clients—some of my best teachers
—L. A. N.

About the Authors

Robert L. Leahy, PhD, is Director of the American Institute for Cognitive Therapy in New York and Clinical Professor of Psychology in the Department of Psychiatry at Weill Cornell Medical College in New York. He is the author or editor of 19 books on cognitive therapy and psychological processes, including the professional books *Cognitive Therapy Techniques*, *Overcoming Resistance in Cognitive Therapy*, and *Treatment Plans and Interventions for Depression and Anxiety Disorders* (second edition), and the popular books *The Worry Cure* and *Beat the Blues before They Beat You*. Dr. Leahy is Past President of the Association for Behavioral and Cognitive Therapies, the International Association for Cognitive Psychotherapy, and the Academy of Cognitive Therapy. He is a recipient of the Aaron T. Beck Award for Sustained and Enduring Contributions to Cognitive Therapy. He has given workshops worldwide and has appeared frequently in the popular media.

Dennis Tirch, PhD, is Associate Director and Director of Clinical Services for the American Institute for Cognitive Therapy, Adjunct Assistant Clinical Professor at Weill Cornell Medical College, and Founder and Director of The Center for Mindfulness and Compassion Focused CBT. He is a Diplomate and Fellow of the Academy of Cognitive Therapy, a Founding Member and President of the New York City chapter of the Association for Contextual Behavioral Science, and a Founding Fellow, Board Member at Large, and Technology Chairperson of the New York City Cognitive Behavioral Therapy Association. Dr. Tirch has coauthored several journal articles and book chapters on cognitive-behavioral, mindfulness-based, and compassion-focused therapies, and three books on mindfulness, acceptance, and compassion. With Robert L. Leahy, Dr. Tirch is involved in an active, ongoing research program examining the role of emotional schema theory in human wellness and psychological flexibility.

Lisa A. Napolitano, JD, PhD, is Founder and Director of CBT/DBT Associates in New York and Adjunct Clinical Instructor in the Department of Psychiatry at New York University School of Medicine. She is Director of CBT Training in China for the Beijing Suicide Prevention Project and past Chair of the International Training Committee of the International Association for Cognitive Psychotherapy. Dr. Napolitano is a Diplomate and Fellow of the Academy of Cognitive Therapy and a Founding Fellow of the New York City Cognitive Behavioral Therapy Association.

Acknowledgments

Robert L. Leahy and Dennis Tirch: We wish to acknowledge the many researchers and clinicians worldwide whose work has influenced us. We would like to thank the following people for their contributions to the field of cognitive-behavioral therapy and emotion regulation: Aaron T. Beck, David Burns, James Gross, John Teasdale, Jon Kabat-Zinn, Leslie Greenberg, Steven K. Hayes, Tom Borkovec, Adrian Wells, Christopher Fairburn, Mark Williams, Zindel Segal, Marsha Linehan, Kelly Wilson, Francisco Varela, Joseph LeDoux, Edna Foa, Marylene Cloitre, Paul Gilbert, Richard Lazarus, Christopher Germer, Kristen Neff, Paul Ekman, and Douglas Mennin. Poonam Melwani has been an invaluable editorial and research assistant throughout this project, and her dedication and attention to detail are greatly appreciated. The many staff members and trainees at the American Institute for Cognitive Therapy over the years have been especially helpful in clarifying and testing many of these ideas. In particular, we would like to thank Laura Oliff and Jenny Taitz. Finally, the editorial staff at The Guilford Press provided support and valuable suggestions for improvement all along the way. Louise Farkas, Senior Production Editor, was especially helpful in the editing process, and Jim Nageotte, Senior Editor, has been a valuable guide from the very beginning. We also are deeply indebted to our wonderful wives, Helen and Jaclyn, and are honored to dedicate this book to them.

Dennis Tirch: I would like to thank all of my teachers in meditation disciplines, particularly Stephen K. Hayes, Richard Amodio, Robert Fripp, Paul Kahn, and Lillian Firestone, as well as fellow travelers in compassion-focused therapy, Russell Kolts, Mary Welford, Choden, and Chris Irons. Of course, I would also like to acknowledge the lessons in wisdom and compassion that I learned from my mother and brother, Janet and John.

Lisa A. Napolitano: I would like to acknowledge with deep appreciation the work of Marsha Linehan and Aaron T. Beck, the two primary influences in my development of techniques to help clients with emotion regulation. I am also indebted to the work of K. Elaine Williams, Anthony Ahrens, and Dianne Chambless. Their extension of the fear-of-fear construct piqued my research and clinical interest in how beliefs about emotions contribute to emotion regulation difficulties. I would like to thank my colleagues at CBT/DBT Associates, who have provided encouragement throughout the project and acted as a sounding board for many of my ideas, in particular, Annalise Caron, Arielle Freedberg, and Samantha Monk. The suggestions and assistance of the editorial team at The Guilford Press, especially Jim Nageotte, Senior Editor, and Jane Keislar, Senior Assistant Editor, are greatly appreciated. Finally, I would like to thank two mentors at Georgetown University, James T. Lamiell and Daniel N. Robinson. Without their genuine interest in and nurturing of my neophyte understanding of psychology, I might have just remained that impressionable young lawyer they first met in the summer of 1996.

Preface

The idea for this book began at a case conference at the American Institute for Cognitive Therapy in New York City, where we were collaborating in discussions about various clinical problems that arise in doing cognitive-behavioral therapy (CBT). One of us (R. L. L.), the director of the Institute, was eager to foster an openness of discussion about how various theoretical orientations or clinical approaches can be utilized for a variety of problems. In discussing clinical dilemmas and roadblocks, our view was that each theoretical approach might have some legitimacy and that to be tied to any one approach might limit the flexibility and, therefore, the effectiveness of the therapist. Since emotion regulation appeared to be a recurrent issue for our patients, we agreed to a joint collaboration. This book is the product of those meetings.

Why "emotion regulation"? Experienced clinicians realize that one of the most troubling experiences for patients is the experience of being overwhelmed by their emotions and not knowing how to cope with their intensity. As a result, some patients turn to problematic ways of coping, such as alcohol or drug abuse, binge eating, purging, blaming other people, compulsive reliance on pornography, rumination, worry, and other self-defeating strategies. Many patients avoid situations that elicit "problematic emotions" or remain passive and withdrawn, further adding to their sense of ineffectiveness and depression. Others blame either themselves or others for their feelings, leading to greater escalation of depression or alienation from important sources of support. Once emotions are aroused and reach a level of intensity that becomes problematic, it may be especially difficult to utilize traditional cognitive techniques for restructuring, thereby promoting further stress. It may also make it difficult to employ behavioral techniques, especially exposure techniques, that involve engaging in behavior that arouses anxiety, since they may further exacerbate emotional turmoil. Developing capacities for tolerating and regulating emotional responses may help patients to broaden the range of behaviors and responses that they have available in times of intense distress. Indeed, more "conventional" forms of CBT may need to await the calming of emotion. These dilemmas are also the focus of this book.

We recognize the importance of the work of many people in the field of emotion regulation and are indebted to the work of others on emotion theory, especially Richard Lazarus, Robert Zajonc, James Gross, Paul Ekman, Antonio Damasio, John D. Mayer, Peter Salovey, Kevin Ochsner, Joseph LeDoux, Jeffrey A. Gray, Joseph Forgas, Nancy Eisenberg, George Bonanno, Susan Harter, and Francisco Varela. For clinical models for intervention, we owe a great deal to Marsha Linehan, Steven K. Hayes, Aaron T. Beck, John M. Gottman, Adrian Wells, Leslie Greenberg, Paul Gilbert, Jon Kabat-Zinn, and many more. As a practitioner's guide, the book cannot do justice to the burgeoning literature in psychology, psychiatry, neuroscience, and other specializations, but we hope that we have given the reader sufficient information to provide some context for the interventions and ideas proposed in this book—and, more important, to activate enough curiosity to seek out additional literature elsewhere.

We have organized many of the ideas in this book around Leahy's emotional schema therapy (EST) model. According to this model, individuals' differences in interpretations, evaluations, action tendencies, and behavioral strategies for their emotions are referred to as "emotional schemas." Some individuals have negative beliefs about their emotions, such as the belief that their emotions do not make sense, will last indefinitely and overwhelm them, are shameful, are unique to them, cannot be expressed, and will never be validated. These individuals are more likely to utilize problematic styles of coping, such as rumination, worry, avoidance, drinking, bingeing, or dissociating. Others have more positive or "adaptive" views of emotion and are less inclined to experience avoidance, are more willing to express emotion, and are more able to obtain validation. Their emotions make sense to them. They are acceptable, not shameful, not unique, not long-lasting, but are viewed as temporary. As a result, such people are less likely to use problematic strategies for coping.

Each clinical chapter is integrated into an emotional schema conceptualization. Thus, acceptance- and willingness-focused techniques (Chapter 6) may help patients to modify their relationship to destructive emotional schemas or may help to modify these schemas themselves. Dialectical behavior therapy techniques (Chapter 4) may help modify the emotion myths that some patients endorse and may suggest more adaptive skills for distress tolerance and emotion regulation. Compassion-focused therapy (Chapter 7) may help patients soothe their emotions and, thereby, modify their experience of fearful and shame-based emotional schemas. Similarly, mindfulness (Chapter 5) may help patients recognize that emotions need not be controlled or suppressed, but can be tolerated and accepted through the deployment of flexible, focused attention in the present moment. Emotional processing and emotional intelligence (Chapter 8) help encourage the observation, differentiation, and use of emotions to achieve greater meaning. EST (Chapter 2) identifies a number of interventions to directly address negative beliefs about emotion, and validation (Chapter 3) helps identify problematic beliefs about receiving support (such as the belief that one must have exact mirroring to get validation). Cognitive restructuring (Chapter 9) and stress reduction (Chapter 10) provide ideas and strategies for coping more effectively, either through behavioral change or cognitive appraisal, so as to lessen the elicitation of difficult emotional experiences.

Although EST is an overarching heuristic or case conceptualization for the book, readers need not adopt the theory to benefit from the use of techniques outlined here. Our view, though, is that therapy is often enhanced by case conceptualization, and not just reliance on sampling one technique after another. Although there are many models for case conceptualization, our view is that EST provides an overarching, integrative model for how the therapist and patient can develop an understanding about the patient's emotional socialization and specific beliefs about particular emotions, a realization of how emotions are tied in with personal relationships, a delineation of problematic coping strategies and beliefs and ways to modify these strategies, and an opportunity to encourage more adaptive, humanizing, and self-accepting beliefs about emotion. As an integrative and open model, EST encourages the use of other conceptualizations and models for intervention. The idea, though, is that interventions help patients learn about and cope with emotion, and this learning—a new model of emotion—is empowering.

It is our hope that this book will help patients to help themselves. We recognize that skilled and experienced therapists will explore novel ways of integrating techniques and ideas and that this openness and flexibility may be part of the adaptation of the therapist to the patient's needs. We are there both to help and to learn from our patients.

We now turn to the first question, "Why is emotion regulation important?"

ROBERT L. LEAHY
DENNIS TIRCH
LISA A. NAPOLITANO

Contents

List of Forms

CHAPTER ONE

Why Is Emotion Regulation Important?

All of us experience emotions of various kinds and attempt to cope with these emotions in either effective or ineffective ways. It is not the experience of anxiety that is the real problem. It is our ability to recognize our anxiety, accept it, use it if possible, and continue to function in spite of it. Without emotions, our lives would lack meaning, texture, richness, joy, and connection with others. Emotions tell us about our needs, our frustrations, and our rights—they motivate us to make changes, escape from difficult situations, or know when we are satisfied. Yet there are many people who find themselves overwhelmed by their emotions, fearful of their feelings, and unable to cope because they believe that their sadness or anxiety prohibits effective behavior. This book is aimed toward all clinicians who help these people cope more effectively with their emotions.

We view emotion as comprising a set of processes, no one of which is sufficient for us to call an experience an "emotion." Emotions, such as anxiety, include appraisal, sensation, intentionality (an object), a "feeling" (or "qualia"), motoric behavior, and, in most cases, an interpersonal component. Thus, when you have the emotion of "anxiety," you recognize that you are concerned that you will not get your work done on time (appraisal), you have a rapid heartbeat (sensation), you focus on your competence (intentionality), you have a dreaded feeling about life (feeling), you become physically agitated and restless (motoric behavior), and you might very well tell your partner that it is a bad day (interpersonal). Because of the multidimensional nature of emotion, clinicians can consider which dimension should be the first focus, choosing among a variety of approaches, each of them represented in this volume. For example, in choosing which techniques to use for which patients, clinicians can consider their technical options on the basis of the presenting problem of the moment. For example, if a patient's struggle with sensations of arousal was most problematic, the therapist might employ stress management techniques (e.g., relaxation, breathing exercises), acceptance-based interventions, emotional schema-focused strategies, or mindfulness. If the patient is confronted with a sense that a situation is overwhelming, the therapist might consider cognitive restructuring or problem solving to put things in perspective and to consider possible modifications of the stressful situation. Thus, emotion regulation may involve cognitive restructuring, relaxation, behavioral activation or goal setting, emotional schemas and affect tolerance, behavioral changes, and modifying problematic attempts to seek validation. In each of the chapters in this volume, we provide suggestions for clinicians in evaluating which techniques might be best for which patients.

Emotions have a long history in Western philosophy. Plato viewed emotions as part of a metaphor of the charioteer who attempts to control two horses: one that is easily tamed and needs no direction and the other that is wild and possibly dangerous. Stoic philosophers such as Epictetus, Cicero, and Seneca viewed emotion as the experience that misled the rational capability, which should always dominate and control decisions. In contrast, emotion and its expression have been highly valued in Western culture. Indeed, the pantheon of Greek gods represented a full range of emotions and dilemmas. Euripides' play *The Bacchae* represents the danger of ignoring and dishonoring the wild and free spirit of Dionysius. Emotion plays a central role in all of the major world religions that stress gratitude, compassion, awe, love, and even passion. The Romantic movement rebelled against the "rationality" of the Enlightenment, stressing the natural, free nature of man, the capability of creativity, excitement, novelty, intense love, and even the value of suffering. In Eastern religious tradition, Buddhist practice discusses emotions that are life affirming and those that are destructive, encouraging the individual to fully experience their range of emotions, while letting go of attachment to the permanence of any emotional state.

WHAT IS EMOTION REGULATION?

Individuals coping with stressful experience will experience increasing intensity of emotion, which, in itself, can be a further cause of stress and further escalation of emotion. For example, a man experiencing the dissolution of an intimate relationship experiences sadness, anger, anxiety, hopelessness, and even a feeling of relief. As these emotions become more intense, he may misuse drugs or alcohol, binge eat, lose sleep, act out sexually, or criticize himself. Once the emotions of anxiety, sadness, or anger have occurred, problematic styles of coping with the emotional intensity may determine whether his stressful life experience spirals into further problematic ways of coping. His emotional dysregulation may lead him to complain, pout, and attack or withdraw from others. He may ruminate on his emotions, trying to figure out what is really going on, which sinks him deeper into depression, isolation, and inactivity. Problematic styles of coping may temporarily reduce arousal (e.g., drinking reduces anxiety in the short term) but may exacerbate emotional coping later. These temporary solutions (bingeing, avoidance, rumination, and substance abuse) may work in the short term; however, the solutions may become the problem.

We define emotion dysregulation as difficulty or inability in coping with experience or processing emotions. Dysregulation may manifest as either excessive intensification of emotion or excessive deactivation of emotion. Excessive intensification of emotion includes any rise of the intensity of an emotion that is experienced by the individual as unwanted, intrusive, overwhelming, or problematic. Increases of emotion resulting in panic, terror, trauma, dread, or a sense of urgency that one is overwhelmed and has difficulty tolerating an emotion would qualify under these criteria. Excessive deactivation of emotion includes dissociative experiences, such as depersonalization and derealization, splitting, or emotional numbing in the context of experiences that would normally be expected to result in some felt intensity or magnitude of emotion. For example, in confronting a life-threatening event, a woman responds with a sense of emotional numbness and reports feeling like she was in another dimension of time and space while observing what seemed like a movie. This deactivation of emotion, marked by derealization, would be viewed as an atypical response to a traumatic event. Excessive deactivation of emotion impedes emotional processing and is part of a coping style of avoidance. However, there may be situations when deactivating or temporarily suppressing an emotion may assist in coping. For example, a first responder to a catastrophic event may be more adaptive by suppressing fear in the short term in order to cope with the situation in the present moment.

Emotion regulation may include any coping strategy (problematic or adaptive) that the individual uses when confronted with an unwanted intensity of emotion. It is important to recognize that emotion regulation is like a homeostatic thermostat. It can moderate emotions and keep them within a "manageable range" so that one can cope. Or the moderation—up or down—may offset things so extremely as to create a situation that is "too hot" or "too cold." Emotion regulation is like any coping style: It depends on the context, on the situation. It is not problematic or adaptive independent of the person and the situation at the present time.

Adaptation is defined here as the implementation of coping strategies that enhance the recognition and processing of useful responses that increase, either in the short term or long term, more productive functioning, as defined by valued goals and purposes held by the individual. Folkman and Lazarus (1988) have identified eight strategies for coping with emotion: confrontive (e.g., assertion), distancing, self-controlling, seeking social support, accepting responsibility, escape–avoidance, planful problem solving, and positive reappraisal. Coping with experience is part of emotional regulation. If the individual copes better—either by problem solving, asserting him- or herself, engaging in behavioral activation to seek more rewarding experiences, or reappraising the situation—his or her emotions are less likely to escalate. Examples of maladaptive strategies in coping with emotion include alcohol intoxication and self-cutting. These strategies may temporarily reduce emotional intensity and even provide a momentary sense of well-being, but they fail to adhere to valued goals and purposes that the individual would endorse. It is assumed here that very few individuals endorse the belief that alcohol abuse and self-mutilation define a valued life. Adaptive strategies might include self-soothing relaxation exercises, temporary distraction during crises, physical exercise, linking emotions to higher values, trumping an emotion with a more pleasant or valued emotion, mindful awareness, acceptance, pleasurable activities, shared intimate communication, and other strategies that assist in processing, coping with, reducing, tolerating, or learning from intense emotions. In each case, the valued goals and purposes are not compromised but may, in some cases, be further affirmed.

THE ROLE OF EMOTION REGULATION IN VARIOUS DISORDERS

In recent years there has been increasing attention to the role of emotional processing and regulation in a variety of disorders. Emotional processing through the activation of the "fear schema" during exposure has been implicated in the treatment of specific phobias and each of the anxiety disorders (Barlow, Allen, & Choate, 2004; Foa & Kozak, 1986). The activation of fear in the treatment of specific phobia allows for new learning and new associations to occur during exposure treatment. Indeed, the use of tranquilizing medications may compromise exposure treatment and prevent new associations from occurring. If one considers exposure as a form of habituation to a stimulus, including habituation to the fearful sensations that occur with initial exposure, then activation of fear is an important experiential factor in the new learning that results through exposure. This new learning includes the recognition that the feared stimulus "predicts" a rise and decline in emotional intensity and that emotional intensity is not to be feared in itself. Intense feelings can be tolerated as they eventually decline in intensity.

Emotion regulation is also implicated in the treatment of generalized anxiety disorder (GAD). GAD is now viewed as primarily a disorder marked by excessive worry and increased physiological arousal (American Psychiatric Association, 2000). Although there are many components to excessive worry (such as intolerance of uncertainty, decreased problem-focused strategies, and metacognitive factors), emotional avoidance has been found to be a key component in the activation and perpetuation of worry (Borkovec, Alcaine, & Behar, 2004). Similarly, rumination (repeated negative thoughts about past or present) has been shown to be a high-risk cognitive style for depression (Nolen-Hoeksema, 2000) and has also been conceptualized as a strategy of emotional or experiential avoidance (Cribb, Moulds, & Carter, 2006). Hayes and his colleagues have proposed that experiential avoidance is a process underlying a variety of forms of psychopathology (Hayes, Wilson, Gifford, Follette, & Strosahl, 1996). Individuals who utilize experiential or emotional avoidance may be at greater risk for psychological problems; however, those who engage in emotional suppression in certain situations may be coping more adaptively. For example, emotional suppression, a form of emotional avoidance, has been identified as a risk factor for heightened emotional difficulties. Individuals instructed to suppress an emotion reported more negative emotions. In contrast, expression of emotion has been linked to improvement in psychological stress such that individuals believe that by journaling emotions over a period of time events make more sense, perhaps helping them process the experience and the emotion better (Dalgleish, Yiend, Schweizer, & Dunn, 2009; Pennebaker, 1997; Pennebaker & Francis, 1996). Indeed, simply activating, expressing, and reflecting on emotion may have ameliorative effects for depression. Depressed individuals who were initially higher on a measure of emotional suppression benefited from a 6-week treatment of expressive writing, which resulted in a reduction of their depressive symptoms (Gortner, Rude, & Pennebaker, 2006). However, in one study emotional suppression was more effective than acceptance in reducing the impact of watching a traumatic event on video (Dunn, Billotti, Murphy, & Dalgleish, 2009). In addition, emotional suppression was not related to binge eating in another study (Chapman, Rosenthal, & Leung, 2009). Moreover, suppression of emotion was associated with reporting a "better day" for individuals high on features of borderline personality disorder (BPD; Chapman et al., 2009). Clearly, there are no absolutes when it comes to emotional processing. Sometimes suppression helps; other times it impairs.

Although eating disorders may be the result of a number of factors (e.g., self-image, perfectionism, interpersonal difficulties, and affective disorders), there is considerable evidence that emotion regulation plays a significant role, with complex cases (marked by a combination of the risk factors just listed) benefiting from a "transdiagnostic" treatment strategy (Fairburn et al., 2009; Fairburn, Cooper, & Shafran, 2003). Part of the transdiagnostic treatment strategy is using emotion regulation techniques to assist patients who resort to problematic coping (bingeing, purging, drinking, cutting) because they do not know what else to do to handle their emotions (Fairburn et al., 2003, 2009; Zweig & Leahy, in press). Further, emotion regulation mediates shame and eating disorders (Gupta, Zachary Rosenthal, Mancini, Cheavens, & Lynch, 2008). Rumination is another strategy that may be used by individuals with eating disorders, as suggested by the work of Nolen-Hoeksema, Stice, Wade, and Bohon (2007).

Emotional suppression can result in decreased efficacy in communication. In one study, participants instructed to suppress their emotions while discussing a difficult topic had increased blood pressure and decreased effectiveness of communication. In addition, participants assigned to listen to speakers who were attempting to suppress emotions also had increased blood pressure (E. A. Butler et al., 2003).

Individuals differ in their "philosophies" about the expression and experience of emotion. In marital therapy, Gottman identified a variety of emotional philosophies that affect how individuals think about, evaluate, and respond to their partner's emotional state. Thus, some partners may view emotion as a burden and, therefore, use a dismissive or even disparaging style. Others may view emotions as an opportunity to get closer to and get to know their partner better and get to help them (Gottman, Katz, & Hooven, 1997). Emotion regulation is also part of anger management, with angry individuals often showing an intense rise in the sensations of activation (pulse rate, physical tension), along with a full range of maladaptive appraisals, communication styles, and physical action (DiGiuseppe & Tafrate, 2007; Novaco, 1975). In fact, the emotional intensity may become so overwhelming for some that self-imposed "time-out" is sometimes the first line of intervention. Finally, emotion dysregulation underlies self-injurious behavior, which is often a negatively reinforced behavior for reducing intense emotion (Nock, 2008). The self-injury releases endorphins, which temporarily decrease the negative emotional intensity of anxiety and depression.

Perhaps the earliest and most comprehensive work highlighting the role of emotion dysregulation in a particular clinical disorder is Linehan's theoretical work on the development of borderline personality disorder (BPD). Linehan (1993a, 1993b) conceptualized BPD as a disorder of pervasive emotion dyregulation resulting from the transaction of a biologically based vulnerability to emotions with an invalidating caretaking environment. The invalidating environment has three defining features. First, it responds in a critical, punitive, or dismissive way to the emotionally vulnerable child, thereby exacerbating the child's emotional vulnerability. Second, it responds erratically to extreme emotional displays, reinforcing them intermittently. Third, it overestimates the ease of problem solving. As a result, the invalidating environment fails to teach skills needed to regulate intense emotions. Consequently, the emotional vulnerable individual may resort to maladaptive emotion regulation strategies such as cutting, bingeing, and overdosing as a way to escape or decrease the intensity of emotions. Central to Linehan's conceptualization of BPD is emotional avoidance. Indeed, she characterizes the individual with BPD as "emotionally phobic." The fear of emotions is thought to derive in part from negative evaluation of emotional experience.

Linehan's conceptualization of BPD as a disorder of emotion regulation informs her treatment approach: dialectical behavior therapy (DBT; Linehan, 1993a, 1993b). DBT is a mindfulness-based behavioral treatment that balances the use of acceptance and change techniques. Within a DBT framework, emotion regulation is conceptualized as a set of adaptive skills, including the ability to identify an emotion, understand emotions, control impulsive behaviors, and use situationally adaptive strategies to modulate emotional responses. An essential part of the treatment is helping patients to overcome their fear and avoidance of emotions and to increase acceptance of emotional experience.

Increasingly, cognitive-behavioral models of psychopathology are being expanded to reflect emotion regulation perspectives. Emotion regulation deficits have been implicated in a range of clinical disorders, including substance abuse and posttraumatic stress disorder (PTSD; Cloitre, Cohen, & Koenen, 2006). Mennin and colleagues have developed an emotion dysregulation model of GAD in which the disorder is characterized by heightened intensity of emotions, poor understanding of emotions, negative reactivity to one's emotional state, and maladaptive emotional management responses (Mennin, Heimberg, Turk, & Fresco, 2002; Mennin, Turk, Heimberg, & Carmin, 2004). Barlow and colleagues (2004) have developed a theory and unified treatment of the mood and anxiety disorders based on emotion regulation theory.

Recent research has examined differential disturbances in emotional processing in GAD and social anxiety disorder (Turk, Heimberg, Luterek, Mennin, & Fresco, 2005). Newer treatment models of GAD call for the integration of emotion-focused techniques (Roemer, Slaters, Raffa, & Orsillo, 2005; Turk et al., 2005).

There are a wide variety of emotion regulation strategies, which may or may not be useful. A recent meta-analysis of emotion regulation strategies across a variety of disorders indicated that the most frequent strategies are rumination, followed by avoidance, problem solving, and suppression; there is relatively less emphasis on reappraisal and acceptance (Aldao, Nolen-Hoeksema, & Schweizer, 2010). This meta-analysis provides important information on the relative utilization of strategies but, of course, cannot argue which strategies might be most *helpful* in changing emotion dysregulation. In any case, the transdiagnostic nature of emotion dysregulation appears to be gaining importance (Harvey, Watkins, Mansell, & Shafran, 2004; Kring & Sloan, 2010).

EVOLUTIONARY THEORY

Darwin (1872/1965) is credited as the originator of the comparative psychology of emotional expression. His detailed observations and descriptions—often depicted in photographs and drawings—indicate the similarity between humans and animals and also suggest universal patterns of facial expression. Emotions are viewed in evolutionary theory as adaptive processes that allow individuals to assess danger (or other conditions), activate behavior, communicate with other members of the species, and increase adaptive fitness (Barkow, Cosmides, & Tooby, 1992; Nesse, 2000). For example, fear, a universal emotion, is an adaptive response to natural danger, such as heights. Fear may freeze the animal in its footsteps, motivate it to escape or avoid, and provide the facial and vocal cues to warn others of impending danger. Negative emotions may be particularly adaptive because they are invoked at times of danger or threat and may require immediate response to ensure survival (Nesse & Ellsworth, 2009). Ethologists have noted that emotions may be displayed in apparently universal patterns in facial expression, posturing, eye gaze, and gestures of appeasement or threat (Eibl-Eibesfeldt, 1975).

Darwin was particularly interested in the facial expressions of various emotions, collecting numerous photographs from people from all social classes (including a "lunatic asylum"). The apparent universal nature of facial expression has been supported by the cross-cultural work of Paul Ekman, who demonstrated that facial expression and perception of expression of basic emotions are found in all cultures, suggesting that there are basic emotions that are universal (Ekman, 1993). Indeed, the natural tendency to express emotions facially makes it almost impossible to hide the emotions that one is actually feeling (Bonanno et al., 2002). Similarly, the difficulty in reading the emotions of others may confer disadvantage for some individuals.

THE VALUE OF EMOTIONS

Emotions assist us in evaluating our alternatives, providing the motivation to make a change or to do something, and tell us about our needs. For example, individuals with brain damage to the centers linking emotion and reason may be able to weigh rational pros and cons but unable to make decisions. Damasio (2005) has referred to emotions as "somatic markers" that tell us what we "want" to do. Although rational approaches to decision making based on utility theory suggest that individuals should or do weigh all the available evidence and make decisions based on trade-offs, research on *actual* decision making suggests that we often rely on heuristics (rules of thumb) and that emotions are one heuristic that is often relied on. This approach is similar to the popular idea of "gut reaction," as reflected in the title of cognitive social psychologist Gerd Gigerenzer's (2007) book *Gut Feelings: The Intelligence of the Unconscious.* Contrary to a rationalist model that gut responses are less valid or reliable, there is increasing evidence that gut responses may often be more effective, quicker, and more accurate (Gigerenzer, 2007; Gigerenzer, Hoffrage, & Goldstein, 2008). Moreover, emotional or intuitive evaluations are often the basis of most moral or ethical judgments rather than complex moral reasoning (Haidt, 2001; Keltner, Horberg, & Oveis, 2006). This view that there are gut responses underlying traditional ethical decision making—or what some might call "wisdom"—suggests that there may be some emotional basis to "wise mind."

Emotions help link us with others and constitute a shared "theory of mind." Individuals suffering from Asperger syndrome or autism are unable to accurately assess the emotions of others, often resulting in awkward and dysfunctional interpersonal behavior (Baron-Cohen et al., 2009). The inability to recognize, label, differentiate, and link emotions to events is called "alexithymia," and is associated with a wide variety of problems, including substance abuse, eating disorders, GAD, PTSD, and other problems (Taylor, 1984). The language of emotion is part of the emotional socialization of children. Families differ in their use of words referring to emotion, distinguishing and labeling emotions, and encouraging discussion of emotions. This "emotion talk" has an effect on later "alexithymic" tendencies, or the ability to recognize and label emotions. Families that talk about emotions are less likely to have alexithymic children (Berenbaum & James, 1994).

The concept of emotional intelligence captures the general nature of emotional awareness and adaptation, suggesting a general trait that has wide-ranging implications for adaptive functioning. Emotional intelligence comprises four factors: perceiving, using, understanding, and managing emotion (Mayer, Salovey, & Caruso, 2004). These abilities are important in intimate relationships; in problem solving, decision making, expressing appropriate emotions, controlling emotions, and in the workplace (Grewal, Brackett, & Salovey, 2006). Throughout the present volume, we describe emotion regulation techniques that address (1) the perception and labeling of emotion, (2) the ability to use emotions to make decisions and clarify values and goals, (3) understanding the nature of emotion by dispelling negative interpretations of emotion, and (4) the manner in which emotions can be managed and contained. Indeed, emotion regulation techniques may be viewed as part of a larger and more integrative approach that recognizes the central role of emotional intelligence. In the current volume, we offer an integrative, overarching theory that incorporates each of these techniques: emotional schema theory, which describes the various interpretations, strategies, and goals that one might utilize to cope with emotions (Leahy, 2002, 2005a). We view emotional schema therapy (EST) as a case conceptualization of the patient's theory about emotion, models of emotion control, and strategies for coping with emotions. We suggest that many contemporary approaches to emotional regulation can be viewed as models of coping with the issues raised by EST. However, readers may use the techniques in this book without incorporating EST as a guiding theory.

NEUROBIOLOGY OF EMOTIONS

Research on the neuroscience of emotion regulation has led to important yet potentially confusing and contradictory findings. Nevertheless, researchers and theorists have recently begun to integrate this literature to provide a comprehensive framework for understanding the neurobiology of emotion regulation. Ochsner and Gross (2007) have offered a theoretical model of the interactive neural systems involved in emotion regulation, based on their review of the literature. Their model integrates both "bottom-up" and "top-down" aspects of emotional processing.

A "bottom-up" model of emotion regulation describes emotions as a response to an environmental stimulus. Certain triggering stimuli in the environment may be seen as possessing inherent qualities that provoke specific emotions in humans, also described as the "emotion-as-stimulus property view" (Ochsner & Gross, 2007). Nonhuman research has demonstrated that the amygdala is involved in learning the prediction of aversive stimuli and the unpleasant experiences that follow exposure to them, while extinction appears to involve activity in the medial and orbital frontal cortices (LeDoux, 2000; Ochsner & Gross, 2007; Quirk & Gehlert, 2003).

"Top-down" emotion regulation models hypothesize that emotions emerge as a result of cognitive processing. Such processing involves discriminating which stimuli should be approached, avoided, or selected for attention in the environment. This also involves an assessment of whether a stimulus will be beneficial or harmful to the individual, particularly in terms of their needs, goals, and motivations (Ochsner & Gross, 2007). Human beings are uniquely qualified to employ language, rational thinking, relational processing, and memory to execute deliberate, conscious emotion regulation strategies. According to Davidson, Fox, and Kalin (2007), findings from nonhuman studies, human neuroimaging research, and lesion studies suggest that a series of interrelated regions of the brain may serve as our emotion regulation "circuitry." These regions include the amygdala, hippocampus, insula, anterior cingulate cortex (ACC), and dorsolateral and ventral regions of the prefrontal cortex (PFC) (Davidson, 2000). Prefrontal activity has been hypothesized to be a central component of emotion regulation in humans, particularly in top-down processing (Davidson, 2000; Davidson et al., 2007; Ochsner & Gross, 2005). Furthermore, relatively left lateralized PFC activity may be involved in a superior capacity to regulate and reduce negative emotions (Davidson et al., 2007).

Ochsner and Gross's (2007) model hypothesizes that both bottom-up and top-down modes of processing are involved in emotion regulation. When a human being encounters an aversive stimulus in the environment, such as a threatening, predatory animal, a bottom-up emotional response may ensue. This response may involve the activation of appraisal systems, including activity in the amygdala, the nucleus accumbens, and the insula (Ochsner & Feldman Barrett, 2001; Ochsner & Gross, 2007).

These appraisal systems communicate with the cortex and with the hypothalamus to generate behavioral responses. A top-down emotional response also may begin with a stimulus in the environment. However, it may be a discriminative stimulus, which suggests that an individual might predict that an aversive stimulus or sensation may be on its way. The stimulus in top-down processing may also be a neutral one that may provoke a negative response in a given context. In such cases, higher cognitive processes are involved in generating a modulated emotional response. These processes involve PFC appraisal systems acting through such structures as the lateral and medial PFC as well as the ACC (Ochsner & Gross, 2007). As such, we can see the potential for interdependence across modes of affective processing, which suggests the possibility that neither mode of processing needs to be viewed as dominant. Indeed, these models of processing may be related in a sophisticated continuum that researchers have yet to fully understand or explain.

PRIMACY: COGNITION OR EMOTION?

A recurring debate in the field is the question of causality: Do emotions have primacy, or do cognitions lead to emotions? Zajonc (1980) proposed that the apprehension of novel or threatening stimuli can occur almost immediately without conscious awareness and that evaluations of the stimuli may follow after an emotional response has been activated. Lazarus, in contrast, argued that appraisals of a situation result in emotional responses and that cognition has temporal primacy over emotion (Lazarus, 1982; Lazarus & Folkman, 1984). As with many dichotomized debates, there is some validity to both positions. Favoring the primacy of emotion over cognition is a considerable body of research demonstrating that some stimuli (such as novel and threatening stimuli) initially bypass the cortical sections of the brain and are almost instantaneously processed by the amygdala outside of conscious awareness. This nonconscious processing of fear affects learning, memory, attention, perception, emotion inhibition, and regulation (LeDoux, 1996, 2003; Phelps & LeDoux, 2005). Linking the rapid "processing" outside of conscious awareness to evolutionary adaptation, neuroscience has attempted to place fear conditioning in the context of adaptive responses to threat that cannot be delayed for conscious processing. For example, the individual is walking along, suddenly becomes afraid, jumps back in alarm, and then *subsequently* says, "That looks like a snake." The conscious awareness of the nature of the stimuli occurs *after* the emotional response. To further complicate the role of conscious awareness, there is considerable evidence that conscious awareness is a poor historian of internal events. For example, if we think of conscious awareness as a bookkeeping process of internal events, there is ample empirical support for its inaccuracy. We are often not aware of the stimulus events that have impacted on our emotional or even cognitive processes (Gray, 2004).

Lazarus (1991) has argued that Zajonc has confused *cognitive* processing with *conscious* processing and that one can have a cognitive appraisal without being conscious of it. Thus, in this model, appraisals may occur immediately and outside of conscious awareness. If one takes this view, then it can be argued that the amygdala does "appraise" stimuli in terms of intensity, novelty, change, looming, or other "relevant" stimulus dimensions. Further, models of the primacy of emotion fail to provide an adequate account of the differentiation of emotions that may be characterized by similar physiological processes. For example, fear, jealousy, anger, and other emotions may be "reduced" to *similar* physiological processes of arousal, but the experience of these emotions is dependent on the appraisal of the threat and the context in which the arousal occurs. I may be afraid of the snake, jealous of my partner's attentions to another, angry at being blocked in traffic, or aroused as I run faster on the treadmill. The underlying physiological sensations may be quite similar, but the appraisal and the context help define the emotion for me.

Bower's network theory of emotion and cognition shares some common emphasis with the Zajonc position. According to this model, emotions, thoughts, sensations, and behavioral tendencies are linked associatively in neural networks. Thus, activating one process activates the others. The network model often utilizes emotional induction to activate the physiological processes and cognitive content that may be linked in the network (Bower, 1981; Bower & Forgas, 2000). Research by Forgas and colleagues indicates that induction of emotion affects judgment, decision making, person perception, attention, and memory—all cognitive processes (Forgas & Bower, 1987). Moreover, induced affect also affects attribution or explanatory processes (Forgas & Locke, 2005). Forgas has further elaborated an affect infusion model, which proposes that affective arousal influences cognitive processing, especially when heuristics (shortcuts) or more extensive processing is activated (Forgas, 1995, 2000). Indeed, people often assess how risky an alternative may be based on their current affective state (Kunreuther, Slovic, Gowda, & Fox, 2002). Arntz, Rauner, and van den Hout (1995) suggest that this emotion heuristic is used as "information" in the assessment of danger in phobic individuals such that they reason, "If I feel anxious, there must be danger." The affect infusion model and the network model proposed by Bower both suggest that emotional arousal may activate specific cognitive biases, which further exacerbate the triggering of further dysregulation. Consequently, the ability to soothe or calm affective arousal should it occur and the ability to modify the negative cognitive biases that are activated by affect should be useful in facilitating emotional regulation.

The foregoing does not resolve the primacy of emotion debate—and, indeed, its resolution may depend on semantic meanings of "appraisal," "consciousness," and "cognitive processing." Nonetheless, there is considerable evidence that emotion and cognition are interdependent and that each can influence the other in what one might view as a feedback cycle. In the current volume, we recognize that these processes are interdependent, and there is no necessity to take a position on primacy to develop useful techniques to help patients.

ACCEPTANCE AND COMMITMENT THERAPY

Acceptance and commitment therapy (ACT) is based on a behavioral theory of language and cognition known as relational frame theory (RFT), which provides a theoretical account of the core processes involved in psychopathology and emotion dysregulation (Hayes, Barnes-Holmes, & Roche, 2001). According to this account, the central cause of emotion-related problems involves ways in which the nature of human verbal processing contributes to "experiential avoidance" (Luoma, Hayes, & Walser, 2007). The term "experiential avoidance" represents efforts to control or alter the form, frequency, or situational sensitivity of thoughts, feelings, and sensations, even when doing so causes behavioral harm (Hayes et al., 1996).

According to RFT, humans learn to relate events and experiences to one another in a relational network throughout their lives and learn to respond to events based, in part, on their relationship to other events rather than merely on the stimulus properties of the event at hand

(Hayes et al., 2001). In this way, one event may come to be associated with any other event. For example, if I were to attend a memorial service by a beautiful lake at sunset, my future experiences of relaxing beside a lake at the end of the day may evoke a sense of sadness. RFT also suggests that when we experience thoughts or mental representations of an event, the stimulus properties of such an event show up in a literalized fashion. For example, when a person with depression experiences the negative thought "Nobody will ever love me," he or she responds emotionally to this thought as though it were real and literal rather than as an event in the mind. This process is referred to as "cognitive fusion" (Hayes, Strosahl, & Wilson, 1999). Given the processes of relational responding and cognitive fusion, we find ourselves in an interesting situation where we can learn to relate any event to any other, and when a mental representation of an event is triggered, we may respond to the stimulus properties of that mental representation as though it were literal.

A natural and reasonable way that humans respond to distressing and difficult situations involves attempts to avoid or escape these situations. This strategy is appropriate and effective for interactions involving our environment. For example, if I fear that a certain cave is dangerous and avoid it, I am that much less likely to be attacked by the hungry predator living in that cave. This is similar to Mowrer's (1939) two-factor theory of acquisition and conservation of fear. Avoidance is reinforced through the reduction of fear, thereby conserving fear of the stimulus. Unfortunately, the nature of human relational responding is such that attempts to avoid, suppress, or eliminate mental events such as thoughts and emotions may serve to actually amplify the distress or upset that is experienced (Hayes et al., 1999). This is easy to comprehend, in that trying to "not think about fear" involves, by definition, thinking about your fear or a feared stimulus, which can evoke fear in turn. In this way, the RFT model suggests that human relational responding and cognitive fusion contribute to experiential avoidance, which, in turn, contributes to emotion dysregulation, psychopathology, and people living lives that are less than rewarding and realized.

ACT suggests that the aim of psychotherapy may be to establish and maintain "psychological flexibility" (Hayes & Strosahl, 2004), or "the ability to contact the present moment more fully as a conscious human being and, based on what the situation affords, to change or persist in behavior in order to serve 'valued ends'" (Luoma et al., 2007, p. 17; see also Hayes & Strosahl, 2004). ACT interventions utilize six core processes, which seek to bring patients into direct experiential contact with their present-moment experiences, to disrupt cognitive fusion, to promote experiential acceptance, to help patients let go of attachment to their narrative construction of themselves, to assist them in coming to terms with what they most value, and to facilitate their commitment to valued directions in their lives. In this way, the overall aim of ACT is a process of emotion regulation and affect tolerance in the service of deeply held, intrinsically rewarding behavioral trajectories. The patients gradually learn to expand their behavioral repertoire in the presence of distressing internal events, which is, perhaps, a core element of any definition of emotion regulation.

REAPPRAISAL

One of the most widely used strategies in coping with emotion is the use of appraisal—or reappraisal. These "cognitive" models are sometimes not considered part of emotion regulation from the viewpoint that appraisals (are presumed to) precede emotion. For example, one can divide emotion-coping strategies into *antecedent* and *response-focused strategies*. An example of an antecedent strategy would be evaluating the stressor as less threatening or as the self as fully capable of coping. Another example of antecedent strategies includes stimulus-control arrangements (e.g., not keeping high-calorie snacks in the house). Cognitive restructuring and problem solving also are examples of antecedent strategies. Examples of response-focused strategies include self-calming, suppression of emotion, distraction, and engaging in pleasurable activities; some of these strategies pose further problems. In a study comparing the two styles, reappraisers coped more effectively, experiencing more positive emotions, less negative emotions, and better interpersonal functioning, with the opposite trend evident for suppressors (Gross & John, 2003). Perhaps the most widely used clinical model for reappraisal is cognitive restructuring, using the many techniques from Beckian cognitive therapy or Ellis' rational emotive behavior therapy (Beck, Rush, Shaw, & Emery, 1979; Clark & Beck, 2009; Ellis & MacLaren, 1998; Leahy, 2003a). There is considerable empirical evidence for the efficacy of cognitive therapy for a wide range of disorders (A. Butler, Chapman, Forman, & Beck, 2006).

Reappraisal includes evaluating the thoughts about a situation that elicit emotional arousal. For example, Beck's model proposes that automatic thoughts occur spontaneously, often going unexamined or evaluated. Automatic thoughts can be categorized as distortions or biases, including mind reading, dichotomous thinking, fortune telling, personalizing, and labeling. These thoughts are linked to conditional rules of assumptions, such as "If someone doesn't like me, then it is terrible" or "I must hate myself if you don't like me." Further, assumptions and automatic thoughts are then linked to core beliefs or personal schemas about self or other, such as viewing the self as incompetent and viewing others as highly critical. Reappraisal models attempt to identify these thinking patterns and alter them through cognitive restructuring and behavioral experiments.

META-EMOTION

Gottman et al. (1996) have proposed that an important component of socialization involves parents' "philosophical" view of emotion, or what they refer to as "meta-emotional philosophy." Specifically, some parents view the child's experience and expression of emotions, such as anger, sadness, or anxiety, as a negative event that must be avoided. These negative emotional views are communicated in parental interactions, such that the parent will be dismissive, critical, or overwhelmed by the child's emotions. In contrast to these problematic emotional socialization styles, Gottman et al. (1996) identified an *emotion-coaching style* that entails the ability to recognize even low levels of emotional intensity, seeing these "unpleasant emotions" as an opportunity for intimacy and support, assisting the child in labeling and differentiating emotions, and engaging in problem solving with the child. Parents who adopt the emotion-coaching style are more likely to have children who are able to self-soothe their own emotions; that is, *emotion coaching* assists in emotional self-regulation. Furthermore, children of parents using emotion coaching are more effective in interactions with their peers, even when appropriate behavior with peers involves the inhibition of emotional expression. Thus, children of parents utilizing emotion coaching are more advanced in emotional intelligence, knowing when to express and when to inhibit expression and knowing how to process and regulate their own emotions (see Mayer & Salovey, 1997). Emotion coaching does not simply "reinforce" a cathartic style in children; rather, it allows them to identify, differentiate, validate, self-soothe, and problem solve. The emotion-coaching style as described by Gottman and colleagues is an extension of the active listening skills and problem-solving strategies advocated by communication-based models of relationship interaction (e.g., N. S. Jacobson & Margolin, 1979; Stuart, 1980).

EMOTION-FOCUSED THERAPY

Emotion-focused therapy (EFT) is an experiential and humanistic therapy that has its origins in attachment theory, emotional neuroscience, and concepts of emotional intelligence (Greenberg, 2002). EFT is an evidence-based, empirically supported therapy. Similar to Gottman's description of effective working with emotions in parenting, in EFT the therapist can also serve as an emotion coach who helps patients to be more effective and adaptive in processing their emotional responses.

In EFT the relationship between the psychotherapist and the patient is itself viewed as serving an affect regulation function through attachment processes (Greenberg, 2007). Several processes can be found in EFT that are also present across third-generation cognitive-behavioral therapy modalities, such as acceptance, contact with the present moment, mindful awareness, the cultivation of empathy, and the activation of attachment-based self-soothing processes. Specifically, the therapeutic alliance in EFT is said to function as a soothing dyad. In this dyadic interaction, with the dynamics of evolved human attachment at work, patients may be able to internalize self-soothing capacities through repeated emotion coaching and experiential learning in therapy sessions. Additionally, the therapeutic alliance may create an environment in which patients may directly and deeply encounter challenging emotions, while learning the skills they need to tolerate distress and effectively regulate their emotional responses (Greenberg, 2002).

Although EFT acknowledges that cognition is an essential component of emotional processing, cognitive control or reappraisal of emotion is not the central process in the EFT model (Greenberg, 2002). The EFT model suggests that emotions may influence cognition just as cognition may influence emotions. Cognitions might be used to affect emotions, but emotions might even be used to change or transform other emotions. EFT suggests that appraisal processes, physical sensation processes, and affective systems activate in an integrated way to evoke the experience of an emotion (Greenberg, 2007). EFT, the concept of emotional intelligence, and EST all hold that emotional experiences involve a high level of synthesized and synchronized activity across human biological and behavioral systems.

EMOTIONAL SOCIALIZATION

Although emotions have been linked to evolutionary theory and emotions appear to be universally experienced, parental socialization does have an impact on emotional awareness, expression, and regulation. Since the publication of Bowlby's (1968, 1973) seminal work on attachment, there has been considerable interest in the importance of secure or insecure attachment on development from infancy through adulthood. Bowlby proposed that the essential component of a secure attachment was the predictability and responsiveness of the parental figure. Bowlby and others suggested that disruptions in the attachment between child and parent can affect the development of "internal working models"—that is, schemas or concepts—about the predictability and nurturance of others. Infants and children lacking a secure attachment are at greater risk for anxiety, sadness, anger, and other emotional problems. There is some evidence that attachment patterns are moderately stable in the first 19 years of life (Fraley, 2002). In a study of adults exposed to a traumatic event (the 9/11 attack on the World Trade Center), those who had secure attachments were less likely to suffer from PTSD (Fraley, Fazzari, Bonanno, & Dekel, 2006). Although early attachment issues have primarily been a focus of object relations theories (Clarkin, Yeomans, & Kernberg, 2006; Fonagy, 2000), attachment processes have also been a focus for cognitive therapists (Guidano & Liotti, 1983; Young, Klosko, & Weishaar, 2003).

Children's understanding of the emotions of others, social competence, positive emotionality, and general adjustment are related to higher parental warmth, higher positive emotional expressivity, and lower disapproval and hostility (Isley, O'Neil, Clatfelter, & Parke, 1999; Matthews, Woodall, Kenyon, & Jacob, 1996; Rothbaum & Weisz, 1994). Negative expression of emotion and less parental warmth are associated with higher incidence of anti-social behavior (Caspi et al., 2004). Eisenberg and her colleagues have found that parental negative expressivity is associated with lower emotion regulation, which in turn is associated with more externalizing problems and lower social competence (Eisenberg, Gershoff, et al., 2001; Eisenberg, Liew, & Pidada, 2001). Thus, emotion regulation mediated the relationship between parental expression and other social capabilities.

There is considerable emphasis on the importance of invalidation in DBT theory as an early contributing factor to the development of emotion dysregulation. In a recent study, deliberate self-harm was associated with retrospective reports of parental punishment and neglect when the child was sad (Buckholdt, Parra, & Jobe-Shields, 2009). Children who had an anxiety disorder were more likely to have parents who expressed less positive affect and more negative affect and who engaged in fewer explanatory discussions about emotion (Suveg et al., 2008). All of these attachment and interpersonal processes suggest that relationship issues and processes are a central component of emotion regulation. This is consistent with the interpersonal model of depression and suicide that proposes that universal needs for belongingness and a sense that one is not a burden to others are vulnerability factors (Joiner, Brown, & Kistner, 2006).

META-EXPERIENTIAL MODELS

Emotions are social cognitive content in themselves; that is, people have their own theories about the nature of their emotion and the emotions of others. In recent years, theory of mind has been proposed as a general social cognitive capacity underlying the ability to understand the emotions of self and others and as an ability that begins development in infancy and early childhood and continues thereafter. One dimension in conceptualizing emotion is the degree to which one believes that emotions are fixed (entity) or changeable (malleable). These dimensions were predictive of adjustment in college. Entity theorists had higher rates of depression, more difficulty in social adjustment, and lower well-being and were less likely to use reappraisal strategies (Tamir, John, Srivastava, & Gross, 2007).

Metacognition is similar to nonegocentric thinking, which was emphasized by Flavell and others in developmental psychology several decades ago (Flavell, 2004; Selman, Jaquette, & Lavin, 1977). Borrowing from Piaget's concept of decentration, nonegocentric thinking entails the ability to stand back and observe the thinking and perspective of others and to coordinate self–other perspectives. Thinking about thinking was the key concept in developmental psychology that reflected the potentially recursive and self-reflective nature of social cognition. When applied to thinking about emotion—in self or other—the concept has "evolved" into theory of mind (Baron-Cohen, 1991), which has importance in both cognitive and psychodynamic models as well as neuroscience (Arntz, Bernstein, Oorschot, & Schobre, 2009; Corcoran et al., 2008; Fonagy & Target, 1996; Stone, Lin, Rosengarten, Kramer, & Quartermain, 2003; Völlm et al., 2006). The metacognitive model advanced by Adrian Wells is the most detailed clinical theory for theory of mind and how metacognitive processes underpin various disorders (Wells, 2004, 2009). For example, chronic worriers believe that they must attend to, control, and neutralize intrusive thoughts and that thoughts confer personal responsibility. The metacognitive model seeks to clarify beliefs about how the mind functions, rather than modify the content of thoughts, and to assist the patient in relinquishing unhelpful strategies, such as attempts to suppress, control, gain certainty, and use reassurance and other "mind-control" methods. Leahy has expanded on this to develop a *meta-experiential model*—called *emotional schema therapy*—that suggests that people differ in their beliefs about the nature of emotion (e.g., controllable, dangerous, shameful, unique to the self) and the necessity of invoking emotion-control strategies such as worry, rumination, blame, avoidance, or substance abuse (Leahy, 2002). The emotional schema model also shares with DBT a recognition of common emotional myths, for example, "Some emotions are really stupid," "Painful emotions are the result of a bad attitude," or "If others don't approve of my feelings, I shouldn't feel the way I do" (Linehan, 1993a). We examine the common dysfunctional beliefs about emotion that may exacerbate emotional coping and illustrate the use of EST and DBT in more effective coping strategies. In the next chapter, we provide an overview of EST, which incorporates the various components of emotional processing and regulation discussed throughout this book, and we propose specific techniques for identifying and modifying problematic interpretations, evaluations, and strategies for coping with difficult emotions.

CONCLUSIONS

Emotion is not one simple phenomenon. It comprises appraisal, physical sensation, motor behavior, goals or intentionality, interpersonal expression, and other processes. Consequently, a comprehensive approach to emotion regulation should recognize the multifaceted nature of emotion and provide techniques that can address any of these processes. That is the purpose of this volume. Moreover, coping strategies vary considerably, and individuals may prefer certain strategies over others. For some, cognitive restructuring may obviate any of the other emotion regulation strategies by modifying the emotional response through reappraisal. In contrast, others for whom intense emotions have already been activated may benefit from a wide range of stress reduction techniques, mindfulness, acceptance, or emotional schema techniques. Some patients may have difficulty with the interpersonal nature of their emotional experience and may benefit from techniques addressed at validation or interpersonal functioning (e.g., learning skills to maintain friendships and social support). Although there may be many zeitgeists within the field of psychology, patients are less interested in the theoretical allegiances of the therapist and more interested in the relevance and effectiveness of the techniques available. Consequently, each of us—representing somewhat different interests and areas of expertise—has attempted to provide the reader with a wide range of techniques that may be tailored to individual patients. As indicated earlier in this chapter, the clinician can assist patients in examining (1) whether the problem allows for modification of the situation either through problem solving, stimulus control, or cognitive restructuring; (2) whether the problem is the increase in arousal and sensations (where stress reduction techniques such as progressive relaxation, breathing exercises, and other self-calming may be useful); or (3) whether the problem is how to cope with emotional intensity once it has arisen, suggesting the usefulness of acceptance, mindfulness, compassion-focused self-soothing, and other techniques. In each of the chapters to follow, we suggest guidelines for "choosing techniques" and relate each technique to relevant alternatives.

CHAPTER TWO

Emotional Schema Therapy

Consider the following situation. Philip is going through a breakup in a relationship. He feels sad, angry, confused, anxious, and a little relieved. He normalizes all of these emotions: "Breakups are difficult and confusing and others might have all of these feelings if they went through a breakup." He is able to express these emotions with a friend, who validates his feelings and encourages him to feel comfortable about having whatever feeling he has. Philip thinks his emotions make sense, he doesn't think he should only feel one way (e.g., angry), and he views his emotions as difficult but tolerable and temporary. In contrast, Edward has a very different view of his own emotions after going through his breakup. He is confused that he has "contradictory feelings"—he thinks he should feel one way (e.g., angry). His emotions don't make sense, and he believes that others would have a different response: They might feel sad or relieved but not angry. He believes that his feelings of sadness and anxiety point to his weakness, a character defect he feels ashamed of. He is afraid of sharing these emotions because he believes that others would not understand, he thinks it's humiliating, and he believes that expressing emotions would open a "can of worms." Edward's negative interpretations of his emotions make him afraid of his feelings, and he turns to drinking, isolating himself, and ruminating. His beliefs and strategies perpetuate his depression.

All of us experience feelings of sadness, anxiety, fear, and even hopelessness. However, an important "next move" in responding to a patient's emotions is, "What do you do, think, or feel *after* you have that emotion? For example, when you feel anxious, do you avoid, escape, binge, blame, ruminate, worry, or drink? Do you seek out support, validation, and expression of your emotions and do you actually experience validation? Do you normalize your emotions, accept them, or do you feel guilty, overwhelmed, and confused?" The consequence of using behavioral strategies such as avoiding and escaping is that the patient reinforces the belief that he or she cannot tolerate his or her emotions, similar to the argument raised in ACT about experiential avoidance (Hayes et al., 1999). If a patient has problematic or negative interpretations of his or her anxiety—and believes that it is overwhelming and out of control—the patient will continue to feel anxious. These behavioral, interpersonal, and cognitive strategies and responses are the components of emotional schemas.

Beck and his colleagues indicate that individuals have a variety of schemas, such as emotional, decisional, physical, and relational, each of which includes a set of rules that direct the individual in specific situations (Beck, Freeman, Davis, & Associates, 2004; Clark, Beck, &

Alford, 1999). Impairment in functioning may be manifested in any one of these schematic processes. Beck has suggested that a superordinate, or organizing, structure stands over and above these schemas (Beck, 1996; Clark et al., 1999). This superordinate structure is referred to as a "mode," including anger, depression, and anxiety modes. The emotional schema model proposes that interpretations of emotions and strategies that are activated to cope with emotion incorporate the evaluation, interpretative, and active mode of adaptation, as implied in the Beck et al. model.

Beck et al. (2004) expanded the cognitive model to focus specifically on a variety of personality disorders that are characterized by various schematic issues and adaptations. According to this model, each personality disorder may be characterized by the specific content of the dominant schema; for example, for the compulsive personality, the dominant schemas are control and rationality. These "overdeveloped" areas are contrasted with the "underdeveloped" areas of emotional expression and flexibility. Beck and Freeman propose that individuals may either attempt to avoid situations that may threaten the schema or attempt to compensate for their fears of the "undeveloped" polarity. For example, the compulsive individual, fearing loss of control, may attempt to exercise extreme control over his or her environment through hoarding and organizing minutia. These extreme attempts at compensation give rise to depression or anxiety when they fail to adequately control the feared polarity.

Because personality disorders are enduring, Beck and associates propose that affected individuals have consistently employed these avoidant and compensatory adaptations, presumably warding off the threat of full exposure to the schema. Thus, individuals with a compulsive personality have warded off confrontation with the experience that they are "really completely out of control" or "really completely irrational and crazy" by avoiding situations that they cannot control or by magical attempts to control their environment.

The schema model of Beck and associates attempts to modify the risk of depression and anxiety in the personality disorders by first conducting a cognitive assessment with the patient (see also J. S. Beck, 2011, for a discussion of cognitive assessment). The patient's automatic thoughts are linked to underlying assumptions and conditional beliefs. For example, the automatic thought "I am losing control" is linked to a conditional belief, "If I do not have complete control, then I have no control." This is then linked to an underlying assumption, "I must be in total control at all times." The underlying core schema is identified as "out of control."

Young (1990) has also proposed a schema model that emphasizes individual schemas, independently of personality disorders. Young has suggested that there are several dimensions of schematic content. Further, he has attempted to integrate a range of theoretical perspectives, such as object relations theory and Gestalt theory, with a cognitive model. According to this model, individuals engage in three adaptations to their "early maladaptive schemas"—avoidance, compensation, or schema maintenance, the latter adaptation simply referring to the fact that individuals may pursue experiences that reinforce their schema. For example, the narcissistic individual may pursue relationships that reinforce her belief that she is special and unique. In the current model proposed in this chapter, we borrow from both the Beck–Freeman and the Young models and attempt to relate these approaches to the issue of emotion regulation.

We refer to "schemas" in the manner proposed by Beck and colleagues (2004). According to that cognitive model, one can have concepts and strategies about others, self, body, feelings, and other specific "objects of experience." Schemas in the cognitive model imply beliefs about coping. In the Beck et al. and the Young et al. models, coping may involve overdeveloped and underdeveloped strategies or avoidance, compensation, or schema maintenance. In the emotional schema model, individuals differ in their interpretations of their emotional experience and may attempt to cope with their emotions through experiential avoidance (e.g., suppression, numbness, avoidance, escape), unhelpful "cognitive strategies" (e.g., overreliance on worry and rumination), seeking social support (either adaptive or maladaptive validation strategies), or other strategies.

In this chapter we introduce a clinical model that focuses on how people conceptualize their emotional experience, what their expectations are, how they judge their emotions, and the behavioral and interpersonal strategies that they employ in response to emotional experience. This model—emotional schema therapy (EST)—is a metacognitive or, we prefer, "meta-experiential" model of emotion whereby emotions are an *object* of social cognition (Leahy, 2002, 2005a, 2007a, 2007b; Wells, 2009). Emotional schemas are individual "philosophies" about emotion, reflecting the influence of Gottman's meta-emotional model (Gottman et al., 1996; Gottman, 1997). Here we focus on the individual's beliefs about the legitimacy of an emotion; his or her need to control, suppress, or express emotion, or tolerance for complexity and self-contradiction. In addition, individuals differ as to the strategies that they believe are required to "cope" with an emotion, with some people accepting emotion, linking emotion to higher values, and seeking validation and others suppressing, escaping, or attempting to numb their emotional experience.

In the following example, consider how we might view someone else's emotion. This person is angry and frustrated and feels hurt because of unpleasant things others have said to him. In one case, we respond to that person by normalizing his emotion ("Many people would feel upset with that"), validating the hurt feelings. We invite him to express these emotions: "Let me know what you are feeling about this. I want to be helpful." We link his emotions to their higher values: "You feel this way because you are conscientious and things matter to you." In this example, we sound like the "ideal validator," inviting the expression of emotion, helping the person label those feelings, and offering a respectful and caring safe relationship for their expression. We have been employing our own emotional "schemas" or concepts and strategies—that the other person's emotions make sense, they need to be validated, and they are linked to higher values.

An alternative response to the other person's emotions could be very different—and very destructive. We might ridicule the person—"You sound like a big baby. Grow up!"—or tell him he is irrational and neurotic. We might tell him there isn't time or energy available to hear all these complaints. Or we might say, "Have a drink" and hope his feelings are dissipated as he becomes more inebriated. The message conveyed by this alternative approach is that this individual's emotions are a burden, annoying, or beneath contempt.

Just as we have conceptualizations and strategies that we use in understanding and responding to the emotions of others (which we call "schemas"), we also have these schemas in responding to our own emotions. For example, Bill's partner has left him. He now feels sad ("I miss her"), anxious ("Will I ever find someone to love?"), fearful ("It's going to be hard being alone"), and even hopeless ("I could be alone forever"). Bill's problem is not the experience of the breakup but rather that he handles his emotions in the most problematic way. He believes his feelings don't make sense ("Why should I be so upset after only a few months of a relationship?"); he thinks these emotions are going to last forever and they will overwhelm him ("My God. How will I be able to work when I'm so anxious and depressed?"); and he thinks a "real man" shouldn't be so upset. He feels ashamed of his feelings, so he won't share them with Roger, his best friend, and thus he will not have a chance to receive validation because he's all alone with his feelings. As he has done many times in his life when faced with problems, Bill turns to drinking as a way to cope.

The emotional schema model is depicted in Figure 2.1, reflecting normalizing and pathological styles of coping with emotion. For example, the normalizing process in the model is that painful and conflicting emotions can be accepted, that they can be expressed and normalized, and that they may reflect the higher values of commitment that is broken in the end of a relationship. Bill could have normalized his feelings and recognized that painful emotions often follow a breakup, that emotions are temporary, and that, in some cases, emotions can point to one's higher values ("valuing a loving relationship"). In contrast, a problematic response to the emotions of sadness and anger might be to pathologize them, viewing them as unique to the self and as lasting indefinitely, overwhelming and impairing, embarrassing or a sign of weakness, or needing to be suppressed or controlled. The problematic coping depicted in Figure 2.1 represents reliance on drinking, binge eating, substance abuse, blaming, rumination, and worry. An emotional schema model proposes that, rather than using avoidance and rumination as strategies, one can use acceptance, behavioral activation, and the development of more meaningful supportive relationships to cope with emotions. Emotional schemas are evaluated by adminis-

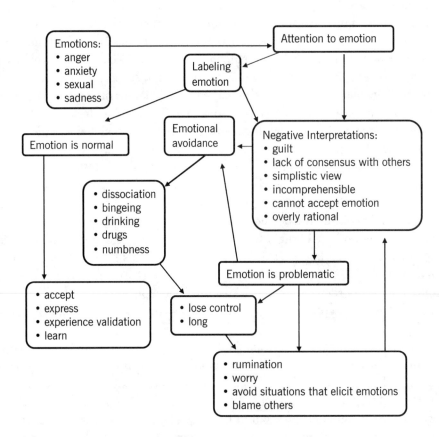

FIGURE 2.1. A model of emotional schemas.

tering Form 2.1, the Leahy Emotional Schemas Scale (LESS), which defines 14 dimensions of emotional schemas.

EST is a form of cognitive-behavioral therapy (CBT) that is grounded in some key principles (Leahy, 2002, 2009):

- Painful and difficult emotions are universal.
- Emotions emerged through evolution, as they provided an adaptive advantage by warning us of danger and telling us about our needs.
- Underlying beliefs and strategies (schemas) about emotions determine the impact that an emotion has on the further escalation or maintenance of an emotion. Thus, catastrophic beliefs about anxiety lead to escalation of anxiety, not dissimilar to the panic model advanced by Barlow, Clark and their colleagues (Barlow, 2002; Barlow & Craske, 2006; Clark, 1986).
- Problematic schemas include catastrophizing an emotion, thinking one's emotions do not make sense, and viewing an emotion as permanent and out of control, shameful, unique to the self, and needing to be kept to the self.
- Emotional control strategies such as attempts to suppress, ignore, neutralize, or eliminate emotions through substance abuse and binge eating help confirm negative beliefs of emotions as intolerable experiences.
- Expression and validation are helpful insofar as they normalize, universalize, improve understanding, differentiate various emotions, reduce guilt and shame, and help increase beliefs in the tolerability of emotional experience.

EST assists the patient in identifying a variety of emotions and labeling them; normalizing emotional experience, including painful and difficult emotions; linking emotions to personal needs and to interpersonal communication; identifying problematic beliefs and strategies (schemas) that the patient has for interpreting, judging, controlling, and acting on an emotion; collecting information, using experiential techniques, and setting up behavioral, interpersonal, and emotional "experiments" to develop more helpful responses to the patient's emotions; and developing new, more flexible, and adaptive beliefs and strategies about one's emotional experience.

EST attempts to make sense of emotion, put emotion into a context of a meaningful life and values worth living by, normalize emotions, and help individuals explore emotional possibilities. Thus, the emotional schema therapist can help patients differentiate the variety of emotions available to them and even explore emotions as possible goals. The purpose is not to eliminate or suppress emotions but to provide constructive and meaningful ways to use emotional experience.

Some therapists recognize that intense emotional expression and experience can be opportunities for deepening therapy—by accessing the "hot cognitions," the core beliefs, and the imagery and memories associated with intense emotions and with significant life events. These therapists would likely endorse the following beliefs (Leahy, 2005a, 2009): "Painful feelings are a chance to form a closer relationship," "I can matter more when the patient is feeling this way," "Painful feelings are part of life," "I can also imagine myself in this situation," "Painful feelings are not permanent," and "I should respect the patient's suffering and pain."

EMPIRICAL SUPPORT FOR THE EMOTIONAL SCHEMA MODEL

There is empirical support for the emotional schema model as related to anxiety, depression, and other forms of psychopathology. The LESS (see Forms 2.1 and 2.2[1]) has adequate internal consistency: Cronbach's alpha for 1,286 participants was .808. A number of the 14 emotional schema dimensions are significantly correlated with the Beck Depression Inventory (BDI) and the Beck Anxiety Inventory (BAI) (Leahy, 2002). In a separate study ($N = 1,363$), a stepwise multiple regression analysis indicated the following order of predictors of depression on the BDI: Rumination, Guilt, Invalidation, Lack of Higher Values, Control, Incomprehensibility, Expression (higher), and Low Consensus. A stepwise multiple regression analysis ($N = 1,245$) of the LESS dimensions on the BAI indicated the following order of predictors: Loss of Control, Incomprehensibility, Rumination, and Expression (higher). Thus, in both multiple regressions, greater expression was associated with greater depression and anxiety, contrary to a catharsis model. In a study of the relationship between a derived measure of negative beliefs about emotion (summing across LESS dimensions), each of the metacognitive factors in the Wells model (Wells, 2004, 2009) were significantly correlated with negative beliefs about emotions, adding to the construct validity of the scale ($N = 1,293$). Further exploration of the independent predictive value of LESS dimensions or metacognitive factors indicated that both theoretical models are supported. Stepwise multiple regression yielded the following order of predictors for the BDI: Rumination, Guilt, Invalidation, Loss of Control, Cognitive Competence/Confidence (Metacognitions Questionnaire [MCQ]), Positive Worry (MCQ; negative), Uncontrollability and Danger of Worry (MCQ), and Expression (negative). These findings on the relationship between the LESS, MCQ, and depression suggest that metacognitive factors of worry may partly be activated because of negative beliefs about emotion. The pattern of predictors in a stepwise multiple regression on anxiety (BAI) also reflect this integrative meta-emotion/metacognitive integrative model: Control, Uncontrollability and Danger of Worry (MCQ), Positive Worry (MCQ; negative), Cognitive Self-Consciousness (MCQ), Comprehensibility, Expression (negative), and Invalidation. An unexpected finding is that positive views of worry are associated with less depression and anxiety. In a study of satisfaction in intimate relationships, every one of the 14 LESS scores is significantly correlated with marital satisfaction (Dyadic Adjustment Scale) ($N = 662$). Again, the multiple regression analysis reflected intriguing findings, especially about the importance of Invalidation. The stepwise order of predictors is as follows: Invalidation, Blame, Lack of Higher Values, Simplistic View about Emotion, Incomprehensibility (higher), and Low Acceptance of Feelings. Given the importance of validation in the prior findings, it is of interest that a stepwise multiple regression of the predictors of validation revealed the following order: Guilt, Low Expression, Rumination, Low Acceptance of Feelings, Blame, Lack of Consensus, and Numbness. These data suggest that validation may modify other emotional schemas, thereby assisting in emotional regulation. This may be why patients who are emotionally overwhelmed seek out validation.

Further support for the importance of Invalidation is reflected in the data on the stepwise predictors of the LESS on the Millon Clinical Multiaxial Inventory (MCMI) Alcohol Dependence subscale: Invalidation, Lack of Higher Values, Simplistic, Blame, Low Consensus, and

---

[1] All forms are in the Appendix at the end of the book.

Numbness. Perhaps alcohol-dependent individuals derive validation, relationship to higher values, differentiation of complex emotions, reduced blame, and consensus from group meetings of Alcoholics Anonymous. An examination of the predictors of higher scores on the MCMI Borderline Personality Disorder dimension revealed the following predictors: Incomprehensibility, Rumination, Invalidation, Numbness, Blame, Simplistic View of Emotion, Loss of Control, Lack of Higher Values, and Need to Be Rational (lower). These data strongly suggest the importance of emotional schemas in psychopathology.

Significant relationships among psychological flexibility, dispositional mindfulness, and emotional schemas have also been found in recent research (Tirch, Silberstein, & Leahy, 2009). In a cross-sectional, observational study, 202 participants who had presented for treatment in outpatient CBT completed measures of psychological flexibility (Acceptance and Action Questionnaire–II; Bond & Bunce, 2000), dispositional mindfulness (Mindful Attention Awareness Scale [MAAS]; Brown & Ryan, 2003), and emotional schemas (LESS; Leahy, 2002). In this group, dispositional mindfulness was significantly correlated with psychological flexibility. All 14 of the emotional schema dimensions were also highly correlated with psychological flexibility and dispositional mindfulness. One possible interpretation of the highly significant correlations among more adaptive emotional schemas, mindfulness, and psychological flexibility is that a possible function of more adaptive cognitive schematic processing of responses to emotions is a greater degree of psychological flexibility and greater receptive attention to and awareness of present events and experiences. Because these correlations do not establish causality or direction in the relationships discussed, it is also possible that a person who presents with a higher degree of mindful awareness and psychological flexibility might report emotional schemas that are more adaptive as well. Indeed, it is likely that these schemas may be interacting processes involved in the establishment and maintenance of psychological flexibility and adaptive emotional functioning.

To examine the differing relationships across emotional schemas, mindfulness, and psychological flexibility, a stepwise multiple regression analysis was conducted. Psychological Flexibility, as a measure of accepting and adaptive behavioral functioning, was used as the dependent variable in this analysis, while emotional schemas related to emotion regulation strategies (Rumination, Expression, Need to Be Rational, and Acceptance of Feelings) and dispositional mindfulness were used as independent variables. Results indicated that the LESS factors of Expression and Need to Be Rational were not sufficiently significant predictors in this regression analysis to be included in the regression model. A model including the LESS factors Rumination and Low Acceptance of Feelings, as well as dispositional mindfulness, as measured by the MAAS accounted for a significant proportion of the variance in psychological flexibility compared with the other LESS factors hypothesized to be involved in emotion regulation strategies. Rumination was included in the first step of this model, followed by Low Acceptance of Feelings and then by dispositional mindfulness. The addition of each of the subsequent variables resulted in a statistically significant change. One possible interpretation of these results suggests that emotion regulation strategies that involve letting go of a ruminative thinking style, the adoption of an open acceptance to feeling emotions as they arrive, and an active attending to what is arising in the present moment do form the foundation of psychological flexibility. The degree to which a person is or is not overly rational or verbally expressive appeared to be less important in maintaining psychological flexibility in this research. Accordingly, the degree to which a meta-experiential stance is less ruminative, more accepting of emotion, and more grounded in receptive awareness of present experiences appears to contribute more to psychological flexibility than the degree of rationality or expressiveness involved in such a stance. This interpretation of these results would accord with the hypothesis inherent in the ACT hexaflex model that acceptance, defusion, and contact with the present moment are important components of psychological flexibility. The research also supported the relationship among the functioning of more adaptive emotional schemas and the ability to respond with flexibility rather than experiential avoidance. EST has aims and conceptual directions in common with several third-generation cognitive and behavioral theories, including the recognition that experiential avoidance may be related to the beliefs about emotion and distress that maintain problematic functioning.

AN OVERVIEW OF EST AND EMOTION REGULATION

Throughout this book we provide a wide range of techniques and strategies for assisting patients in coping with emotion. One can approach each chapter and choose to utilize the techniques as he or she feels is necessary. However, we believe that an integrative model of emotion regulation can be provided by EST that can assist the clinician in selecting the more relevant techniques and incorporating them in a more meaningful conceptualization that helps in understanding the patient's overall theory of emotions, including evaluations, predictions, and coping strategies. Thus, DBT techniques that improve the moment or allow one to "ride the wave" of an emotion address the belief that emotions need to be controlled or eliminated or that they are dangerous. Acceptance techniques that allow for committed action to valued goals address the belief that one needs to escape from emotion in order to get things done. Cognitive restructuring allows the patient to learn that changing interpretations of events can modify emotional responses, thereby conferring a greater sense of efficacy when experiencing an "unwanted" emotion. Stress reduction techniques that provide for reduction of autonomic arousal (e.g., progressive relaxation or breathing exercises) assist in learning that one can cope with an emotion and gradually reduce the intensity. Clarification of validation strategies that may not be helpful—or those that are helpful—assist the patient in using social support more effectively. In each case, we try to introduce techniques in light of the emotional schema issues that they may address.

We suggest the overall view of emotion regulation encompassed by an emotional schema model as presented in Figure 2.2. This model is not exhaustive, but it does suggest that a variety of strategies or techniques may be utilized. Problematic strategies include avoidance, suppression, and rumination/worry. (Of course, we could add many other problematic strategies such as blaming, numbing, dissociation, and substance abuse.) More helpful strategies (discussed in the chapters to follow) include modifying emotional schemas (in this chapter), acceptance and mindfulness, reducing arousal, problem solving, behavioral activation, cognitive restructuring, and adaptive behaviors seeking social support.

How can the clinician choose? There is no hard and fast rule. However, one issue is whether the antecedent event—the trigger for the emotional response—is amenable to cognitive reappraisal or problem solving. If so, then these strategies may be the first line of intervention. Indeed, even avoidance may be useful, such as deciding to avoid an abusive relationship. Behavioral activation may also be a valuable strategy if changing passivity and isolation can

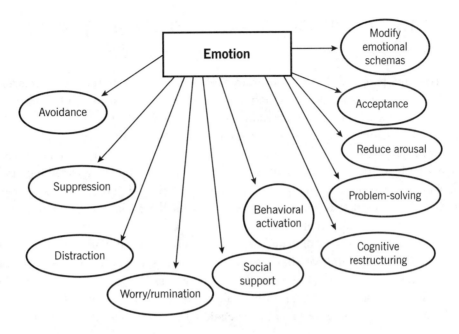

FIGURE 2.2. Strategies of emotion regulation.

lead to more rewarding experiences that can change emotion. In this case, the clinician may evaluate whether isolation, passivity, or responding to dysphoria with depressogenic behaviors is the problem. In the event that the patient feels overwhelmed by emotion, a variety of techniques may be helpful, including those described in Chapter 4 covering DBT and techniques described in the sections on acceptance, mindfulness, and stress reduction. Problematic interpretations of emotions may be addressed with the emotional schema model as well as the DBT discussion of emotional myths, including socialization about the meaning of emotions. Patients who hate themselves because of the way they feel may benefit from compassionate mind training, cognitive restructuring, or EST. Finally, one of the most powerful predictors of depression (and suicide) is problematic styles of interpersonal relating, which we identify in Chapter 3 on validation resistance. Quite often patients who feel overwhelmed with emotion may have idiosyncratic theories about validation or problematic styles of seeking validation. Our experience has been that exploring these interpretations while maintaining a compassionate, accepting, and nonjudgmental stance is an essential component for most patients experiencing emotional dysregulation. Thus, the clinician can determine which specific "presentation" of emotion dysregulation needs to be addressed and can implement the relevant techniques as described here. Our hope is that these techniques can then be related to modifying the patient's problematic theory of emotion and assist in developing a more adaptive set of interpretations, evaluations, and strategies to enhance emotional resilience.

EST is grounded in the key principles we discussed and makes use of a range of intervention techniques. In the rest of this chapter, we describe specific techniques related to interpretations, evaluations, attributions, and strategies related to emotion. With each technique we offer a description, specific questions to pose to patients, interventions to try, an illustrative example from a therapy session, homework suggestions, ideas for dealing with likely challenges and problems that often arise with these techniques, and cross-references to other techniques.

TECHNIQUE: IDENTIFYING EMOTIONAL SCHEMAS

Description

As we discussed, people differ in their awareness, recognition, differentiation, interpretation, and evaluation of, and strategies for, emotional experience. The first step in helping the patient understand emotional schemas is to introduce the model—and the schematic—that is the basis for the model. Negative interpretations of emotions contribute to the fear or intolerance of emotion, thereby leading to a sense of dysregulation, to being overwhelmed by emotions, and to employing problematic strategies, such as worry, rumination, bingeing, drinking, and acting out, to suppress or terminate emotional experiences. The LESS (Form 2.1), as we mentioned earlier, is a 50-question self-report scale that allows for the evaluation of emotional schemas along 14 dimensions: Invalidation, Incomprehensibility, Guilt, Simplistic View of Emotion, Lack of Higher Values, Loss of Control, Numbness, Need to Be Rational, Duration, Low Consensus, Acceptance of Feelings, Rumination, Expression, and Blame. The individual items are shown in Form 2.2; reverse-scored items are marked by parentheses. The scale can be reversed for specific items so that all scores that are positive reflect a negative view of emotion. Each dimension is weighted by the number of items on that specific subscale or dimension. Currently, there are no norms for the LESS.

Question to Pose/Intervention

"All of us have emotions of various kinds at different times. We all may have feelings of sadness, anxiety, fear, anger, hopelessness, happiness, helplessness, joy, confusion, or other emotions. I am going to ask you to complete a questionnaire that assesses how you think and respond to your emotions." The patient is given a copy of the LESS, which can be scored for 14 dimensions of emotional schemas (see Form 2.1). After the patient has completed the LESS, the therapist continues. "Let's look at how you think and respond to your emotions. You might have some difficulty, for example, in labeling an emotion—even noticing it—and recognizing that you might have a wide variety of emotions. And you might have some negative interpretations of these emotions—that they are shameful, not normal, that you are alone with these feelings. Or you might try to suppress these emotions by doing certain things that might make matters even worse in the long run but might help suppress an emotion for a short period of time. These interpretations that you have and the behaviors or strategies that you use we will call 'emotional schemas.' They are like your theory about your own emotion and your beliefs about how to handle emotion."

Example

Therapist: I saw on the questionnaire that you thought your emotions don't make sense to you, and that you thought no one really understands the way you feel. Can you tell me about which emotion that is?

Patient: I don't know why I feel so sad at times and then numb at times. It's hard to explain, and I don't think anyone is interested anyway.

Therapist: Yes, that must be hard to have those feelings and to feel you can't share them. When are you feeling sad?

Patient: When I come home to my apartment and I walk in and a feeling of sadness and dread comes over me.

Therapist: What would have made you feel better when you got home?

Patient: I'd feel better if I had someone to care for who cares for me.

Therapist: So your sadness is related to feeling lonely, not connected to someone, and that matters a great deal to you?

Patient: Yes, I used to be married to someone I loved, but he died and now I feel so lonely.

Therapist: So, when you feel lonely and sad, do you also think this feeling is going to go on and on, never end?

Patient: Yes, it seems like my whole life at times.

Therapist: And what do you do at times to handle this sadness?

Patient: I have a drink and then another one until I feel numb.

Homework

If the patient has not completed the LESS, then he or she can complete it as part of his or her homework. In addition, the patient can look over the figure that depicts the emotional schema model (Figure 2.1) and his or her responses on the LESS, and list some specific examples of thoughts and behaviors that represent his or her emotional schemas. For example, the therapist can suggest examining how emotional schemas about shame or guilt over emotion have impacted the patient's life or how beliefs about the duration and uncontrollability of emotion have led to problematic coping strategies, such as drinking, bingeing, or rumination.

Possible Problems

Although many patients find the schematic quite illuminating and informative, some may argue that their emotions are real and that they are based on a realistic assessment. The therapist can indicate that all emotions are real because they are experienced by the patient, and that the issue is not whether the emotions are valid but rather how one interprets and responds to them. For example, one can have a physical injury and can experience significant pain but can also view the pain as normal, temporary, and treatable.

Cross-Reference to Other Techniques

Labeling and differentiating emotions, emotion logs, and activity scheduling can be helpful. Identifying typical emotional myths can also be helpful. Similarly, Linehan (1993b) has identified a number of common myths about emotion which we review in Chapter 4 on emotional myths.

Forms

Form 2.1: Leahy Emotional Schemas Scale
Form 2.2: Fourteen Dimensions of the Leahy Emotional Schemas Scale

TECHNIQUE: LABELING AND DIFFERENTIATING
OTHER POSSIBLE EMOTIONS

Description

As we have mentioned in the Emotion-Focused Therapy section in Chapter 1, labeling emotions is a key part of processing experience. By labeling an emotion, the individual is able to recall the emotion and recognize the context in which it arises. People with alexithymia who have difficulty labeling emotions also have difficulty linking emotions to experience, recalling their emotions, and processing emotion. Alexithymia has been viewed as a "meta-emotional" deficit reflecting difficulties recalling emotions or identifying situations that give rise to emotions (Taylor, Bagby, & Parker, 1997). Overall levels of anxiety are positively related to alexithymia (Culhane & Watson, 2003; Eizaguirre, Saenz de Cabezon, Alda, Olariaga, & Juaniz, 2004). In a study of 85 combat veterans, alexithymia was predictive of PTSD (Monson, Price, Rodriguez, Ripley, & Warner, 2004), while in another study alexithymia was found to be essentially a *symptom* (i.e., emotional numbing) characteristic of PTSD (Bandura, 2003). Alexithymia is related to maladaptive coping with anxiety, such as drinking and the search for perfectionism (Lundh, Johnsson, Sundqvist, & Olsson, 2002; S. H. Stewart, Zvolensky, & Eifert, 2002).

There are two parts to differentiating emotions. One is the classic emotion-focused technique in which we distinguish between primary and secondary emotions, for example, "If you weren't feeling angry, would you possibly be feeling anxious about this?" (Greenberg & Watson, 2005). However, a second technique is also possible: to imagine other emotions that one *could have* but does not currently have. This creates the possibility of flexibility in emotional response.

Question to Pose/Intervention

"It sounds like you are angry about this, but there could be an entire range of emotions that you might also have—but you might not have them right now. For example, is it possible that in a situation like this someone else might be indifferent, amused, curious, challenged, or even relieved?" The therapist can direct the patient to a checklist of possible emotions. "Are there any emotions here that someone could have about this situation? Would any of these emotions be preferable to you than the one you are having now?"

Example

Karen was upset that she wasn't invited to dinner by some of her friends. The therapist validated her feelings, but asked Karen to examine other emotions that one could have about the situation.

Therapist: You said you felt "upset" but I wonder if you could be more specific about your feeling.

Patient: I don't know. I felt my heart racing and tense. Just upset.

Therapist: Sounds like it was bothering you. What could the emotion be that you were feeling?

Patient: I guess I was feeling hurt.

Therapist: OK. And that must have felt pretty bad, too. And was there another feeling that you also could be having about this? Try to imagine what it felt like, that heart racing, tense, upset. Think about not being invited to the party.

Patient: I guess I was feeling sad, too.

Therapist: OK. And why were you sad, do you think?

Patient: I felt I wasn't cared for. No one wanted me around.

Therapist: And thinking that no one wanted you, at that time, was there another feeling that you also could have been having?

Patient: I felt angry. I was really angry that they would treat me that way.

Therapist: OK. So we can see that you had a lot of different feelings about this. You started by saying you were upset, which seemed a little vague—and then you said you were hurt, and then we can see that you also felt angry. And your heart was racing and you felt tense.

Patient: Yeah. Those were the feelings I had.

Therapist: I wonder if anyone could look at this situation and imagine having feelings other than feeling hurt, sad, and angry.

Patient: But don't I have a right to have these feelings?

Therapist: Yes, but you might consider additional ways of feeling and thinking, not to invalidate your right to your feelings, but to expand the range of experiences that you might be able to have.

Patient: I guess that I could also be feeling anxious because I worry that people don't like me and I won't be included in other things.

Therapist: Yes, I can see how that feeling could make sense, too. Are there other possible ways that someone might feel about this—perhaps not even the way that you are feeling?

Patient: I guess there are some people who might not care at all.

Therapist: How would those people think about it so that they didn't care?

Patient: They might think that they had better things to do with their time.

Homework

The patient can be given the checklist of emotions from Greenberg's emotion-focused therapy manual (Emotion Log, see Form 2.3). In addition, the patient can monitor and label emotions for specific situations and identify the variety of thoughts that are associated with those emotions. It is important to identify both thoughts ("I am a loser") and emotions evoked by these thoughts ("sadness, hopelessness"). This allows the therapist to make the important distinction between a thought that can be open to restructuring and an emotion that may be regulated using other techniques. Additionally, the therapist can ask the patient to list "alternative" emotions that others might have about the situation in order to create a possible range of emotions that can become "targets" or "goals" in therapy (see Form 2.4). For example, less unpleasant emotions, such as indifference, could be identified, along with the thoughts that would give rise to these new emotions. This exercise opens up flexibility of response to emotions and situations and suggests different ways of thinking and coping.

Possible Problems

Some patients confuse a thought ("There is nothing that I can do") with an emotion ("sadness" or "helplessness"). In some respects this may be inevitable, because many emotions entail cognitive appraisals. However, the therapist can help the patient distinguish thoughts from emotions by indicating that an emotion is a feeling (e.g., sad, anxious, angry), while a thought is a belief about reality (e.g., "I cannot do anything to help myself"). Thoughts can be examined in terms of the evidence, while feelings are by their nature true statements about one's subjective experience.

Cross-Reference to Other Techniques

The therapist can assign activity schedules to help the patient identify how emotions may vary with the situation.

Forms

Form 2.3: Emotion Log
Form 2.4: Possible Emotions Someone Could Have in This Situation

TECHNIQUE: NORMALIZING EMOTION

Description

In cognitive therapy for obsessive–compulsive disorder, a key element is helping patients realize that intrusive thoughts (often of an unwanted or bizarre nature) are quite common among the nonclinical population. Metacognitive therapy has been very helpful in assisting patients in reevaluating the nature of intrusive thoughts by helping them realize that one is not responsible for thoughts, thoughts don't necessarily lead to action (thought–action fusion), and one does not have to control or suppress thoughts (Clark, 2002; Wells, 2009). In EST, normalizing a range of emotions—often ones that are unwanted—can help patients process these feelings in their lives and reduce their fear and guilt about the way they feel. Patients feel less alone, better understood, and less "pathological" if they know that many other people might have similar emotions in a given situation, especially with specific beliefs about the situation. Normalizing an emotion helps validate patients.

Question to Pose/Intervention

"It sounds like you think that your feelings are unusual, maybe even strange, and that others might not have these feelings. Let's take your feeling of [jealousy, anger, anxiety]. Have you known other people with these feelings? Are there songs, poems, novels, or stories in which people have these feelings? Could you ask some of your friends if they have had these feelings?

Do you think your friends are weird, unusual, or abnormal because they have these feelings? Why not?"

Example

Sandra was feeling jealous that her partner had dinner with his ex-girlfriend. The therapist attempted to normalize feelings of jealousy.

Therapist: It sounds like you are feeling jealous but you also are feeling bad about being jealous. Why is that?

Patient: I don't want to be one of those neurotic jealous girlfriends.

Therapist: So it sounds like you are equating feeling jealous with being neurotic. But I wonder if you have talked to any of your girlfriends about Victor having dinner with the ex-girlfriend.

Patient: Well, some of them say they understand. In fact, one of them said she'd be even more pissed off than me. And one of my friends said, "Don't worry. He chose you."

Therapist: Well, it sounds like feeling jealous is something that could be normal. It's a painful feeling, I know, but you seem to think that there is something wrong with you that you have this feeling.

Patient: I'm worried that Victor will think I'm insecure.

Therapist: It's possible to have jealous feelings because you are human. Almost everyone feels jealous at times. But it also might point to the fact that things matter.

Patient: What do you mean?

Therapist: Well, imagine that your boyfriend said to you, "I decided it's completely OK with me if you go out and have dinner with any of your ex-boyfriends. I won't even ask you about it."

Patient: I'd think he's screwing around.

Therapist: So, jealousy might simply be a feeling that we have when people matter to us.

Homework

The patient can list the specific emotions that he or she considers "abnormal" and the advantages and disadvantages of thinking that these are "normal" feelings. The patient can conduct a survey and ask friends if they or anyone they know has ever had a specific emotion that the patient views as abnormal (e.g., envy, jealousy, anger). The patient can list any songs, poems, stories, or novels that depict these emotions. For example, if the patient has feelings of jealousy, he or she can identify songs about jealousy or literature that depicts jealousy (e.g., Shakespeare's *Othello*). They can do a Google search linking the specific emotion with the genre to determine who else has felt this emotion. The patient can complete Form 2.5 (Costs and Benefits of Thinking My Emotions Are Abnormal) to evaluate what the advantages and disadvantages are of believing that his or her emotions are abnormal. Some patients believe that pathologizing themselves will help them change. This can be examined through cognitive restructuring, which is described in Chapter 9. In addition, normalizing emotions can be achieved by asking others about their emotional experiences, using Form 2.6 (Survey of Other People Who Have These Emotions). Many patients find that others not only have many of the same emotions that they have, but that those people can also suggest different possible emotions, thoughts, and coping strategies that have been helpful.

Possible Problems

Some patients may conclude that because others have had the same emotion it means they have to be stuck in that emotion. The therapist can help patients recognize that emotions may be temporary, depend on the circumstances, which are ever changing, and depend on the coping mechanisms that they use.

Cross-Reference to Other Techniques

The self-validation exercises may help normalize emotions. Also, identifying emotional myths is relevant.

Forms

Form 2.5: Costs and Benefits of Thinking My Emotions Are Abnormal
Form 2.6: Survey of Other People Who Have These Emotions

TECHNIQUE: SEEING THAT EMOTIONS ARE TEMPORARY

Description

One of the fears that people have is that their painful emotions are unending and will pervade their entire day. This then makes them want to get rid of the emotion, which usually results in greater frustration, anxiety, and intolerance of emotion. By using the technique of finding that emotions are temporary, patients are instructed in taking a mindful observing stance toward their emotion and recording the different emotions and their intensity during the course of the day. This allows them to see that a full range of positive, negative, and neutral emotions occur and that emotions are like worries: They change and dissipate.

Question to Pose/Intervention

"Sometimes we are afraid of our feelings because we think that they will go on forever or last indefinitely. But it may be that your emotions are temporary—they may change moment to moment. Have you noticed that feelings you've had in the past that you don't have at this moment? Have you noticed your feelings change even while we are talking? Does the intensity of your feeling increase and decrease? Are there specific things that you are doing or thinking that are related to your feelings fluctuating? What are those things?" The therapist can ask the patient what the consequence would be if he or she really believed that feelings are temporary. Would he or she be less afraid of those feelings, less likely to use problematic strategies to handle those feelings?

Example

Therapist: Your feelings of loneliness seem to really bother you. You said before that you were thinking, "I'm always lonely." That's a strong feeling about a feeling.

Patient: Yeah. When I go home to my apartment and I walk in, I get this sense that I will be overwhelmed with the loneliness, and then I think I am going to be lonely forever.

Therapist: That's a scary thought to think you would be lonely forever. But let's check this out and see what the facts say. For example, even during the course of the evening last night, were there other feelings that you had beside loneliness?

Patient: I decided to watch television and I got intrigued with this program.

Therapist: So you had the feeling of being intrigued. Any other feelings watching the program?

Patient: It was exciting toward the end—it was a rerun of *Law and Order*.

Therapist: That's one of my favorite programs, too. And beside the show, were there any other feelings that you had?

Patient: Well, I felt relaxed when I took a bath and put on some music. I felt a little dreamy.

Therapist: OK. So we can see that your feelings of loneliness subsided during those other times and that you had other feelings. Does that suggest that feelings can be temporary? Maybe they change moment to moment.

Homework

The self-help assignments for this technique include completing an activity schedule on which activities, thoughts, and feelings—and the intensity of feelings—are charted. This helps the patient realize that feelings vary with activities, time of day, thoughts, and other situational factors. The patient can also complete a cost–benefit analysis for believing that feelings are temporary and develop a list of plans for how to aim for other feelings (and not get stuck in a feeling). The patient can use Form 2.7 (Activity Schedule, Emotions, and Thoughts) and Form 2.8 (Costs and Benefits of Believing That Emotions Are Temporary) to evaluate how emotions change and the consequences of recognizing that emotions change. For example, the Activity Schedule, Emotions, and Thoughts from can illustrate that a certain emotion and its intensity may ebb and flow with activities, thoughts, relationships, and even time of day or night, thereby revealing that emotions are not fixed or permanent. In addition, the patient can examine the costs and benefits of realizing the transient nature of emotion, freeing him or her from the belief that an emotion is "forever."

Possible Problems

Some patients believe that claiming emotions are temporary minimizes the pain that they experience and invalidates their emotional suffering. The therapist can indicate that part of therapy is the dialectic between change and validation, between actively moving forward while validating what has happened in the past.

Cross-Reference to Other Techniques

Validation exercises and self-validation as well as compassionate mind exercises can be helpful.

Forms

Form 2.7: Activity Schedule, Emotions, and Thoughts
Form 2.8: Costs and Benefits of Believing That Emotions Are Temporary

TECHNIQUE: INCREASING ACCEPTANCE OF EMOTION

Description

Many patients with emotion regulation difficulties believe that they have to "get rid" of an emotion, very much like worriers or obsessive patients who believe that they have to eliminate intrusive thoughts. They often fear that the emotion will overwhelm them, incapacitate them, or will go on indefinitely; therefore, there is a sense of urgency in eliminating the emotion. Just as thought suppression or unhelpful thought control strategies are unsuccessful and add to the sense of being overwhelmed and controlled by unwanted and intrusive thoughts, emotion suppression strategies and a sense of urgency add to the struggle within oneself that adds to further emotion dysregulation.

Acceptance of an emotion does not imply that one believes the emotion is a good or bad experience, but only acknowledges that it is an experience that one is having for this moment in time. Acceptance of the emotion can help divert the patient from a sense of urgency and futile attempts to rid oneself of feeling.

Question to Pose/Intervention

"I can see that you are having difficulty accepting that you are anxious [sad, angry, jealous]. What are the advantages and disadvantages of accepting these feelings? What do you think would happen if you did? What thoughts, behaviors, ways of interacting with others or other strategies would you then give up on? If you accepted that you have a feeling right now, could you also imagine focusing on other behaviors, experiences, and relationships that might be helpful? For example, if you accepted that you were anxious and said, 'I know I am feeling anxious right at this moment,' could you also—at the same time—say, 'I will also do some things that can be rewarding'?"

Example

The patient felt lonely when she returned to her apartment and felt a sense of panic that she had to get rid of the feeling of loneliness.

Therapist: I can understand that this feeling of loneliness feels very painful for you, and I notice that this seems to precede your desire to drink. Are you feeling you can't accept that feeling of loneliness?

Patient: I want to get rid of that feeling. I want to numb myself.

Therapist: Yes, and that is one strategy that many of us try—to get rid of a feeling, to get to feeling numb, feeling nothing. It's as if we are saying, "I can't accept and tolerate that feeling." But what has the consequence been for you of getting rid of a feeling rather than accepting it?

Patient: I'm drinking too much and I am afraid of being alone.

Therapist: What if you were to imagine your emotion—your feeling—of loneliness as a visitor that shows up and is just there. Kind of like a guest at a large dinner party and there are many other guests. "Lonely feelings" is the character who shows up.

Patient: That's an interesting image. It's like one of my in-laws.

Therapist: Yeah. That's a way of viewing this. You already accept that in-law and maybe you are polite and respectful. But you don't make it the entire focus of the party. There are other guests and other things to do.

Patient: That sounds a little odd—to think about a feeling like a guest. But I can try to think of it that way.

Therapist: Another technique that could be helpful is to imagine that the emotion comes into your body and you feel it. Like that feeling of loneliness—where do you feel it in your body?

Patient: It's a heavy feeling in my chest and a down feeling going into my stomach and I feel tired but a little jittery, like I have to get out.

Therapist: It sounds like a feeling of being defeated but wanting to run away from that feeling, so you feel jittery, maybe a little agitated.

Patient: That sounds right.

Therapist: OK. So let's imagine that this feeling comes to your chest and you are feeling it and now you just surrender and let it come over you, and it's like water going over the stones in a stream and you are the stones and the feeling washes over you and goes down the stream. And then another gentle wave of feeling comes and goes over and it is past and it is gone.

Patient: This is like I am the stones in the stream? Hmm. I always want to get rid of the feeling and now I imagine it washing over me.

Therapist: But you are the stones, impassive, strong, watching the feeling, seeing it go over and past and through the water and the river continues.

Patient: This feels very relaxing.

Therapist: So when you are in your apartment and the feeling of loneliness comes, you can say to yourself, "I don't have to get rid of a feeling. I can accept it, tolerate it, and welcome it in—as the guest that shows up."

Patient: It's a very different way of experiencing this for me.

Therapist: Yes, not accepting what comes leads you to struggle against yourself. And then you might also say to this emotion, "You are here again. Welcome once more and have a seat while I get on with the other things that I need to do." And then you just do things for yourself that are rewarding and pleasurable.

Patient: But what will happen to the feeling of loneliness?

Therapist: It may still be there, but perhaps it is more in the background. You aren't focusing on it all the time because you are now focusing on things that matter, that are pleasurable.

Homework

The chapter on rumination in Leahy's *Beat the Blues Before They Beat You* (2010) provides a number of ideas of how to handle recurring, intrusive thoughts and feelings. The patient can practice surrendering to the sensations of the feeling, imagining the feeling as water that flows over a rock, and observing the feeling as it comes and goes. Form 2.9 (How to Accept Difficult Feelings) can be assigned. Examples of how to accept feelings include the following: "Don't fight the feeling, allow it to happen. Stand back and observe it. Imagine that the feeling is floating along and you are floating along next to it. Watch it go up and down, come and go, moment to moment."

Possible Problems

Some patients believe accepting an emotion is equivalent to surrendering to suffering. In a sense there is a surrender of the struggle against an emotion, but acceptance does not mean one does nothing to feel better. Accepting that it is raining does not mean I leave my umbrella behind. Recognizing, acknowledging, and building space for a variety of emotions helps put them in perspective of a larger meaning and potential in life. Attentional deployment exercises can help the patient recognize that one can be aware of something without getting stuck in it. For example, a patient reported feeling anxious, and he was asked to describe all the colors of books in the office. As he did so, his anxiety decreased. This indicated that he could be momentarily aware of the anxiety but redirect attention elsewhere. Acceptance does not imply inflexibility or being stuck in the emotion at the moment. The therapist can indicate that one can accept feeling anxious at the present moment while engaging in behavior that can lead to a change in that emotion. Furthermore, acceptance does not imply rumination; in fact, rumination is a form of experiential avoidance. For example, accepting that I am sad can imply that I do not need to ruminate about it with unanswerable questions such as, "Why is this happening to me?" Acceptance can follow this sequence: "I accept I am sad. I know that is how I feel. But I can engage in other behaviors that can lead to valued goals."

Cross-Reference to Other Techniques

Any of the mindfulness exercises can be incorporated with this technique. Acceptance and willingness exercises are also useful.

Form

Form 2.9: How to Accept Difficult Feelings

TECHNIQUE: TOLERATING MIXED FEELINGS

Description

Anxious people often have difficulty tolerating uncertainty. Indeed, Dugas, Ladouceur, and their colleagues have advanced a treatment for generalized anxiety based on increasing tolerance of uncertainty among worried patients (Dugas & Robichaud, 2007; see also Wells, 2009). In fact, intolerance of uncertainty also underlies maladaptive evaluation of obsessive intrusions and drives ruminative processes of thinking. Individuals activate a strategy of worry or rumination in order to reduce their uncertainty, equating uncertainty with negative outcomes and a sense of irresponsibility. Having mixed feelings—or ambivalence—is an emotional manifestation of uncertainty, because individuals experience potentially conflicting feelings about people, experiences, or the self. This ambivalence may generate anxiety and a sense of "confusion" as these individuals search for "what I really feel." However, "univalent" feelings—that is, feelings that only "go one way" ("I really like him" or "I really don't like him")—may be unrealistic, because people (and experiences) often provide considerable complexity, situations change, people change within those situations, and consistency of traits may be less likely than the impact of situations. Indeed, Mischel's rejection of "trait psychology" in favor of "person–situation" conceptualizations may be more empirically valid (Dugas, Buhr, & Ladouceur, 2004; Mischel, 2001; Mischel & Shoda, 2010).

There are advantages in tolerating ambivalence, ambiguity, and uncertainty. First, dispositional inferences may be less accurate in predicting behavior than contextual or situational descriptions. Thus, if dispositions or traits are actually "myths," then ambivalence and ambiguity may be more realistic. An individual's behavior may depend more on the situation or context than on fixed traits. Second, by focusing on variability and context, there are more "degrees of freedom" in regard to behavioral flexibility. For example, if I know that you might respond more favorably given a different perception of situational contingencies, then I might consider rearranging the reward structure to benefit you (and to get what I want from you). Our research shows that one of the main predictors of marital dissatisfaction is being unable to tolerate mixed feelings (Leahy & Kaplan, 2004).

The technique of accepting mixed feelings assists the patient in differentiating feelings, viewing them in a dialectical manner (balanced and conflicting), while increasing recognition that "mixed feelings" may simply reflect greater awareness of the complexity, truth, and realities of human nature. Indeed, one question to raise is whether feelings are "contradictory" or "complementary." For example, one can argue that red and blue complement each other or that certain notes in a musical score may complete the melody. They do not contradict each other; feelings are not like logical statements. Viewing emotions as linear and logical experiences in the phenomenology of mind may obscure the fact that emotions tap into different perceptions, needs, and nuances.

Question to Pose/Intervention

"Are there advantages to accepting mixed feelings? Are there disadvantages? What are they? Is it possible to think of mixed feelings as reflecting simply *knowing more*? Aren't people complicated, and so mixed feelings could be simply a reflection of the complexity of human nature? Do other people have mixed feelings? Do you have mixed feelings about your friends or family members, and could they have mixed feelings about you? Is the difficulty with mixed feelings a reflection of your perfectionism? If you accepted or tolerated mixed feelings, would you worry or ruminate less?"

Example

A young woman was experiencing mixed feelings about her fiancé, recognizing that there were qualities about him she found irritating but other qualities that she highly valued. She complained that she didn't know how she "really felt."

Therapist: You seem to find it hard to recognize that you are having mixed feelings about Dave, and I was wondering why mixed feelings are hard for you to tolerate.

Patient: Maybe there is something that I am missing. If I am having mixed feelings, then maybe I am making a mistake.

Therapist: Well, it's important to feel that you are making the right decision for yourself. But it seems that you are equating mixed feelings with "making a mistake." [The therapist and patient then examine the positives and negatives about Dave as a partner and she weighs them out as 80% positive and 20% negative.] It sounds that it's 80–20 in Dave's favor. How does that feel to you?

Patient: I know that he has a lot of positives. He's a great guy, the best I've been with. But should I make a decision with mixed feelings?

Therapist: You are equating mixed feelings with a bad alternative. Can you imagine any major decision in your life that won't have pros and cons? Are there any friends whom you have had for a long time who you don't have some mixed feelings about?

Patient: I guess you're right about that. But they're friends, not someone I might marry.

Therapist: Do you think that married people don't have mixed feelings?

Patient: I know my parents do. And they've been married for 35 years.

Therapist: You could also think of mixed feelings as reflecting the fact that you know someone well. Being able to accept, tolerate, and be nonjudgmental might be a different way of looking at it.

Patient: But if I accept this, doesn't that mean I am settling?

Therapist: But whenever we make important decisions, aren't we settling for the balance of the pros and the cons. Aren't we saying, "On balance, it looks pretty good, although it's not perfect."

Patient: I guess Dave has some mixed feelings about me as well.

Therapist: Maybe that's because you know each other and you simply can see that people are complicated and that's OK, too.

Homework

The patient can complete Form 2.10 (Examples of Mixed Feelings) and Form 2.11 (Advantages and Disadvantages of Accepting Mixed Feelings).

Possible Problems

Some patients believe that tolerating mixed feelings renders them confused and ultimately helpless. The assumption is that there is only one way to feel about things and that this one way must be discovered. A useful analogy to challenge this assumption is that of painting. Is there one color that should comprise the entire painting, or is the painting richer, more meaningful, more emotional with many colors?

Cross-Reference to Other Techniques

Form 2.3 (Emotion Log) helps identify a variety of feelings in the same or different situations. Also, monitoring how thoughts and feelings vary with automatic thoughts can be a helpful way of illustrating that thoughts and feelings change and can be mixed together.

Forms

Form 2.10: Examples of Mixed Feelings
Form 2.11: Advantages and Disadvantages of Accepting Mixed Feelings

TECHNIQUE: EXPLORING EMOTIONS AS GOALS

Description

Greenberg and Safran have described how some emotional experiences are primary and others are secondary (Greenberg & Safran, 1987, 1990). For example, patients may present with feelings of anger, but underlying the anger may be feelings of anxiety, which may be seen as less tolerable or more threatening. In the emotional schema model, emotions can become goals in themselves, thereby freeing individuals from the sense of "getting stuck in a feeling." We often sense that our feelings "happen to us," as if a feeling is a wave that comes over us and envelops us. This sense of being a victim of their own feelings can make patients fearful of allowing a feeling to exist and may lead them to struggle against an emotion that they think they need to get rid of. There is no a priori reason why the emotion they are experiencing currently need be the only emotion that can occupy their field of experience. Patients who are feeling angry about one event might consider exploring feelings of appreciation about other events. Frustration can yield to curiosity.

Just as we can make choices regarding the food we eat at a buffet, we can also make choices as to the emotions we are going to aim for today. Similar to the DBT technique of improving the moment (Linehan, 1993a, 1993b), with EST we can also decide which emotions to "go for" (Greenberg & Safran, 1987; Leahy, 2010). EST recognizes the importance of positive psychology, especially the role of positive emotions in buffering us against stress. In Form 2.12, we have included the 10 most important positive emotions that have been identified by Fredrickson (Fredrickson & Branigan, 2005; Fredrickson & Losada, 2005).

The following may be helpful to the patient in identifying emotions as goals: (1) recognition of choice ("You can decide if you want to experience and focus on the current emotion or see if there is a way to have another emotion," "What would be the advantages of having a different

emotion—about something entirely different in your life—rather than the current emotion?";
(2) setting an emotion as a goal ("Which emotion would you like to create for yourself? Happiness, curiosity, appreciation, fear, confusion, challenge, gratitude?"); (3) activating memories and images ("Let's take the emotion of 'pride.' Close your eyes and try to recall a moment in your life when you felt proud of doing something"—Therapist uses imagery induction to guide the patient through memories, images, thoughts, sensations, and feeling); alternatively family "scrapbooks" of photographs can be used to bring back other memories); (4) using activity to make the emotion real ("Let's imagine that over the next week you were going to try to catch yourself or other people feeling proud. What would be some examples of this? What are some things that you could do—even very small things that you might do—to catch some examples of yourself feeling proud?") In addition, traditional activity scheduling can assist the patient in recognizing that other emotions occur dependent on the activities engaged in.

Question to Pose/Intervention

"I notice you are feeling [emotion] right now and this is disturbing you. It makes sense that this feels bad right now. But I am wondering if we might put that feeling up on a shelf for a few minutes and consider other emotions you might want to have." For example, the therapist could say, "You are feeling frustrated about being blocked on this. What if you were to aim for feeling indifferent? What would you have to think to feel indifferent?" Or "This particular [event] has been upsetting for you. Let's put that up on the shelf for a few minutes and think about other things in your life. For example, imagine you were trying to think of something that you could be appreciative of [have gratitude for]. What kinds of thoughts and images go with that?"

Example

Bill was angry and frustrated with his colleagues, whom he described as petty and unfair. They were "blocking" him from pursuing his goals.

Therapist: You seem stuck in this feeling of anger and resentment, and who could blame you for that? They haven't treated you fairly. But this feeling of being stuck is making you feel trapped.

Patient: Yeah, I keep going over and over about this. Angry, frustrated. I can't get past it.

Therapist: Let's recognize for now that you will have those feelings of anger about this. But I'd like to try a different exercise today—let's aim for a different set of feelings about this. You can put the anger up on a shelf for a few minutes and see if there are other ways to feel that could also make sense.

Patient: I'm not sure what you mean.

Therapist: Well, two other feelings come to mind about these people. One is a feeling of indifference and the other a feeling of curiosity. What if either or both of those feelings were the way you felt?

Patient: I'd be a lot less angry.

Therapist: Yeah, and less stuck. OK. So, let's imagine that you wanted to go –with all your heart—for true indifference. The "I don't really care what they think" attitude. What would be some thoughts that might lead you to the peace and freedom of true indifference?

Patient: I guess I'd realize that they are what they are, they won't change, and I can still get almost everything done. I didn't need them before and I don't need them now. I mean, why should I really care about their view on this? It's not like I really look up to them.

Therapist: OK, sounds like you are reaching a plateau of indifference. And how would you aim for curiosity about this? For example, what if you were to try to figure out some strategies that you could use to cope with this? Develop curiosity about your alternatives?

Patient: I guess I could figure out how to get around them. Try to figure out some alternative way of solving the problem. I could think about how this makes sense from everything I have heard about this organization and these people. When I think about it, I might think, "Why should I really be surprised?

Therapist: How does curiosity work for you?

Patient: It works OK. But I think I prefer indifference.

Therapist: OK, then your emotional goal is indifference.

Homework

Homework can consist of identifying alternative, more pleasant, or rewarding emotions and compiling a list using Form 2.12 (Looking for Positive Emotions). Greenberg's Emotion Log can be employed as an example. The patient then can list activities or thoughts that can produce these emotions and complete Form 2.13 (Emotional Goal Inventory), which asks the patient to develop a "narrative" that can lead to a new emotion. Again, this exercise increases the range of flexibility of emotional experiences and helps patients realize that they are not stuck in an emotion and that they do not need to ruminate about where they are stuck.

Possible Problems

Many people believe that emotions happen to them: "How can I make emotion a goal if it's simply something that I feel (or something that comes over me)? I have no control over my feelings." This sense of helplessness about emotion can be examined by monitoring how emotions change with behavior and thoughts, using the activity schedule or a daily record of dysfunctional thoughts. In-session exercises that guide the patient through imagery induction, meditative or mindful breathing exercises, or compassionate mind exercises can demonstrate how new emotions can become more salient.

Cross-Reference to Other Techniques

Activity scheduling, compassionate mind exercises, and mindful breathing can be used.

Forms

Form 2.12: Looking for Positive Emotions

Form 2.13: Emotional Goal Inventory

TECHNIQUE: MAKING ROOM FOR EMOTION

Description

Patients frequently believe they can have only one emotion and have to choose between this emotion or another—they can't have both. This then leads to struggles with one's own emotional experience and attempts to suppress emotions or to numb emotions with bingeing, purging, drinking, or taking drugs. Using the technique of "making room for emotion," the therapist can introduce the idea of a larger "life space of experience." One's emotional world can become larger and provide a context in which emotions are contained and counterbalanced.

Question to Pose/Intervention

"We often get very focused on one painful emotion and think that we can't stand it because the pain is so great. But emotions exist in a context of other things in your life. What would be the advantages and disadvantages of accepting this emotion for right now, without trying to eliminate it? What are the other emotions and meanings in your life that can be larger and more meaningful to you than the feeling that you are having?"

Example

The patient was a man in his 60s whose wife had died after a long illness. Months later he felt that he couldn't get over it and worried how he would be able to cope.

Therapist: So, it sounds like losing Tricia after all these years still wears on you.

Patient: Yeah. I can't seem to get over it. I realize it was a long period of cancer, eating away at her and, in a sense, it was a blessing. But I can't seem to get past it. It's been 6 months now.

Therapist: Tricia was your wife for almost 40 years, and a lot of meaning and love and memory are contained in your experience of her. I wonder if it really is necessary to *get over it*.

Patient: But how can I get on with my life?

Therapist: One way of thinking about this—and it can be painful to feel these things—is to say, "I never have to get over this." In fact, I might even say to you, "I hope that you will still be capable of feeling sad when you think of losing her. I hope you still can be open to that loss." But I would add that I hope that you can build a life large enough in meaning that it can contain that loss. And that you can remember her with the wonderful and happy moments and still be open to the sadness that she is gone. And, in that way, you never lose her in your mind.

Patient: (*crying*) That is very helpful to me. Yes, I have been trying to get over it.

Therapist: It's not always about eliminating suffering. It's about living a life worth suffering for. And at this moment you are suffering because it has been worth it.

Patient: Thank you.

Therapist: And to ask yourself, with her memory with you now, what she would want you to do with your life.

Patient: She would want me to live my life.

Therapist: And maybe by living your life and keeping her memory within you that the loss is still there but less painful because there are so many other emotions along with the loss. There is the joy of her memory and the meaning of your life. Your life can contain that loss.

Homework

The patient can complete Form 2.14 (Additional Meanings in Life) and Form 2.15 (Possible Emotions That I Can Also Have).

Possible Problems

Many patients believe that sad emotions must be eliminated lest they overwhelm them and make life unbearable. This self-protective strategy to suppress or eliminate emotions only makes emotions more feared. Patients can identify sad or anxious experiences that no longer bother them, such as the loss of a friendship, loss of a pet, or failure to achieve a goal. The therapist can ask whether the passage of time, while building new meanings in life, has allowed these previously difficult experiences to be incorporated in life.

Cross-Reference to Other Techniques

Other helpful techniques include Greenberg's Emotion Log (Form 2.3), identifying emotions to aim for (Form 2.13), compassionate mind exercises, and activity scheduling.

Forms

Form 2.14: Additional Meanings in Life
Form 2.15: Possible Emotions That I Can Also Have

TECHNIQUE: CLIMBING A LADDER OF HIGHER MEANING

Description

Emotions give meaning to our experiences. Without emotion we would be frozen in indecision, unable to make a choice between alternatives. Painful emotions can reflect the events that matter to us and shed light on the meaning and values that underpin our existence. The technique of "laddering" is derived from personal construct theory and allows patients to clarify the higher values that emotions and experience give rise to (Cohn & Fredrickson, 2009). The concept of laddering allows patients to find the higher meaning that they may want to preserve or respect in the painful emotion that they experience at the present time. Laddering also can help clarify higher order (superordinate) constructs or values that may give emotional importance to everyday experiences, sometimes in a manner that can be destructive. For example, laddering can lead to the higher order value of perfectionism, which can undermine experience. However, in the current context, laddering is used as a way of accessing the higher values that may make difficulties worth enduring. Although personal construct theorists use laddering or pyramiding in specific ways, in the current context we are focusing on "climbing a ladder of meaning" to focus on the positive implications of realizing the satisfaction of a need.

Question to Pose/Intervention

"We are often upset or frustrated because we feel our needs and values are not being realized. Let's take your current situation. You are upset [other emotion] because of the [current situation]. But let's imagine that you were able to get that need met. Let me ask you to complete each sentence with whatever comes first to your mind. 'If I got [this need met], that would be good because it would mean [what about me, life, the future]? And if that happened, it would be good because it would mean. ... ' Let's say you feel sad about a relationship breakup. Doesn't this mean you have a higher value that's important to you, for example, a value of closeness and intimacy? Doesn't this value say something good about you? If you aspire to higher values, doesn't this mean you will have to be disappointed at times? Would you want to be a cynic who values nothing? Are there other people who share your higher values? What advice would you give them, if they were going through what you are going through?"

Example

The patient was a widowed woman with a history of alcohol abuse. She claimed she would get high before arriving at her apartment because she otherwise would feel overwhelmingly sad when she entered the apartment.

Therapist: If you weren't high when you opened the door to your apartment, what would you feel?

Patient: I'd feel really sad. And empty.

Therapist: And what are you thinking when you walk in and you feel sad and empty?

Patient: I'm all alone. I have no one.

Therapist: Yes, it's hard for you feeling alone without someone. I wonder, if you walked in and you had someone, that would make you feel better because you would think what?

Patient: I'd think, "I have someone to care for."

Therapist: OK. And it would make you feel good to have someone to care for because it would mean what for you?

Patient: That I'm not alone—that I can share my life with someone.

Therapist: And if you had someone to share your life with, that would feel better because it would mean what for you?

Patient: That I can give my love to someone.

Therapist: And the reason you want to give your love to someone is that …

Patient: I'm a loving person.

Therapist: So you have climbed a ladder of meaning from loneliness and emptiness to being a loving person. And that is an important source of meaning in your life. And here is the dilemma in our lives: that sometimes it is painful that things matter to us, but not to have meaning, not to be a loving person, would be the true emptiness. And you are a loving person.

Patient: Yes, I am.

Therapist: And that is a value to hold on to. It may be painful. But you don't have to feel bad about feeling bad, because your pain comes from a good place. It comes from caring and loving, and that is the person you are.

Patient: But it's frustrating.

Therapist: Yes, it is. But there are other ways of being a loving person. There are people in your life to love and there is you to love. Maybe you can also think about being a loving person toward yourself.

Patient: I've never thought of it that way.

Homework

Patients can list the higher values that they aspire to. Then they can identify the sadness, anxiety, stress, anger, or other difficult emotions they are experiencing and examine how they might be related—or not—to those higher values. If they are not related to higher values, then patients can examine what behaviors will help achieve the experience of those values. Patients can identify and clarify their values by completing Form 2.16 (Relationship to Higher Values) and Form 2.17 (VIA Survey of Character Strengths). The VIA identifies and assesses 24 character strengths that can be identified as values, personal traits, or goals that one can use to structure life choices. Examples include creativity, curiosity, love of learning, open-mindedness, bravery, persistence, integrity, vitality, kindness, social intelligence, citizenship, fairness, leadership, forgiveness/mercy, modesty/humility, prudence, self-regulation, appreciation of excellence and beauty, gratitude, hope, humor, and spirituality.

Possible Problems

Listing the higher values and emotions to which one aspires may create a sense of momentary loss and failure for some patients. The therapist can help patients realize that disappointment and frustration can be positive motivations to aspire to more important values and goals. Using the negative feeling as a reminder that authentic and meaningful goals can empower individuals in overcoming the obstacles that they foresee. Patients who focus on rumination and regret when their important values and goals are not currently realized may be reminded that rumination is a way of avoiding real choices in the real world. Moreover, goals and values such as loving-kindness do not necessitate an intimate partner. One can direct these values and emotions toward strangers and friends, toward pets, and, of course, toward oneself.

Cross-Reference to Other Techniques

Many of the compassionate mind techniques may be helpful in generating an openness to more positive and empowering values. Also, activity scheduling and planning positive activities may assist in realizing important values and goals.

Forms

Form 2.16: Relationship to Higher Values
Form 2.17: VIA Survey of Character Strengths

CONCLUSIONS

The emotional schema model draws on a social cognitive model of implicit theory of emotion—that is, patients' beliefs about the meaning, causes, need to control, and implications of emotional experience. Negative beliefs about emotions further complicate the experience of "feeling bad," leading patients to a recursive and escalating dysregulation of feeling bad about feeling bad. Modifying these emotional schemas can assist patients in normalizing, temporarizing, accepting, and giving up unhelpful strategies of emotional avoidance, suppression, or other maladaptive coping behaviors, such as binge eating, self-injury, or substance abuse. Similar to the recognition of emotional myths in Linehan's work, the emotional schema model helps patients elaborate their implicit theory of emotion (and its regulation) to develop a more realistic and adaptive model of emotional experience.

CHAPTER THREE

Validation

A number of theories stress the importance of validation, empathy, and emotional connection in the therapeutic process. Rogers (1965) emphasized unconditional positive regard, Kohut (1977) proposed that mirroring and empathic failures are often inevitable components of the therapeutic relationship, and a variety of other contemporary experiential and cognitive-behavioral approaches emphasize empathy and compassion (Gilbert, 2007; Greenberg & Safran, 1987; Leahy, 2005a; Linehan, 1993a; Safran, Muran, Samstag, & Stevens, 2002). Empathy refers to either the identification or shared experience (mirroring) of an emotion that another person has ("I see that you are upset" or "I feel the sadness that you are feeling"), validation refers to finding the truth in the feeling ("I can see why you are upset because you were hoping to get that, but you didn't"), and compassion is the attempt to soothe and comfort the other ("I see that you are upset and I hope that I can make you feel cared for and loved").

Validation, empathy, and compassion (responding to, reflecting, soothing, and connecting to the emotions of another person) are processes that originate in the infant–parent interaction, with parents (often mothers) attuned to the cries and discomfort of their infants. In his attempt to challenge the drive-reduction model of psychoanalytic theory, Bowlby proposed that infants are innately predisposed to form and maintain attachment to a single figure, and interruptions in the attachment bond will activate behavioral systems that seek completion until attachment is secured. Bowlby's ethological model of attachment stressed the evolutionary implications of attachment in establishing proximity to adults who could protect, feed, and socialize the infant in appropriate behaviors (Ainsworth, Blehar, Waters, & Wall, 1978; Bowlby, 1968, 1973). Attachment theorists further elaborated this model to emphasize the importance for the infant or child in establishing a sense of *security* in attachment, not simply proximity (Sroufe & Waters, 1977). This security entails the predictability of the responsiveness of the caregiver for the child. Although some have argued for some continuity between early attachment and adult attachment styles, others have disputed the validity of these claims (Fox, 1995; van IJzendoorn, 1995).

Ainsworth and others have differentiated various forms of attachment styles, including secure, anxious, avoidant, and disorganized. Other classification systems that have been employed differentiate three types: secure, avoidant, and ambivalent (Troy & Sroufe, 1987;

Urban, Carlson, Egeland, & Sroufe, 1991). Research on attachment styles suggests that early childhood attachment is predictive of social functioning in middle childhood and early adulthood, specifically peer relationships, depression, aggression, dependency, and social competence (Cassidy, 1995; Urban et al., 1991).

Bowlby proposed that security in attachment is enhanced through the development of *internal working models* or cognitive representations of the attachment figure. Specifically, an internal working model for a securely attached infant would imply that the caregiver will respond to cries of distress, will be responsive in soothing the infant through reciprocal interactions, and will be predictable in providing positive rather than punitive interactions (Main, Kaplan, & Cassidy, 1985). The assumption guiding attachment theory is that these internal working models, established in earlier childhood, will affect subsequent attachment experiences with other individuals in the person's life. It is this responsiveness, as described by Bowlby and others— that marks the early foundation of validation schemas. Extensions of the internal working model are reflected in a number of cognitive models of early maladaptive schemas (Guidano & Liotti, 1983; Smucker & Dancu, 1999; Young et al., 2003).

Validation is reflective of attachment issues. First, during the process of forming and maintaining attachment during early childhood, the rudiments of empathy, mirroring, and validation include the caregiver's responsiveness to the child's distress, which reinforces the child's mental representation—"My feelings make sense to others." Second, responsive soothing of the child's feelings by the caregiver encourages the child to believe, "My distressed feelings can be soothed." Initially, it is proposed that this "soothing" occurs through the caregiver's attention and reassurance but later is "internalized" by the child in self-calming and optimistic self-statements, similar to Bowlby's idea of internal working models, in this case the internal representation that one's feelings make sense and can be calmed. Third, the child's communication of feelings to the caregiver becomes an opportunity not only for expressing feelings but for the caregiver to link emotional states to external events that "cause" the feeling—"You're upset because your brother hit you." This attempt to comprehend the cause of feelings and to share them with the caregiver can also assist in differentiating these feelings—"It sounds like you are angry and hurt"—and in constructing a theory of mind that can be applied to both self and others. Indeed, without an adequate theory of mind, the child will be impaired in showing empathy, validation, and compassion toward others and will be unable to soothe her own feelings and the feelings of others (Eisenberg & Fabes, 1994; Gilbert, 2007, 2009; Leahy, 2001, 2005a; Twemlow, Fonagy, Sacco, O'Toole, & Vernberg, 2002).

Patients may exhibit a variety of attachment styles in therapy: secure, anxious, avoidant, or disorganized. The anxious attachment style is characterized by clinging behaviors and need for reassurance and reflects fears that validation will not be obtained. Moreover, individuals with anxious attachment styles may have idiosyncratic beliefs about validation (e.g., "You have to feel what I feel to understand me") and may fear that the therapist will become critical or withdrawn. Nevertheless, these anxious individuals will still seek out validation and eventual attachment to the therapist. In contrast, the avoidant attachment style will be reflected in wariness and distance, avoiding closer contact and openness in the therapeutic relationship. Individuals with a disorganized attachment style may have difficulty identifying needs or may escalate the expression of these needs for fear that they will not be heard and, therefore, never be met. These attachment styles, therefore, may be activated when emotions escalate, leading to attempts to regulate emotions through problematic interpersonal styles of validation seeking. Emotion regulation is affected by a patient's perception that she is validated or not, and beliefs about validation (e.g., "You have to agree with me entirely") or self-defeating attempts to seek validation that may be problematic (e.g., escalation of complaints, yelling, dramatic displays, withdrawal) may heighten and prolong emotional dysregulation. As indicated in Chapter 2 on EST, perception of validation is one of the key predictors for depression, substance abuse, marital conflict, and borderline personality disorder. In the current chapter, we review some common problems in emotion dysregulation that are reflected in self-defeating or problematic validation strategies that may inadvertently lead to further emotional escalation.

TECHNIQUE: VALIDATION RESISTANCE

Description

Experiencing and receiving validation, empathy, and unconditional positive regard are key elements in a variety of theories. Rogers emphasized a nonjudgmental, nondirective unconditional positive acceptance of the patient, Bowlby described how attachment systems and a secure base can help with the integration of emotion and self-identity, Kohut described the role of mirroring and empathic failures in therapy, Greenberg emphasized emotional processing and empathy, Safran described the therapeutic alliance and healing ruptures, and Linehan proposed that invalidating environments are a key factor in the emergence of borderline personality disorder and emotion dysregulation in general. Indeed, one might argue that validation is a transtheoretical and transdiagnostic process that can be relevant across a variety of disorders. Given the importance of validation, it is not surprising that emotionally dysregulated patients may often feel invalidated in therapy and in their lives outside of therapy.

Leahy has proposed that noncompliance or resistance in therapy may often result from beliefs in the failure to obtain validation and the activation of problematic standards and strategies for seeking validation (Leahy, 2001). For example, patients who are distraught by their emotions may have problematic criteria for validation, such as the belief that the other person needs to agree with everything that is said, needs to feel the same pain and suffering in order to understand or be helpful, or needs to hear every detail about every emotion and thought to "really understand" (Leahy, 2001, 2009). This technique introduces the issue of invalidation in therapy and can serve as a source of information for examining patients' problems in finding validation.

Question to Pose/Intervention

"Feeling validated—that someone understands and cares—is an important part of therapy and of life in general. Are there times with me that you don't feel validated? Could you tell me some examples? Are there times you do feel validated? What examples can you tell me about? Sometimes we believe that someone doesn't validate or care unless they say or do something. Do you have any standards for feeling validated? When you don't feel validated, what do you do next?" The therapist can explore examples of escalation, complaining, repeating, attacking, pouting, self-injurious behavior, and other problematic strategies.

Example

The patient was a woman going through a breakup with her boyfriend. She was feeling sad and angry and became frustrated with the therapist, who was suggesting some ways of coping with her feelings.

Therapist: This is a really hard time for you right now, and I can see that you are frustrated with what we are talking about. Can you tell me what you are feeling and thinking about our discussion today?

Patient: It seems that you are trying to get me to change the way I think about this. But it hurts me right now, and I don't know if you really understand that.

Therapist: That would make sense, that it is upsetting if I don't understand. I'm sorry that I'm not connecting here. Can we talk about that? Would that be OK?

Patient: Yeah.

Therapist: What did I say that made you feel I don't understand how hard it is?

Patient: You were trying to get me to do things to help myself, like see other people and do activities and that sort of thing.

Therapist: So, did you think that when I was talking about changing some of these things somehow your feelings got left out?

Patient: Yeah. I have a right to feel upset—to feel sad.

Therapist: I agree with you. That's one of the real dilemmas in therapy—trying to find change but being able to stay with the feeling, respect the way you feel, and validate how hard it is. Sometimes I'm not the best at doing that, so it may feel like I don't understand or care.

Patient: Yeah. I feel so bad right now it's hard to get through things. It's hard for me.

Therapist: Here is the dilemma for us—at least for me. I am hoping that I can help you feel better but you may get stuck with that bad feeling and think I don't care if we talk about change. How can we do that—talk about change and respect your feelings? Maybe there's something that I can be doing better—something different?

Patient: Well, actually, what you are doing now is helping me.

Therapist: Could we say that when I am validating you it feels better for you? OK. That's a good thing for me to remind myself to do much more of. Let me know when I'm not validating you. But how about the change?

Patient: I do want to change. Well, maybe we can talk about change.

Therapist: How about this? We talk about change, I really try to connect with your feelings, validate you, maybe ask if you feel understood and validated and cared for, and talk about more change—if that's OK with you.

Patient: OK.

Therapist: It's a deal?

Patient: Yes.

Homework

There are many possible homework assignments to address validation issues. First, monitor examples of feeling validated and not feeling validated. Second, list examples of "what I do" when someone doesn't validate me. The therapist can identify in session some problematic styles of responding to invalidation, such as complaining, escalating, attacking, pouting, or withdrawing. Patients can list specific examples of how they responded "successfully" when not validated, for example, saying "I'm not getting my point across effectively," "I'm not feeling understood here," or "I wonder if you could give me some support on this." The therapist can assign Form 3.1 (Examples of When I Feel or Don't Feel Validated) to chart the examples mentioned previously.

Possible Problems

Patients with validation resistance are particularly sensitive to the impression that the therapist views their feelings as neurotic or unimportant. Even focusing on validation, for some, can "feel" like invalidation: "You're saying that I'm too sensitive. I'm not. This really hurts!" The therapist can sensitively validate the feeling of being invalidated, reflect that it's hard to feel that one's feelings are not important to the therapist (or to anyone), and ask for instruction: "It seems that I am not connecting with the way you are feeling. I am sorry for that. I need to learn from you how to make that connection. Would you be willing to help me? If you were me—talking to you right now—what would you say that would make you feel really validated, cared for, and supported?" The therapist can do an empty-chair role play with the reversal of roles (therapist becomes patient and vice versa).

Cross-Reference to Other Techniques

The therapist can work with patients to identify more adaptive strategies to deal with invalidation.

Form

Form 3.1: Examples of When I Feel or Don't Feel Validated

TECHNIQUE: IDENTIFYING PROBLEMATIC RESPONSES TO INVALIDATION

Description

Some patients may employ ultimately self-defeating styles of seeking validation, such as rumination (repeating the same negative thoughts and feelings, hoping that others will validate them), catastrophizing (exaggerating their problem so that others "get the message" and "understand how bad it is"), attempts to elicit feelings in the therapist ("If you feel bad, then you will understand how bad I feel"), distancing (either "I won't trust you until you prove that you can be trusted" or "You need to come to me to show you care"), or splitting the transference ("I'll show you. My other doctor understands me better than you do. Prove to me you care more than she does") (Leahy, 2001; Leahy, Beck, & Beck, 2005).

Some of these strategies are reminiscent of disrupted attachment styles discussed by Bowlby and others. The problem with complaining, ruminating, escalating, punishing, and pouting is that they inevitably lead to more distancing by others—more invalidation—and more claims that one is truly invalidated. Helping patients identify these problematic strategies may decrease self-induced negative life events and help improve the therapeutic collaboration.

Question to Pose/Intervention

"There are a lot of times when we feel that other people don't understand us, when we may believe we are not being heard, not being validated. This might upset you at times and lead you to feel angry, sad, anxious, all alone. And then when you don't feel validated, you might respond in various ways. For example, you might withdraw or you might get hostile—perhaps there are times that you might criticize the other person. Or you might try other things. It might be worth examining what you do or say when you feel invalidated and see if these responses are working for you."

Example

Therapist: I noticed that you said that your friend didn't understand you and then you got angry with her and told her she was selfish. You must have been upset. What did you think you would accomplish by telling her she was selfish?

Patient: I wanted her to understand how bad I felt. I wanted her to feel as bad as I do.

Therapist: So, it seems you were thinking that, "Maybe if she feels as bad as I do, then she might validate me."

Patient: Yeah. I know it sounds crazy. But I get really upset when people don't understand me.

Therapist: I guess we could think of two parts to that: first, why it gets you so upset and, second, what you do when you are upset. Can we take the second part and look at what you do?

Patient: Sure.

Therapist: You know we all get frustrated when we aren't understood because feeling cared for and validated are really important. It's part of being human, isn't it. (*Patient nods.*) And there are things that we might do when we are not validated that could cause things to get even worse. Even though you might be looking for validation, it might make matters worse if you yell at your friend.

Patient: I know. But I don't know what else to do.

Therapist: That's why we are talking about this. I've found that a lot of people seem to use some problematic ways of responding to not getting validated. For example, some people complain over and over—or raise their voice—because they feel that they aren't being heard. Others might withdraw and pout, hoping that someone will notice and soothe them. You might also threaten people if you got really upset, or you might leave or even threaten to hurt yourself. These are ways of crying for help, because you feel so badly at the time.

Patient: Sounds familiar.

Therapist: The first thing in helping yourself is to look at the things you might do or say when you feel you are not being helped. This could help you use some other behaviors—things that we can go over together—to handle those feelings.

Homework

Patients can complete Form 3.2 (Problematic Ways of Getting People to Respond to Me) and monitor their verbal and physical responses over the next week when not validated. They can also examine how others respond: Do they generally give validation, become argumentative, or distance themselves? Patients can list the pros and cons of each of these strategies and examine whether they are truly accomplishing the goal of being understood.

Possible Problems

Some patients experience this technique as critical and invalidating—blaming themselves for feeling bad and not getting validation from others. Again, the therapist might acknowledge that any examination of validation issues will seem invalidating, because therapy involves both validation of feelings and the search for change. The therapist can assist patients in recognizing that developing better strategies to handle difficult emotions validates that there are important emotions involved.

Cross-Reference to Other Techniques

Other useful techniques include the vertical descent about invalidation and examples of validation resistance.

Form

Form 3.2: Problematic Ways of Getting People to Respond to Me

TECHNIQUE: EXAMINING THE MEANING OF INVALIDATION

Description

Leahy (2001, 2005a, 2009) has described a number of interventions to use with validation resistance. The therapist can first accept the patient's "resistance" rather than equate it with dysfunctional thoughts or lack of motivation. In addition, the therapist can shift from the current impasse in therapy to examining the history of invalidating environments, while eliciting the thoughts and feelings that were generated by these other invalidating experiences. Current experiences of invalidation can also be examined. Vertical descent can be used to elicit the underlying thoughts and feelings when one is not validated. For example, one patient had the following string of thoughts: "If you don't validate the way I am feeling, then you don't care. If you don't care, you can't help me. If you can't help me, then I am hopeless—and I might as well kill myself." This can often lead to general schemas about self and others, such as "My feelings don't matter. People are critical. They can't be trusted." By expanding the discussion of invalidation, the patient will begin feeling more validated. That is, the patient will realize that the therapist understands that he or she doesn't feel understood and that they are exploring together the meaning and consequences of this perception. Finally, acknowledging that the therapist may never be able to quite appreciate all of the pain and suffering—may never really be able to validate completely—can help the patient recognize that "empathic failures" are shared by patient and therapist and that, at least in this sense, the patient feels validated. As one patient said, "Now you understand." Validation can also prove to be paradoxical, for example, acknowledging dilemmas ("It's a hard balance in what we do—to look for change but validate the feelings that you really have"), expanding the criteria and scale for validation ("Perhaps there are degrees of validation—and maybe we can examine that together—but there may never be that complete validation that we hope for. We can try to get as close as we can together.")

Question to Pose/Intervention

"When we feel invalidated, it might have some special meaning for us. Sometimes we can accept it and think that other people are not perfect, perhaps they have other things on their mind, or that they might not have enough information to understand us. But at other times we might think that they don't care, that they are dismissing us, or that they might be critical of us. We can look at what it means to you when you don't feel validated and how this feels to you."

Example

Therapist: It sounds like you feel that I am not hearing what you are saying. I understand that your friend didn't include you in the dinner and that you are really upset.

Patient: You are trying to tell me that I shouldn't feel this way. These are my feelings.

Therapist: Your feelings are very important. But I also noticed a number of times that you get really upset with me and disappointed that I do not understand you, and that seems to be something we can talk about.

Patient: OK. But don't tell me how to feel.

Therapist: All right. Let me ask you what it might mean to you if I don't validate you. Could you help me understand you better? For example, when you think I don't understand and validate you, what kinds of thoughts does that trigger for you?

Patient: I think that you just don't care. You are trying to get me to do your thing.

Therapist: I can see where that would upset you. And if you thought I was trying to get you to do my thing, what does that make you think?

Patient: That you will never understand me and never be able to help me. And if you can't help me, then I must be hopeless.

Therapist: So when I don't understand you, it means that things are hopeless for you and that I am simply trying to control you.

Patient: Now you understand.

Homework

The therapist can assign the vertical descent technique for feeling invalidated: "What does it mean to you when you are not validated?" In addition, the patient can list his or her beliefs about what validation means—what are the criteria for being validated? Examine the automatic thoughts, using vertical descent procedure, to not feeling validated by listing the advantages and disadvantages of having these criteria for being validated. For example, the perfectionistic rule "You must understand every feeling I have" can be examined for costs and benefits. The cost might be that one continues to feel invalidated and, thereby, not supported. The benefit might be that one gains an idealized, supportive relationship. The patient can review whether this rule has worked for him or her or has created more conflicts and disappointments. Relevant homework includes completion of Form 3.3 (My Beliefs about Validation) and Form 3.4 (Vertical Descent for When I Do Not Feel Validated). The vertical descent of what it means not to be validated (e.g., "If you don't validate me, then you can never help me") can be examined in terms of accepting imperfection in others or developing more adaptive ways of making one's frustration known (e.g., "I think you may have missed this particular point").

Possible Problems

Some patients may have difficulty working with the vertical descent exercise or identifying beliefs about validation. They may be so emotionally distraught that they have difficulty distinguishing a thought and feeling: "I feel awful. That's what I think." Using some of the cognitive restructuring techniques might be helpful in distinguishing between thoughts and feelings. In some cases, patients' intensity of emotion may need to be reduced through mindfulness or relaxation exercises before vertical descent can be used. Many patients may believe that using vertical descent is another invalidation, an attempt to prove that they are irrational. This can be examined as part of the beliefs that patients have about being questioned, and the pros and cons can be examined. Moreover, asking about the meaning of invalidation and the feelings that go with it can be interpreted as a way in which the therapist expresses interest and respect for the emotions that are presently experienced.

Cross-Reference to Other Techniques

With any vertical descent, the therapist might also include several of the cognitive restructuring techniques, such as the semantic technique, advantages and disadvantages, and examination of the evidence. Role playing both sides of the "beliefs" or identifying the advice that one would give a friend can help put these thoughts in perspective. Other useful techniques may include viewing events along a continuum, acceptance, and mindful observation.

Forms

Form 3.3: My Beliefs about Validation

Form 3.4: Vertical Descent for When I Do Not Feel Validated

TECHNIQUE: DEVELOPING MORE ADAPTIVE STRATEGIES TO DEAL WITH INVALIDATION

Description

Some patients who feel invalidated adopt a variety of maladaptive strategies for seeking validation, including rumination, perseveration of complaints, escalating intensity of emotion, punishing other people, trying to cause the therapist to feel what they feel, pouting, withdrawing, and threatening self-harm. Because it is inevitable that all of us will feel invalidated at some time—and patients with emotion regulation problems often present with this issue—it is essential to find more adaptive strategies to deal with invalidation. The issue that arises for patients is that there is some emotion of intensity that is not validated. Alternatives to seeking validation—or perfect validation—might include assertion, mutual problem solving, acceptance, putting things in perspective, distraction, self-soothing, and other emotion regulation techniques. In this section we examine alternatives that might be used.

Question to Pose/Intervention

"When you feel invalidated, it triggers certain thoughts and feelings, and you might respond in ways that could be helpful or not helpful. Let's take a look at what you could do that might be helpful to you—helpful in soothing your own feelings and getting your needs met—even when you don't get validated. This way you can rely more on yourself for getting your emotions where you want them to be."

Example

Therapist: I can see that there are a number of times you feel invalidated with your friends and with me, and I wonder if we might figure out whether there is something you could do that might help you cope with these experiences.

Patient: Why should I have to cope? Why can't people see things the way I am seeing them?

Therapist: It would be great to have that, but I wonder if that is something that will only make you feel more alone, more frustrated.

Patient: I seem to be pissed off a lot. Maybe something can help. I don't know.

Therapist: Well, what if we had a set of strategies that you might use when you are feeling invalidated? Would that be a start?

Patient: It might be. What do you have in mind?

Therapist: I was thinking of a number of things that you might consider when you don't feel validated. We can talk about each one. But right now I was thinking of learning how to ask for help more effectively. We can talk about that. Or we can talk about accepting that others will disappoint you some of the time. Or we could talk about how you could validate yourself rather than rely on others. Or we could figure out ways that you might solve problems that you are facing rather than look for reassurance.

Patient: That's a lot to do.

Therapist: The more tools that you have to handle those emotions when you are not validated, the better off you might be. It's hard not to feel validated, and so it might be helpful to have some way to cope with that experience when it happens to you.

Homework

The patient can list all of the alternative techniques that he or she can use when he or she does not feel validated. Many of these techniques are included in this book, so the list could be quite extensive. These include acceptance, mindful observation, costs and benefits, vertical descent, and learning how to validate others who validate you. The patient can complete Form 3.5 (What I Can Do When I Am Not Validated).

Possible Problems

For some patients, asking them to imagine alternatives to getting validation may seem invalidating. They may believe that this is dismissive of their emotion and feel a sense of being victimized and blamed for their feelings. The therapist can address this by examining the pros and cons of having alternatives to validation—to what extent would this be helpful in soothing one's own feelings. If this could help in soothing feelings, then it recognizes that the feelings are important and, therefore, the technique is not invalidating.

Cross-Reference to Other Techniques

Other techniques that are useful include learning how to validate others, acceptance, cost–benefit analysis, and validating the self.

Form

Form 3.5: What I Can Do When I Am Not Validated

TECHNIQUE: HOW TO HELP OTHERS VALIDATE YOU

Description

Patients with validation problems often believe that others should know what the rules are for validating them. They may engage in mind reading ("You know I need validation. Why aren't you doing that?"), personalizing ("You are wrapped up in your own issues, that's why you aren't listening"), shoulds ("You should agree with me that it is awful"), or catastrophizing ("It's terrible that you aren't seeing things my way"). As a result, patients may fail to recognize that others might need some guidance on how to connect, how to validate. One can look at this as an example of mutual problem solving, a technique that is quite helpful in couples therapy. In helping others help themselves, patients can identify what specific behaviors might be helpful for others. However, patients also can indicate how they experience the problem of feeling misunderstood and how this can contribute to unneeded conflicts.

Question to Pose/Intervention

"It seems that a lot of times you are expecting others to know how you feel and how to make you feel understood and validated. Perhaps this can be unrealistic because other people often don't know how we feel and what we need. The good news is that you can help them help you. Just as you can help me help you in therapy by telling me what you need, you can do the same with other people. I like to think of this as mutual problem solving. What this means is that we both might be contributing to the problem—either because of what we think, do, or communicate. So, you might approach other people with the idea that 'It seems like I am not feeling understood, and it might be that you are trying but it isn't working for me. Perhaps part of this is the way I express myself or the way I think about validation. Maybe I can figure out better ways of thinking of support and better ways of expressing myself. But it might be that it would be helpful to me, if I am not feeling understood, to simply tell you, calmly, "I'm not feeling heard here and I wonder if you could rephrase what you hear me saying".'"

Example

Therapist: Sometimes other people don't know what we need them to do, and that's a great opportunity to use some problem-solving skills. For example, there may be times that other people are not validating you and you get angry. But rather than get angry, you might gently and politely give them some ideas of how they can help you feel understood.

Patient: That sounds good. I don't feel understood a lot of the time.

Therapist: Other people can't read our minds or know what we need. If you went into a restaurant, you would have to tell the waiter what you wanted. You wouldn't expect him to guess it right. So the same thing is true with getting validation. Let's think of some ways in which people might validate you better.

Patient: They could listen.

Therapist: Listening is important. But some people make you feel heard better than other people. What if we said, "I am feeling right now that I am not getting my point across, so I wonder if you could rephrase what you hear me saying." That way, other people can tell you directly what they hear.

Patient: That sounds good.

Therapist: But that might not be enough. You might also ask them if they can validate any of the thoughts and feelings that you are having—just simply reflect that they can understand why I feel the way I feel.

Patient: OK. I'm all for that.

Therapist: But if you want it to be mutual—and we are talking about mutual problem solving—you can add that you might be contributing to the problem of not being understood. For example, you might say, "I know that at times I don't feel validated, and part of it is that my emotions get so intense I have a hard time feeling heard. And then I might think that if other people don't agree with me completely they don't care. So, I know I need to change some things, too."

Patient: That's a lot to keep in mind, but I think it would help.

Homework

The patient can complete Form 3.6 (Adaptive Things to Say or Do When I Feel Invalidated) and look for opportunities to use mutual problem solving and to respectfully ask for help and reinforce others.

Possible Problems

Many patients with validation problems believe that others should understand what their needs are without being told. This is a variation of the belief that "my partner should read my mind." The therapist can help illustrate the difficulty in this by asking whether the patient is able to read the minds of others. If not, does that mean that the patient does not care for his or her friends? In addition, the therapist can ask the patient what the advantages are of coming up with new ways of responding to invalidation. Would this assist in emotion regulation?

Cross-Reference to Other Techniques

Other techniques that can be useful include building better friendships, vertical descent for invalidation, challenging invalidation thoughts, and monitoring examples of invalidation and validation.

Form

Form 3.6: Adaptive Things to Say or Do When I Feel Invalidated

TECHNIQUE: OVERCOMING INVALIDATION OF THE SELF

Description

Some patients invalidate themselves and undermine their "right to have their feelings." This perpetuates a sense of guilt or shame about emotion and further adds to the sense that one's emotions make no sense, that there is nothing one can do to soothe emotions, and that one cannot express emotion or receive validation. Typical responses include unwillingness to talk about their needs, viewing needs as weakness, using CBT as a defense against needs ("I chose CBT because I thought we wouldn't have to deal with all of that family stuff" or "I thought it was rational"), apologizing for needs ("I must sound like a baby"), inability to process information about needs ("I don't understand what you are saying" [when talking about emotion, trauma, or difficulties]), dissociation, attempts to lower expectations ("Maybe I'm expecting too much out of my marriage"), and somatization (the patient focuses on physical complaints but will not talk about emotion) (Leahy, 2001, 2005a). For example, patients may withdraw, feeling that their needs are not important or are a sign of weakness or fearing that they will be humiliated if they describe their emotions. Some patients have difficulty attending to their needs and emotions, sometimes "spacing" out (dissociating) or failing to recall discussion of their emotions. Similar to the "hot spots" in imagery work, the therapist may want to attend to the way in which patients talk about or experience the discussion about needs (Holmes & Hackmann, 2004). For example, one patient, when describing her history of depression, suicidal attempts, and substance abuse, had a smile on her face as if she were describing something trivial or even amusing that happened to someone else.

Question to Pose/Intervention

Questions can focus on the "disconnect" between patients' suffering and their presentation of their problem. Examples include the following: "You seem to have a lot that has made you unhappy, but you don't have much feeling when you talk about it" or "You seem to minimize your feeling when you talk about it"). "Why would that be?" Other specific questions could be, "It seems that you sometimes deny or minimize your right to have a feeling—saying [example], 'Maybe I'm expecting too much' or 'I must seem like a real neurotic [complainer, whiner, baby, etc.].'" Follow-up questions include "Why do you think you invalidate (or minimize) yourself this way? What are the advantages of minimizing your feelings? Where did you learn that your feelings don't matter?"

Minimizing needs and feelings may also be a major component of patients' relationships. This can be explored by asking, "Have you been in relationships where your needs have not been met? Where you have been secondary? Where your rights are not important? Do you choose people who don't meet your needs? Have you found that people don't respond well when you talk about your feelings? Are those people more self-centered? Could there be more compassionate people whom you might look to?"

Example

Therapist: I noticed when you were talking about some of these terrible things that have happened to you that you actually had a smile on your face, as if they didn't really bother you.

Patient: Really? I didn't notice.

Therapist: I guess my experience of that in listening was that you were conveying on some level, "These things don't matter." I wondered, then, if you feel a little awkward talking about your needs and the bad things you've gone through.

Patient: I don't want to sound needy.

Therapist: What would it mean to you if you did sound needy?

Patient: It's pathetic. I don't want anyone to feel sorry for me.

Therapist: So, talking about hurt feelings, painful experiences, might make someone feel sorry for you and that would make you pathetic? In your family—with your mother or father—when you had needs, how did they respond to them?

Patient: They told me to get over it. They had their own problems.

Therapist: There was no place for your feelings and needs. I wonder if in your life now that you don't really share your feelings with other people because of that.

Patient: People don't want to hear about your problems.

Therapist: That sounds like the message you got from your family. Maybe one way of coping has been for you to deny that you had needs or that you were in pain.

Patient: I don't know what you mean.

Therapist: Maybe you deny that you really are unhappy, keep it to yourself, keep yourself from recognizing that you have a need to be cared for, respected, accepted, and loved. Just try to convince yourself that these are not real needs for you.

Patient: If I had those needs, they wouldn't be met.

Further discussion with the patient revealed how she feared acknowledging these needs because she believed it would only lead to more disappointment and sadness. She viewed her needs and her past as a sign of being "damaged goods" and relied on marijuana, alcohol, and purging to "get rid of feelings."

Homework

Patients can identify examples of how they minimize their needs or invalidate themselves. For example, "List any example in the past or present when you tried to convince yourself or others that your needs were not important. List the advantages and disadvantages of minimizing or denying your needs. Which needs do you think are ones that you should minimize? Why? Are there some things that you say or do to minimize your feelings? For example, do you apologize for your feelings, make fun of yourself, or refrain from talking to people about what you feel? Do you space out sometimes, can't really pay attention? Does this have anything to do with having uncomfortable feelings?" Patients can complete Form 3.7 (Examples of Minimizing My Needs). The therapist can inquire, "Would you minimize the needs or suffering of a friend? Why not? Would it sound invalidating, cruel, or dismissive? What alternative, compassionate, and validating things would you say to a friend? Is there some reason why you might not say these things to yourself rather than minimize your needs?"

Possible Problems

Some patients believe that validating themselves is equivalent to self-pity. The therapist can indicate that pity implies one's feelings are pathetic as opposed to viewing one's feelings as having importance and value. Validation gives recognition to one's right to feelings and the truth of the feeling that one holds. Other patients believe that they do not have a right to self-validation because they view themselves as unlovable and defective. These thoughts can be examined using cognitive restructuring techniques, or the therapist can use compassionate mind techniques to help build the capacity for self-care. Moreover, learning how to accept feelings, link feelings to higher values, and recognize the universality of the feelings one has can help encourage patients in self-validation.

Cross-Reference to Other Techniques

Compassionate mind and cognitive restructuring can also be helpful.

Form

Form 3.7: Examples of Minimizing My Needs

TECHNIQUE: COMPASSIONATE SELF-VALIDATION

Description

Considerable research shows that the perception of empathy and validation in the therapeutic setting is a strong predictor of improvement. The technique of compassionate self-validation provides patients with the opportunity to direct loving and caring validation toward their own emotion. Derived from Gilbert's "compassionate mind therapy," self-validation with loving kindness can provide patients with a sense of emotional support and self-care that can feel soothing and supportive and can reduce self-loathing tendencies (Gilbert, 2009, 2010).

Question to Pose/Intervention

"We often feel better when someone else validates our feelings and when they show that they understand and that they care. We call this 'compassionate validation'—the kind of loving kindness that a good friend or someone who really cares can give you. Have you ever experienced that kind of closeness and care from someone? What would it be like if you could be that compassionate, loving friend to yourself? So that when you felt down you could turn to yourself with validation, say that you understand and care, and give yourself that kind of warm, loving emotional support?"

Example

Therapist: I can see you are feeling sad about these feelings of loneliness that you have. Sometimes in our lives we have the experience that someone really cares about our feelings, really is able to touch us with their warmth and their compassion. Have you ever had anyone like that?

Patient: Yes, my grandmother was like that. She was so loving, so tender, and gentle.

Therapist: It would be great if you had someone like that to talk to—to share your feelings with. But that's not always possible. But it is possible to be compassionate toward yourself, to direct tenderness and love toward your painful feeling, toward the part of you that hurts.

Patient: But how do I do that?

Therapist: Imagine that you are your grandmother now and you are directing those compassionate, loving feelings toward you. What would that voice sound like?

Patient: It would be soothing, loving.

Therapist: And what would that voice say?

Patient: It would say, "Don't worry about being alone. I'm always with you. I love you. Think of me when you are feeling down."

Therapist: How does that feel?

Patient: I have mixed feelings—feeling sad because she has died but feeling a little relieved because I remember her warmth and I can feel a little of it.

Therapist: Perhaps you could try finding some time to get in contact with directing compassion and validation toward yourself using the image of your grandmother. It's one way of being able to be alone with yourself in a way that feels connected to caring about yourself.

Patient: That would be good if I could do that.

Therapist: Imagine your grandmother with you when you are feeling down or feeling lonely and she is directing that loving kindness toward you. Can you get an image in your mind of her face, her eyes, her hair and imagine the soft, gentle quality of her voice? And she is soothing you and making you feel loved and cared for. I wonder if you could set aside 15 minutes each day for compassionate kindness toward yourself.

Patient: I feel a sense of peace coming over me as we are talking.

Homework

The patient can complete Form 3.8 (Compassionate Self-Validation) and practice compassionate kindness toward the self.

Possible Problems

Many people who are self-loathing may be reluctant to direct compassion toward themselves. They often think that they don't deserve to be kind to themselves since they sometimes hate themselves. They may think, "I am letting myself off the hook" or "I must be pathetic to need this." Others have ambivalence about "compassionate figures" because they may have suffered punishment by people who they thought loved them (Gilbert & Irons, 2005). It may be helpful to externalize the compassion toward someone else. For example, "Imagine you had a friend who you cared for and he was self-critical and you wanted to support him. What are some compassionate things that you might say to him?" Often by externalizing compassion toward others, patients can realize that even strangers can merit compassion, that giving compassion is also soothing, and that if they can be kind toward others there is no harm in being kind toward their own self. In regard to ambivalence toward the attachment figure, the therapist can help patients explore the experiences that give rise to legitimate ambivalence and help them recognize that by becoming one's own source of self-compassion and validation they can create a safe "haven."

Cross-Reference to Other Techniques

Any of the compassionate mind techniques can be used here.

Form

Form 3.8: Compassionate Self-Validation

TECHNIQUE: BUILDING BETTER FRIENDSHIPS

Description

One of the predictors of recurrent depressive episodes is problematic styles of interaction (Joiner et al., 2006; Joiner, Van Orden, Witte, & Rudd, 2009). Patients with validation issues or emotion dysregulation problems often have difficulty in interpersonal relationships. They may complain, demand, escalate, act entitled, punish others, and show little gratitude or appreciation for the help that they get. As a consequence, their interpersonal styles may result in further rejection, followed by anger, depression, and hopelessness. Thus, emotional dysregulation may be partly a result of problematic interpersonal strategies in seeking support. In this section, we identify some common issues that can help build better relationships—not only friendships but a community of support and meaning in patients' lives.

Question to Pose/Intervention

"Many times when we are upset we might fail to recognize the impact that we are having on other people. It's important to get support—but it's also important to give support. Just as we need our friends, they need us. We have examined some ways of asking for validation, using some mutual problem solving and changing some of the rules that you might have for feeling validated. Now we can look at how you might build better friendships. This might require taking an honest look at whether you might be a 'downer' too much of the time, perhaps not realizing that it's also important to edit or shorten what we complain about. It's also important to show appreciation to friends, reward them, acknowledge when they are doing a good job for us. Let's take a look at some examples of how things could be better with friends."

Example

Wendy complained that she felt invalidated and criticized by her friend, Maria. In examining the nature of their relationship it appeared true that Maria was critical. However, Wendy had other friends who were supportive.

Therapist: I can see why it felt bad to you that Maria was critical of you. When we open up to friends we want to feel that they support us, not criticize us. Is Maria often like that?

Patient: Not always. But she is more like that than my other friends are.

Therapist: So, there are friends who are more supportive of you. Who are they?

Patient: Linda and Gail are really good. I can tell them anything.

Therapist: I wonder if you might focus more on sharing feelings with them than with Maria.

Patient: That's probably a good idea.

Therapist: You know, sometimes we feel worse when we open up to the wrong person at the wrong time. So now you have an alternative to Maria. [The therapist also recognizes that Wendy was not always effective in her style of communicating and receiving validation.] Sometimes when we express our feelings and seek validation, we can do it in a skilled way or in a way that is not as skilled. I know that there were times in the past when I would just complain and complain, not recognizing how the other person was experiencing it. Not that they didn't care. But that I needed to "edit" what I was saying.

Patient: I can go on for quite a bit with my complaining. I think it turns people off.

Therapist: I was like that with one of my friends a number of years ago. And he was trying to be supportive. So I tried to learn from my experience. What I learned was that I could limit the amount of things I say and not repeat myself too much, and continue to thank the person who is validating me. I thought of calling this "validate the validator."

Patient: Yeah. I wonder if my friends think I'm doing a dump on them. Just dumping all my feelings.

Therapist: Well, friends are there, you know, to give support. But I realized from my experience that my friends needed support from me when they were supporting me.

Patient: That makes sense.

Therapist: I found it helpful to tell my friends, "I know that I am complaining and I know you have been kind listening to me. I just want to tell you that I really appreciate that. And I am also doing some things to help myself. You've been a good friend during a difficult time."

Homework

The chapter "How to Make Friendships More Rewarding" in Leahy's (2010) *Beat the Blues Before They Beat You* describes dysfunctional styles in interacting with friends and specific suggestions on improving getting support. This chapter can be assigned to patients who are having difficulty getting and receiving validation. The patient can complete Form 3.9, which lists some specific targets for change in order to receive validation. The therapist can have the patient practice editing his or her message to others, setting limits on complaining, describing positives to friends in the context of complaining, and "validating the validator" (i.e., "If someone validates you, tell them, 'I appreciate all the support you are giving me'").

The patient can be asked for examples of feeling validated by others: "Are there some people who accept and understand your feelings? Do you have arbitrary rules for validation? Do people have to agree with everything you say? Are you sharing your emotions with people who are critical? Do you accept and support other people who have these emotions? Do you have a double standard? Why?"

Possible Problems

As indicated earlier, some patients manifest unrealistic standards for validation, expecting that every thought and feeling they have will be "mirrored" by others. These can be examined and tested for costs and benefits, and new, more realistic standards of validation can be identified.

Cross-Reference to Other Techniques

Techniques that can be included are learning to ask for help and helping others help you.

Form

Form 3.9: How to Be More Rewarding and Get Support from Your Friends

CONCLUSIONS

Many patients with emotional dysregulation issues may resist using self-help techniques because they view them as invalidating. As we discussed in the previous chapter on emotional schemas, patients need to believe that others care about and understand their feelings. The primary role of empathy, mirroring, and validation in attachment and throughout relationships across the life span is a key element in a variety of theories. However, some patients may have idiosyncratic rules for validation and may demand and seek validation through problematic strategies and behaviors. Balancing validation with change is a key dialectic in therapy, but addressing validation issues up front may often be difficult. Many patients escalate their claim that they are being criticized for their feelings or are misunderstood. The therapist needs to be aware that these patients are stuck in a validation trap, which can become a useful focus for therapy.

CHAPTER FOUR

Identification and Refutation of Emotion Myths

"Emotion myths" is a term used in dialectical behavior therapy (DBT) to refer to erroneous beliefs about emotions (Linehan, 1993, 1993b). Linehan notes the tendency of individuals with borderline personality disorder (BPD) to negatively evaluate their emotional responses. In addition to believing that emotions are uncontrollable, patients with BPD are inclined to believe that their emotions are unending. These beliefs likely contribute to the fear of emotions and pervasive emotional avoidance that characterize this disorder (Gratz, Rosenthal, Tull, Lejuez, & Gunderson, 2006; Yen, Zlotnick, & Costello, 2002). Further, many of the clinical problems prevalent in BPD, such as substance abuse (Grilo, Walker, Becker, Edell, & McGlashan, 1997), dissociative disorder (Wagner & Linehan, 1998), and bulimia (Paxton & Diggins, 1997), involve emotional avoidance as prominent associated feature.

Research provides preliminary evidence that emotion myths promote the use of maladaptive emotion regulation in both Axis I and Axis II disorders. Campbell-Sills, Barlow, Brown, and Hofmann (2006) and colleagues found that emotion myths such as "feeling sad is wrong" and "showing negative emotions is a sign of weakness" were associated with increased use of suppression in the anxiety disorders. Similarly, Mennin, Heimberg, Turk, and Fresco (2002) found that the appraisal of negative emotions as unacceptable was associated with increased worry, an emotionally avoidant activity. In a study of emotional schemas among the personality disorders, Leahy and Napolitano (2005) found that individuals with BPD endorsed the beliefs that negative emotions are unacceptable and incomprehensible. In a subsequent study, they found that individuals with BPD and other personality disorders characterized by negative beliefs about emotions were more likely to engage in worry, an emotionally avoidant activity (Leahy & Napolitano, 2006). Emotion myths can be considered a narrow part of the broader construct of emotional schemas, which refer to concepts, evaluations, action tendencies, and interpersonal and coping strategies that are employed to cope with emotion (Leahy, 2002). More behavioral than cognitive, DBT does not make emotion myths a primary focus of the treatment of emotion dysregulation. Unlike EST, DBT is not based on a metacognitive model of emotion. Nevertheless, DBT is a rich source for deriving techniques that can be used to challenge inaccurate beliefs about emotions, which is a primary focus of EST.

Some of the emotion regulation techniques employed in DBT are common to other cognitive-behavioral therapies, most notably changing interpretations to change emotions or decrease emotional intensity. From a DBT perspective, the individual with BPD is highly prone to nondialectical or dichotomous thinking. Investigations of dichotomous thinking in BPD support this conceptualization (Napolitano & McKay, 2005; Veen & Arntz, 2000). Extreme evaluations of self, other, and the environment are theorized to contribute to extreme emotional responses as well as to instability in emotions, behavior, identity, and relationships. Accordingly, helping the individual with BPD to develop a more dialectical, less extreme thinking style is an important target of treatment.

DBT differs from other types of CBT in its presentation of a model of emotions to patients. This model, based on the work of Gross and others, describes emotions as complex patterned responses to events that unfold over time (Ekman & Davidson, 1994; Gross, 1998a, 1998b). The model is designed to facilitate the understanding of emotions, a key aspect of emotion regulation. It also provides the information needed to challenge erroneous beliefs about emotions. Emotion regulation strategies can be used at different points of the emotional experience, including before and after the event that prompted the emotion (Gross, 1998a, 1998b). Importantly, the model differentiates emotional experience from emotional expression. The conflation of emotional expression and experience can contribute to the fear of emotion and emotional avoidance. DBT stresses that emotion regulation is a set of skills that the individual is not born with but rather learns in the context of his or her environment. These skills include, but are not limited to, the ability to label an emotion, link it to a prompting event, increase or decrease its intensity, inhibit acting on it, and limit contact with emotional stimuli or triggers.

The mindfulness component of DBT teaches patients to assume a nonjudgmental stance toward their emotions, which promotes acceptance of them and the willingness to experience them. The nonjudgmental stance toward emotions is designed to counteract the tendency to negatively evaluate or judge emotions. Such judgments can generate additional emotions, compounding the emotional experience (Greenberg & Safran, 1987; Linehan, 1993b). The negative evaluation of emotion can also contribute to habitual emotional avoidance (Campbell-Sills et al., 2006; Hayes et al., 2004; Mennin et al., 2002). It has been hypothesized that the beneficial effects of mindfulness on emotion regulation are attributable to non-reinforced exposure to previously avoided emotions. Mindfulness practice is thought to provide a context in which patients can develop new less negative associations with the experience of emotions and old associations are extinguished (Lynch, Chapman, Rosenthal, Kuo, & Linehan, 2006).

In addition to providing patients with a theory of emotions, DBT teaches them about the function of emotions. By highlighting the utility of emotions, DBT provides "emotionally phobic" or emotionally avoidant patients with an incentive to experience emotions. The approach outlined in this chapter entails first helping patients to identify emotion myths as well as their potential origins. We then present psychoeducation and exposure-based techniques to help patients challenge these beliefs.

TECHNIQUE: IDENTIFYING EMOTION MYTHS

Description

DBT helps patients to identify the "emotion myths" that may be contributing to problems in emotion regulation as well as the potential origins of these myths. There are numerous ways to identify emotion myths. Patients can review the emotion myths handout from the *Skills Training Manual for Treating Borderline Personality Disorder* (Linehan, 1993b) to see which of these beliefs they endorse. Alternatively, patients' erroneous beliefs about emotions may emerge on Beck et al.'s (1979) Dysfunctional Thought Record. For example, a patient may have the automatic thought "I'm weak" in response to feeling sad. Upon questioning by the therapist, he or she may explain, "It's weak to feel sad." Emotion myths may also be spontaneously expressed in session. They can also be elicited with the therapist's questioning about patient's in-session behavior. For example, if a patient refuses to discuss something upsetting because he or she believes the rest of the day will be ruined, it suggests the possibility of an inaccurate belief about the duration of emotions. Or if the patient apologizes for expressing emotions, it suggests beliefs about the unacceptability of emotional expression.

After helping patients identify emotion myths, DBT employs psychoeducation, mindfulness, and exposure-based techniques to help them challenge these beliefs. In addition to providing patients with a theory of emotions, DBT teaches them about the function of emotions. With increased understanding of the functionality of emotions, emotionally avoidant patients may become more accepting of their emotional experience.

Question to Pose/Intervention

"What we believe about emotions affects how we handle them. For example, if I believe that anxiety lasts forever, it makes sense that I would try to avoid or block it. Unfortunately, a certain amount of anxiety is inevitable, and my efforts to block or suppress it may only prolong or intensify it. The fact is that no emotion lasts forever; they are all temporary. It's possible that you have some inaccurate beliefs about emotions that are contributing to your difficulties in handling them."

Example

Therapist: How do you feel about your husband's affair?

Patient: Truthfully, I try not to think about it. He's not a bad person. These things happen every day, right?

Therapist: I don't know that they do. But assuming that's the case, for the sake of argument, what does that mean to you?

Patient: It means I have no reason to be upset. How do you think I should feel?

Therapist: I don't think there's any one way you should feel. Any number of emotional reactions to learning about an affair are possible. How do you feel right now as we're discussing it?

Patient: (*crying*) Incredibly sad. I'm sorry. I didn't mean to cry.

Therapist: Why are you apologizing?

Patient: I don't want to impose my feelings on you.

Therapist: Why do you think you're imposing on me by crying?

Patient: People don't want to deal with negative emotions. You're supposed to be happy.

Therapist: I don't find your sadness an imposition at all. I feel privileged that you are sharing it with me. But it sounds like you believe it's unacceptable to express sadness to others and that you should seem happy all the time.

Patient: Yes. Doesn't everyone believe that?

Therapist: Actually, not everyone believes that. Depending on the context, such as work, it may not be effective for you to express sadness. But with a friend or your therapist, it's acceptable. I don't think it's possible to seem happy all the time. I think we should focus on learning more of your beliefs about emotions [Therapist hands patient Form 4.1: Emotion Myths.] This is a list of some of the more common inaccurate beliefs about emotions. Look it over and see if you subscribe to any.

Homework

Patients can review the Emotion Myths list (Form 4.1) as homework and endorse those beliefs they agree with. They can also record other beliefs about emotions that come to mind. Challenges to the beliefs can be formulated with the therapist's help in the next session, and experiments can be designed to test them out.

Possible Problems

Patients who strongly endorse emotion myths may resist the idea that they are erroneous. Such resistance can be handled by providing factual or scientific information about emotions or designing experiments to test emotion myths. However, the therapist should balance the use of these change strategies with validation, communicating to patients that their belief makes sense in light of their experiences. For example, the therapist could tell a patient with panic disorder that it is understandable she believes that to be anxious is to be out of control. However, the therapist should also discuss that anxiety can be experienced at lower levels of intensity that feel less uncontrollable. Further, feeling out of control is not the same as being out of control.

Cross-Reference to Other Techniques

Related techniques include presenting patients with a model of emotions and a theory of emotions. Other related techniques are described in Chapter 2 on EST, such as identifying beliefs about the duration, controllability, uniqueness, and value connection of emotions. It is also helpful to design in-session experiments when possible to test the patient's beliefs about emotions. The technique of observing and describing emotions nonjudgmentally is a form of exposure to emotions that may also weaken emotion myths.

Form

Form 4.1: Emotion Myths

TECHNIQUE: IDENTIFYING THE ORIGINS OF EMOTION MYTHS

Description

Before challenging their beliefs about emotions, it is helpful for patients to understand the contexts in which these beliefs were learned and strengthened. By highlighting their developmental origins, the therapist is emphasizing that emotion myths are beliefs rather than facts. In the section on "The Role of Emotion Regulation in Various Disorders" in Chapter 1, the role played by the invalidating environment in the development of emotion dysregulation was discussed. In addition to not teaching necessary emotion regulation skills, the invalidating environment provides fertile ground for erroneous beliefs about emotions. If the environment persistently ignores emotions, it may teach patients that their emotions are unimportant. Alternatively, if the environment punishes emotions, they may learn that their emotions are unacceptable.

Question to Pose/Intervention

"Many of the beliefs that interfere with emotion regulation were learned in the invalidating environment. How our parents responded to our emotions as we developed can influence our beliefs about emotions and how they should be handled. If your emotions were met with disapproval, you may have learned that emotions are unacceptable. If your emotions were ignored, you may have learned that they are unimportant, and tend to dismiss them."

Example

Therapist: You said that feeling sad is selfish. Why do you say that? Where does that belief come from?

Patient: Growing up, my father always said that I had been given every advantage and every reason to be happy. He said that I was selfish to feel sad.

Therapist: So your father taught you your belief about sadness. How do you think this belief affects your response to sadness?

Patient: I shut the sadness down.

Therapist: Does that work?

Patient: Not really. I still feel it.

Therapist: Often, attempts to block emotions only intensify them. Did you know that sadness is a basic emotion? That we're born with the capacity for it?

Patient: You're saying it's normal to feel sad. I hadn't thought of it that way—as something we're born with.

Therapist: If you thought sadness was just another emotion, would it change how you handle it?

Patient: I'd probably let myself feel it.

Homework

For homework, patients can be asked to write about experiences that contributed to the development of their emotion myths. Also, they can review Form 4.2: Basic Facts about Emotions.

Possible Problems

Patients may be reluctant to identify their parents' contribution to their emotion myths because they believe it is effectively blaming them for their problems. The therapist can handle this by emphasizing that parental invalidation can be inadvertent. Despite the best of intentions, parents can fail to understand their child's emotional needs. Further, although patients may not have caused their problems, they are responsible for fixing them.

Cross-Reference to Other Techniques

Related techniques include explaining the role of the invalidating environment in contributing to emotion dysregulation and emotional socialization.

Form

Form 4.2. Basic Facts about Emotions

TECHNIQUE: PRESENTING THE PATIENT WITH A THEORY OF EMOTIONS

Description

To help patients challenge emotion myths, the therapist needs to provide information about emotions. In refuting the belief that certain or all emotions are unacceptable, it is helpful for patients to learn that humans are born with the capacity for basic emotions. These include anger, joy/happiness, interest, sadness, fear, and disgust (Izard, 2007). Although humans are born with a biological readiness for guilt and shame, these emotions require further cognitive development and, as a result, emerge later than infancy. To challenge erroneous beliefs about the duration of emotions, patients need to know that emotions are temporary phenomena. Like waves, emotions reach a peak intensity and ebb. Patients also need to learn the distinction between moods and emotions. Unlike emotions, moods lack a clear focus or readily identifiable prompting event. They are diffuse and may last for days, months, or years (Batson, Shaw, & Oleson, 1992). In DBT, patients learn that emotions can be self-perpetuating. For example, an event that triggers sadness may be followed by the recall of other sad events, perpetuating the emotion. If the emotion persists for days, it then becomes a mood.

Question to Pose/Intervention

"Emotions are an integral part of being human. We are born with the capacity for several emotions, including sadness, anger, joy, disgust, interest, and fear. We are also born with a capacity for guilt and shame, although we don't experience these emotions until later in life because they require more cognitive development. All the other emotions are combinations of these or are learned. Emotions are time-limited experiences that occur in response to an identifiable event. They are like waves, reaching their peak intensity and then ebbing. However, they are self-perpetuating. For example, something happens to trigger a wave of anger in me, and in my anger I recall other things that I am angry about, each setting off another wave of anger. A mood, unlike an emotion, lasts for days or weeks. A mood is more long-lasting than an emotion and generally cannot be linked as reaction to any one event."

Example

Therapist: You said that you're afraid to feel sad because you don't want to be depressed. Is that right?

Patient: Yes, I was depressed 3 years ago, and I don't want to go back into the abyss.

Therapist: Sadness and depression are two different things. Sadness is an emotion and depression is a mood.

Patient: What's the difference?

Therapist: Emotions are like waves, and they ebb after reaching their peak intensity. Moods last from weeks to months or longer. It's possible to experience sadness without becoming depressed. Can you think of any examples of when you've felt sad but didn't become depressed?

Patient: Well, that movie I saw last weekend made me cry, but I didn't become depressed. I forgot about it by the time I got back to my apartment.

Therapist: Great example. Your sadness passed without becoming a mood. The next time you find yourself unwilling to experience sadness because you believe it will lead to depression, remember the difference between a mood and an emotion.

Homework

The therapist can give patients the Basic Facts about Emotions sheet (Form 4.2) to review after the session.

Possible Problems

Patients may be skeptical of the theory of emotions. Such skepticism can be handled by emphasizing the scientific basis of the theory and providing references to the relevant literature. Alternatively, they may acknowledge the validity of the theory but report that their emotion myths persist. The therapist should point out that their emotion myths would not be expected to change merely by reviewing this information. Rather, this information provides a basis to refute these beliefs each time they come to mind. Additional techniques, such as experiments to test the beliefs, are likely needed to effectively challenge these beliefs.

Cross-Reference to Other Techniques

Related techniques include presenting patients with a model of emotions and experiencing one's emotions as a wave.

Form

Form 4.2: Basic Facts about Emotions

TECHNIQUE: PRESENTING THE PATIENT WITH A MODEL OF EMOTIONS

Description

This model enables patients to conceptualize their emotional experiences and provides a framework for describing them. According to the model, emotions are complex-patterned responses to events that unfold over time (Gross, 1998b; Gross & Thompson, 2007; Linehan, 1993a; Linehan, Bohus, & Lynch, 2007). The process of emotion consists of a sequence of events. The sequence begins with a psychologically relevant situation. Typically, the situation is external to the individual (i.e., something that happened in his or her environment). However, the prompting event for an emotion can also be internal (i.e., a thought, image, or another emotion). Certain factors, such as lack of sleep or hunger, can increase vulnerability to these events and to emotional arousal. Next in the sequence, the individual appraises this event, which encompasses a determination of its importance and relevance. The appraisal determines the particular emotion that is experienced as well as its intensity. As a general rule of thumb, more extreme interpretations lead to more extreme emotions. For patients who are prone to extreme interpretations, an important emotion regulation technique is modifying interpretations.

Importantly, DBT's model of emotions differentiates emotional experience from emotional expression. After the appraisal of the event, brain and body changes occur, which are part of the emotional experience. Neurochemical changes may lead to changes in the body. For example, if the situation is appraised as dangerous, the individual experiences racing thoughts, increased heart rate and respiration, increased muscle tension, and decreased blood flow to extremities. Action tendencies or action urges are also part of emotional experience. For fear, a common action urge is to run. These action tendencies can be modulated or inhibited. Part of the emotional experience includes sensing these changes and the action urge.

The expression of emotion includes whatever actions are taken as well as what is said, facial expressions, and body posture. The model emphasizes that the expression of emotion can be inhibited. Patients' conflation of the expression and the experience of emotion can contribute to their fear of emotion and emotional avoidance. The next step in the process of emotion is labeling the experience with a name such as sadness or joy. Last, the model points out that emotions have aftereffects on thought processes, behavior, and physiology. In DBT patients are taught that "emotions love themselves" or that they can be self-perpetuating. For example, the aftereffects of sadness may include fatigue, withdrawal, and the recollection of other sad events. In this way, the aftereffects would perpetuate sadness. However, the aftereffects of one emotion can also give rise to different emotions.

Question to Pose/Intervention

"Contrary to perception, emotions always begin with a prompting event, which can be internal or external. In other words, emotions can be triggered by your own thoughts and feelings or by things that are happening in your environment. Certain factors make us more vulnerable to prompting events, such as lack of sleep or hunger, or other emotion-inducing events that have already happened. Additionally, as the model for describing emotions [Form 4.3] shows, most emotions entail an interpretation of the prompting event. Exceptions include fear prompted by encountering a ferocious animal or joy prompted by the sight of someone you love. Your interpretation determines which emotion you have as well as its intensity. Each emotion is accompanied by physiological changes and brain changes as well as an urge to do something. Emotions can be expressed through body language, facial expression, and actions taken. However, they may not be expressed at all. Last, emotions have aftereffects. These can maintain the current emotion or lead to another."

Example

Therapist: You've mentioned that emotions tend to creep up on you. I'd like to go over this diagram with you [referring to Form 4.3].

Patient: It looks complicated.

Therapist: It is. Emotions are complex-patterned responses. They may feel like they come from nowhere. But looking at the diagram, it's clear that they always begin with a prompting event. There's usually an interpretation of this event that affects the type and intensity of the emotion you experience. A more extreme interpretation prompts a more extreme emotional response.

Patient: What do these boxes represent?

Therapist: The first box describes the emotional experience that includes brain changes, changes in your body, and an urge to do something. The second box describes the ways emotions can be expressed: body posture, facial expression, and action taken.

Homework

Patients can review the model for describing emotions presented in Form 4.3.

Possible Problems

Patients may have difficulty understanding the model. It is recommended that the therapist check patients' understanding of the model in the therapy session. This can be done by having them describe an emotion that they have experienced in keeping with the model. Patients who routinely block emotions and frequently report emotional numbness may have difficulty describing the physical changes that accompany their emotional experience. The therapist should encourage such patients by stressing that awareness of the physical impact of emotions can be cultivated with practice.

Cross-Reference to Other Techniques

Related techniques include observing and describing emotions, performing experiments to test beliefs about emotions, differentiating the action urge from the action taken, and experiencing the emotion as a wave.

Form

Form 4.3: Model for Describing Emotions

TECHNIQUE: TEACHING PATIENTS ABOUT THE FUNCTION OF EMOTION

Description

It is not unusual for individuals who have problems regulating their emotions to see emotions as useless. This view of emotions provides little incentive to experience them and justifies their avoidance. Educating patients about the functions of emotions can increase their willingness to experience them. The identified functions of emotions include facilitating decision making, preparing and motivating patients to take action, providing information about the environment, communicating, and influencing others (Gross, 1998b). Another function of emotion is self-validation (Linehan, 1993b). An emotion is self-validating when it is communicates information to the self. For example, emotions may be used as evidence that one's perception or experience of the situation is correct (e.g., one feels angry because the situation is unjust and, therefore, one has good reason to be angry). When taken to the extreme, self-validation results in emotions being treated as facts. For example, the individual might reason, "I'm fearful; therefore, the situation is dangerous."

Identifying the function of emotion is also helpful in determining why particular emotions persist contrary to the individual's wishes. For example, if the patient complains of lingering anger, it is important to determine whether it is motivating, influencing others, or self-validating. To the extent that an emotion serves a function, the patient may be reluctant to let go of it.

Question to Pose/Intervention

"Each of our emotions has a function or a purpose. For example, if we are angry and we express it, the anger's function may be to communicate to others that their behavior is unacceptable to us. This may influence them to change their behavior. Alternatively, our anger may motivate us to take action to change an unjust situation. Sometimes are emotions can be self-validating. We feel angry because we have reason to be angry. Emotions can also help us decide what is right and wrong for us. The next time you experience a strong emotion, ask yourself what the function or functions of the emotion is."

Example

Therapist: You said that when you discovered the basement was flooded you became frantic, and then you got upset with yourself for feeling that way.

Patient: I know. It's stupid. It didn't change anything. I think I overreacted.

Therapist: What did you do when you felt frantic?

Patient: I ran down to the basement and moved all the boxes containing family memorabilia upstairs. I didn't get to all of it though. A lot of stuff was destroyed.

Therapist: It sounds like being frantic motivated you to act quickly. Is it fair to say that, in that way, feeling frantic was useful to you?

Patient: Yeah, I guess. But what about the sadness I felt about the stuff that was destroyed? What's the point of that? It seems like a waste of time.

Therapist: Well, sometimes our emotions communicate to us a sense of what we value. Do you think your sadness could have been doing that? What would it have meant if you had felt happy to see family memorabilia destroyed?

Patient: Maybe my sadness was communicating to me that I value my family and the experiences I had with them growing up. I guess if I were indifferent to them or hated them I'd be happy to see all that stuff go.

Therapist: The next time you catch yourself calling an emotion stupid or pointless, I'd like you to think about the function of the emotion.

Homework

Patients can review Form 4.4, which summarizes the functions of emotions.

Possible Problems

Patients may confuse the function of an emotion with its justification. For example, someone with an anxiety disorder may assert that chronic fear has no function in the absence of actual danger. This can be handled by explaining that although the fear is not justified, its function may still be to motivate or prepare one to take action against a perceived threat, even if the perception is erroneous. Another potential problem is the tendency to assume that each emotion has only one identifiable function and the therapist knows better than the patient what this function is. It is important to emphasize that identifying the function of an emotion is somewhat subjective and that the same emotion can have multiple functions.

Cross-Reference to Other Techniques

Related techniques include observing and describing emotions, reviewing the model of emotions, and providing psychoeducation about emotions.

Form

Form 4.4: What Is the Function of Emotion?

TECHNIQUE: OBSERVING AND DESCRIBING EMOTIONS

Description

Fundamental to emotion regulation is an awareness of one's emotions and the ability to describe and label them. In this exercise, patients observe and describe their emotions nonjudgmentally and one-mindfully or with full awareness. These observations are recorded using Form 4.5. Many individuals with emotion regulation problems attempt to avoid emotional experience. They tend to have a negative view of emotions and erroneous beliefs about emotions. Further, deficits in the ability to tolerate emotions may lead them to act impulsively in an effort to escape them. The observing and describing of emotions exercise counteracts the tendency to avoid emotions. In this sense, it is a form of exposure to emotional experience. Because it is practiced with a nonjudgmental stance, observing and describing of emotions is also designed to promote emotional acceptance, counteracting a negative view of emotions. In recording their emotional experiences, patients are asked to note the precipitant for their emotions as well as their interpretation of precipitating events. It is important that patients develop the skill of linking emotions to precipitating events. This skill helps to demystify emotional experience. Observing and describing exercises also help patients to become mindful of the action urges that accompany emotions. This awareness decreases the likelihood of impulsively acting on these urges. Many patients who employ blocking strategies to handle their emotions are out of touch with the physiological aspects of emotion. Observing and describing counteracts these blocking tendencies by having patients describe physical changes that accompany emotions. Patients who use blocking or numbing as emotion regulation strategies tend to mask their facial expressions or lack an awareness of them. Observing and describing exercises increase patients' awareness of their facial expressions or lack thereof, as well as other nonverbal expressions of emotion such as body posture.

Question to Pose/Intervention

"The first step to regulating our emotions is to have an awareness of them as we experience them. In other words, I can't regulate my anger unless I'm aware that I'm experiencing anger. Only with an awareness of my urge to attack when I'm angry do I have the choice not to act on it. When we're out of touch with our emotions, we may become aware of them only after we've acted on them—after we've said some angry words or slammed a door. However, awareness of emotions is a skill that can be developed only with practice. One way to cultivate this skill is to practice observing and describing emotions. This exercise is done nonjudgmentally and with full awareness or one-mindfully."

Example

Patient: I'm anxious. My mood has been low and I think I'm headed back into a deep, dark depression.

Therapist: You say you're feeling low. Can you be more specific and tell me what emotion you're feeling?

Patient: I don't know. I've been feeling really bad since Saturday for some reason.

Therapist: Let's see if we can't demystify this. What was going on Saturday?

Patient: Well, I was supposed to have a date with someone I met online, but he never called to confirm.

Therapist: What emotions did that kick up?

Patient: I just felt like I wasn't good enough and that I would never meet anyone.

Therapist: Those are your thoughts about his not calling. What emotions were you feeling?

Patient: I think I was feeling sad. I wasn't sure at the time.

Therapist: How were you feeling before Saturday?

Patient: Pretty good. I went to an art opening at a friend's gallery. School was good this week.

Therapist: As we're talking, it's becoming clear that your mood took a downward turn on Saturday, and it looks like the missed date was the trigger. Are you still feeling anxious?

Patient: I feel better now. This makes sense. I didn't understand why I was feeling bad before and I was scared.

Therapist: I think you need to work on identifying emotions and linking them to triggers so they aren't so mysterious and frightening. I also think you need to become more aware of them as they're happening. What do you think?

Patient: I agree. But how?

Therapist: I'd like you to practice observing and describing your emotions.

Homework

Patients should be instructed to fill out Form 4.5 (Observing and Describing Emotions) for particularly intense or long-lasting emotions over the coming week. If patients report that they do not feel any emotions, they can be instructed to complete the work sheet at a particular time of the day or describe an emotion that they have experienced in the past. Observing and describing emotions can also be done after an in-session induction of emotions.

Possible Problems

Patients may have difficulty observing and describing an emotion if they are experiencing more than one emotion simultaneously. It is recommended that a separate form be used for each emotion.

Cross-Reference to Other Techniques

Related techniques include mindfulness, differentiating the action urge from the emotional experience, practicing a nonjudgmental stance toward emotions, and experiencing emotion as a wave.

Form

Form 4.5: Observing and Describing Emotions

TECHNIQUE: NONJUDGMENTAL STANCE TOWARD EMOTIONS

Description

Many patients with problems in emotion regulation judge their emotions negatively. These judgments, in turn, can prompt other emotions or secondary emotions (Linehan, 1993b). For example, an individual might appraise his experience of joy as an indication of naïveté, which could lead to self-contempt. Secondary emotions compound the emotional experience and often make identification of the primary emotion difficult. Further, negative evaluations of emotions may promote the suppression and avoidance of emotions. By assuming a nonjudgmental stance toward emotions, patients cultivate acceptance of emotional experience. Acceptance of emotional experience does not mean that one condones feeling sad, only that one acknowledges the sadness. To accept emotions is to acknowledge them nonjudgmentally as they arise.

Question to Pose/Intervention

"When we judge our emotions, we generate additional emotions or secondary emotions. For example, if I feel sad and then judge my sadness as a weakness, I may feel angry with myself. If I then judge my anger as dangerous, I could end up feeling fearful. Now, I'm feeling sadness, anger, and fear. Notice how each of my judgments compounded my emotional experience. If I hadn't judged my emotions, I'd just be feeling sad. Not judging my emotions doesn't mean I have to see them positively. I don't have to feel happy about being sad, I just acknowledge it. The first step to practicing a nonjudgmental stance toward emotions is to become mindful or aware of your tendency to judge your emotions. You may notice that you are more inclined to judge some emotions than others. When you become aware of these judgments, try to let them go."

Example

Therapist: I see on your thought record that when your boyfriend didn't call you had the thought, "He doesn't care," and you felt sad. But then you had the thought, "I'm a loser to feel this way." What feeling did that thought kick up?

Patient: Anger at myself and disappointment.

Therapist: So you started out with just sadness. But then you judged your sadness and ended up feeling sad, angry, and disappointed. What do think would have happened if you hadn't judged your sadness?

Patient: What do you mean?

Therapist: If you had just let yourself feel sad without criticizing yourself for it.

Patient: I wouldn't have felt those other emotions—anger and disappointment. I would have just felt sad.

Homework

The therapist can have patients practice a nonjudgmental stance toward their emotions over the coming week. If this seems overly broad, they can jointly decide to focus on one or two particularly problematic emotions. Alternatively, patients can focus on not judging their emotions in particular contexts. Patients should be instructed that the first step to assuming a nonjudgmental stance is to bring judgments of their emotions into awareness. Their judgments can be recorded using Form 4.6: Practicing a Nonjudgmental Stance toward Emotions. Patients should be urged not to judge their judging. Instead, when they become aware of a judgment, they should practice letting it go.

Possible Problems

Resistance to practicing a nonjudgmental stance toward one's emotions may stem from erroneous beliefs about the nature of emotions. For example, a patient may refuse to acknowledge or accept sadness because she believes that emotions are of indefinite duration. Beliefs underlying the resistance can be elicited in session by asking the patient what she believes would happen if she did the homework. These beliefs can then be challenged with information about the nature of emotions and by examining evidence that supports and contradicts these beliefs from the patient's prior experience with emotions. Resistance to practicing a nonjudgmental stance may also derive from the perception that the therapist is asking the patient to condone her negative feelings or to feel positively about having them. This can be handled by reiterating that the task is merely to acknowledge emotions as they arise without positive or negative evaluation. The therapist should emphasize that accepting an emotion does not mean condoning it.

Cross-Reference to Other Techniques

Related techniques include meditation, psychoeducation with facts about emotions, and observing and describing emotions.

Form

Form 4.6: Practicing a Nonjudgmental Stance toward Emotions

TECHNIQUE: DIFFERENTIATING ACTION URGES AND ACTIONS TAKEN

Description

The fear of experiencing emotions may stem from the belief that it necessarily entails action. For example, a patient may attempt to block his anger because he believes that the experience of this emotion necessarily involves attacking others. To challenge this belief, it is necessary to differentiate the action urge that accompanies an emotion from the actions taken. Continuing the prior example, it is possible to experience the urge to attack verbally and yet remain silent. This distinction between the emotional experience and emotional expression is made in the model of emotions that DBT presents to patients. However, it is recommended that the therapist highlight this distinction to be sure that patients grasp it.

Question to Pose/Intervention

"Every emotion is accompanied by an urge to take some action. For example, when we are angry, the urge is usually to attack verbally or physically. However, that urge is not always acted upon. There may be times that you are angry, and rather than attack, you simply remain quiet. The urge to take action is part of the experience of emotions. Acting or not acting on this urge is part of the expression of emotions. It's possible to experience an emotion without acting on it, although sometimes it may be challenging."

Example

Therapist: You say that you're afraid to let yourself get angry?

Patient: Yes, I'm afraid of what I might do.

Therapist: What do you think you would do?

Patient: I would lose control, start screaming, or throw things.

Therapist: You might. But then again, you might not. Do you usually do those things when you get angry?

Patient: No.

Therapist: Feeling the urge to throw things and scream is part of the experience of anger. When we're angry, we have the urge to attack. Just being aware or mindful of these urges decreases the likelihood that you'll act on them impulsively. This awareness creates a window of opportunity to respond differently to the urge. Without awareness of the urges, there isn't this window.

Homework

Patients can use Form 4.5 (Observing and Describing Emotions) to record the urges that accompany emotional experiences and the actions that are part of emotional expression.

Possible Problems

On the basis of their history of impulsively acting on their emotions, some patients have learned to conflate emotional experience and expression and are understandably skeptical of the distinction between them. This can be handled by highlighting the distinction in emotions that are less problematic for the patients. For example, a patient being counseled for anger management would be instructed to monitor his action urges and actions taken when experiencing fear rather than anger.

Cross-Reference to Other Techniques

Related techniques include observing and describing emotions, practicing mindfulness of emotions, and experiencing emotion as a wave.

Form

Form 4.5: Observing and Describing Emotions

TECHNIQUE: EXPERIENCING AN EMOTION AS A WAVE

Description

Some individuals believe they must use a technique whenever an emotion arises to decrease its intensity. Some may believe that emotions last indefinitely, and therefore they must be stopped or blocked as they arise. Alternatively, others feel compelled to amplify or intensify their emotional experience. It is important for the therapists to teach these patients that another option is simply to step back and experience the emotion as a wave. This technique is essentially mindfulness of the current emotion. By describing emotions as waves, the therapist is communicating that they are time-limited phenomena and do not last forever.

Question to Pose/Intervention

"Emotions are like waves. [Therapist draws a wave.] They reach their peak intensity and then ebb. Individual emotions last from seconds to minutes. They will pass as a function of time if you don't try to block them and instead let them run their course. Blocking them will only make them persist. Just step back and experience them as waves. Don't try to push them away if they are unpleasant or prolong them if they feel good. Just ride the wave. Each wave lasts from seconds to minutes. But emotions are self-perpetuating. If I think of something sad, I experience a wave of sadness. This may predispose me to recall another sad thing, which kicks up another wave of sadness, and so on."

Example

Therapist: How was your mood this week?

Patient: Not good. I got really anxious on Friday before my race. I tried the deep breathing you taught me, but it didn't work.

Therapist: When you say it didn't work, what do you mean?

Patient: It didn't get rid of the anxiety. In fact, I felt like I was getting worse.

Therapist: That must have been frustrating. But that technique is intended to take the edge off of the anxiety, not get rid of it. I get the sense that when you feel anxiety coming on you feel compelled to stop it.

Patient: Yeah. What else am I supposed to do?

Therapist: One option is to do nothing. Emotions are like waves. They reach their peak intensity and then fall without your doing anything.

Patient: They don't feel like waves. They seem to go on forever.

Therapist: I think that's because you try to block the emotion when you first sense it. If that fails, I think you get more anxious because you believe you need to stop it.

Patient: Yes, that's true. I'm afraid of what will happen if I don't stop it.

Therapist: But you don't have to stop it. If you let the emotion run its course, it will subside on its own. Would you be willing to try that?

Patient: Maybe. I don't think it will work.

Therapist: Well, remember you're not trying to get rid of the emotion. Note how intense your sadness becomes and how long it takes before it falls. Maybe a good place to start is to practice with an emotion other than anxiety.

Homework

The therapist can instruct patients to practice this technique during the week when they have occasion to experience a particular emotion, using Form 4.7 (Experiencing Your Emotion as a Wave), as a guide. Alternatively, patients can be instructed to create an opportunity for practicing this technique by inducing emotions.

Possible Problems

Resistance may stem from beliefs about the duration of emotions and skepticism that emotions will ebb as a function of time. The therapist can suggest that patients practice with positive emotions or emotions of low intensity. Alternatively, the therapist might also practice this technique with patients during the therapy session.

Cross-Reference to Other Techniques

Related techniques include observing and describing emotions and emotion induction.

Form

Form 4.7: Experiencing Your Emotion as a Wave

TECHNIQUE: EMOTION INDUCTION

Description

Emotional avoidance is problematic because it maintains the fear of emotions. It is reinforced by an immediate short-term decrease in distress that increases the likelihood of avoidance recurring. For this reason, patients may be committed to overcoming emotional avoidance but nonetheless continue to engage in it. Emotional avoidance includes escape behaviors such as distraction, the use of prescribed and nonprescribed drugs, bingeing, and other impulsive behaviors. The induction of emotions both in and out of session provides patients with the opportunity to experience emotions and practice emotion regulation techniques. By encountering emotions, patients can obtain information needed to challenge their emotion myths and overcome their fear. Music, movies, pictures, and conversation topics can be used to induce emotions. For example, the therapist could instruct patients to listen to a piece of music that they find emotionally evocative and attend to the experience, observing the rise and fall of the emotion.

Question to Pose/Intervention

"Continually avoiding emotions strengthens our fear of them. We miss the opportunity to test our beliefs about emotions or learn that we can handle them. When I avoid my emotion, I may decrease my distress over the short term. This reduction in distress makes it more likely that I will avoid emotions in the future. In other words, it reinforces avoidance. One way to end the cycle is to willingly encounter my emotions. I could wait until something emotional happens, or I could be more proactive and create an emotional experience. For example, I could listen to a piece of music that I find sad and let myself experience the sadness. I could notice where I feel it in my body and how intense it is, and observe its rise and fall."

Example

Therapist: Did you practice observing and describing emotions this week?

Patient: I'll be honest. I intended to practice because I know it would be good for me. But whenever I felt an emotion coming on, I avoided it. It seemed almost automatic.

Therapist: OK, that makes sense. Your avoidance of emotions decreases your distress, and the reduction in distress increases the likelihood you avoid again. In other words, your tendency to avoid emotions has been strengthened.

Patient: How can I stop avoiding?

Therapist: Well, one way to break the cycle of avoidance would be to induce an emotion in session. You could bring in a piece of music that triggers intense emotions for you. You could listen to it in here and bring your awareness to what you are feeling. I can help you to keep your awareness on the emotions you would feel. What do you think?

Patient: That's a great idea. Let's try it next week.

Homework

For homework, patients can be instructed to select something to be used in the emotion induction (i.e., music, picture, conversation topic). After an emotion induction has been completed in the session, patients can induce emotions outside of session, using Form 4.8 as a guide, and practice experiencing the emotion as a wave.

Possible Problems

Patients may be reluctant to experience negative emotions. In this case, the emotion induction can be focused on creating a positive emotion. Patients who engage in pervasive emotional avoidance may have difficulty selecting emotionally evocative material for the induction. In this case, the therapist should make suggestions.

Cross-Reference to Other Techniques

Related techniques include experiencing an emotion as a wave and observing and describing emotions.

Form

Form 4.8: Emotion Induction Record

TECHNIQUE: DESIGNING EXPERIMENTS TO TEST EMOTION MYTHS

Description

One of the most powerful ways for patients to challenge their emotion myths is to test them empirically. Experiments can be conducted during the therapy session or outside of the session for homework. Before conducting the experiment, it is important that patients identify the hypothesis to be tested and specify the degree of confidence in the prediction. After conducting the experiment, patients should record the actual outcome and note whether it confirms or disconfirms the prediction. The therapist should explain to patients that the tendency to discount outcomes that contradict emotion myths serves to maintain these erroneous beliefs. For this reason, it is important to focus awareness on the actual outcome of the experiment. For example, a patient may have the inaccurate belief that sadness lasts indefinitely. Using the emotion induction technique described previously, this belief can be tested in session.

Question to Pose/Intervention

"One way to evaluate the accuracy of your beliefs about emotions is to test them out. Often, we have a tendency to believe something despite evidence to the contrary. This is because we're not keeping track of the evidence that contradicts or supports our belief. For example, we could design an experiment to test your belief that sadness lasts indefinitely. Before we begin the experiment, you need to specify what you think will happen and how confident you are in your prediction. We can then create an opportunity to experience sadness in the session and note exactly what happens."

Example

Therapist: You've said you'd rather not discuss the conflict you're having with your mother. Why is that?

Patient: Well, I have to go to class this evening, and I need to be able to focus.

Therapist: So, it sounds as though you're predicting that if we discuss the conflict now, you won't be able to focus in class this evening.

Patient: Exactly. I don't want to talk about it. I'll become sad and it will ruin the day, maybe even the week.

Therapist: Well, then it makes perfect sense that you don't want to discuss it. If I believed the emotion of sadness lasted an entire day or even a week, I wouldn't want to talk about something that would trigger sadness either.

Patient: Are you saying my belief is wrong?

Therapist: Why don't we test it out by conducting an experiment?

Patient: How would we do that?

Therapist: We could discuss the argument that you had with your mother and monitor how long the sadness lasts and whether it ruins the day. But before we conduct the experiment, I need you to predict on a scale of 0 to 100 how sad you think you'll become and how confident you are in your predictions.

Homework

For homework, patients can be instructed to design and conduct other experiments about emotions and record the results.

Possible Problems

Emotionally avoidant patients may be reluctant to conduct experiments outside of session. In this case, the therapist should conduct in-session experiments more frequently. Alternatively, patients may report that they have conducted experiments but have not completed the Experiment Record (Form 4.9). In this case, the therapist should emphasize the importance of recording actual outcomes as a way to offset the tendency to discount information that is inconsistent with their beliefs.

Cross-Reference to Other Techniques

Related techniques include experiencing the emotion as a wave, observing and describing emotions, and emotion induction.

Form

Form 4.9: Experiment Record

TECHNIQUE: OPPOSITE ACTION

Description

One of the most effective ways to attenuate the intensity of an emotion is to act counter to the action tendencies that accompany it (Izard, 1971). This principle underlies the exposure-based treatment of phobias, in which patients approach rather than avoid the feared object, and as a result fear attenuates. The facilitation of action tendencies not associated with the emotion that is disordered is a key component of Barlow's unified treatment for negative affect syndrome. The principle of opposite action has also been utilized by Beck and colleagues in the behavioral activation treatment of depression. Rather than giving into the urge to withdraw that accompanies sadness and hopelessness, patients who are depressed are encouraged to become active. The principle of opposite action was expanded by Linehan in DBT to address a broad range of emotions, including shame and anger. In DBT, patients are taught the technique of opposite action as an emotion regulation strategy. By acting counter to the action urge associated with any emotion, patients can attenuate its intensity provided that it is not justified (i.e., there is no good reason to feel fear). With proficiency in the use of opposite action, patients collect evidence to contradict the beliefs that emotions are uncontrollable or never ending.

Question to Pose/Intervention

"Every emotion is accompanied by an action urge or the urge to do something. When we are angry we feel like attacking. When we act consistent with that urge, we maintain or strengthen the emotion. However, when we act opposite to the urge, we decrease the intensity of the emotion. This is the technique of opposite action. It works most effectively when an emotion is not justified, that is, it does not fit the facts of the situation. In other words, if an animal is truly dangerous, your fear will not decrease by approaching it. An exception to this rule is anger. Even if you are justifiably angry with someone else, you can decrease your anger toward him by using opposite action."

Example

Therapist: So you say you felt guilty after asking a question in class today. Why do you think you felt guilty?

Patient: I don't know. I don't like to take up class time with my stupid questions. I felt like I was imposing. I only did it because it was homework to practice being assertive.

Therapist: But aren't you a member of the class too? Aren't you entitled to ask questions like any other student?

Patient: I know it doesn't make sense. But I feel guilty about a lot of things for no particular reason.

Therapist: Remember how we discussed that every emotion has an action urge? What do you have the urge to do when you're feeling guilty?

Patient: Sneak. Hide.

Therapist: What do you think happens to your guilt when you give in to the urge to sneak around or hide?

Patient: It increases?

Therapist: That's right. And by acting opposite to those urges, you can weaken the guilt you're feeling. In other words, the more you ask questions in class, the less guilty you'll feel about intruding on class time. Are you willing to give it a try?

Homework

Patients can be asked to practice opposite action over the coming week with the target emotion and take note of changes in the intensity of the emotion, using Form 4.10 (Opposite Action).

Possible Problems

Resistance to this intervention may stem from the misinterpretation of opposite action as a directive to be phony or fake. It is important to emphasize that opposite action is a behavioral technique that patients can use at their discretion to decrease the intensity of various emotions. Masking an emotion and acting opposite to its action tendencies are different. For example, the task in opposite action with fear is not to pretend that one is not afraid. Rather, the patient is mindful of her fear and the urge to run but makes a deliberate decision to approach.

Cross-Reference to Other Techniques

Related techniques include explaining the model of emotions, mindfulness practice, and meditation.

Form

Form 4.10: Opposite Action

CONCLUSIONS

More behavioral than cognitive in its approach, DBT does address cognitive contributions to emotion dysregulation. In particular, erroneous beliefs about emotions or emotion myths are viewed as contributing to the use of maladaptive emotion regulation strategies. Identifying and changing erroneous beliefs about emotions are not a primary focus of DBT but are central to an EST approach, which is based on a metacognitive model of emotion. Both theory and research suggest that beliefs about emotions can negatively impact emotion regulation. Accordingly, to address emotion regulation difficulties effectively, it is recommended that the therapist help patients identify erroneous beliefs about emotions and target them for change. To that end, DBT is a rich source for techniques. As in other mindfulness-based treatments (which we discuss in more detail in Chapter 5), in DBT, developing a nonjudgmental awareness of emotions is a foundational emotion regulation skill. The nonjudgmental stance of mindfulness counteracts the tendency to negatively evaluate emotions. Mindfulness is also a form of exposure and can provide a context for the development of less negative associations with the experience of emotions. However, DBT is distinguished from other mindfulness-based treatments and cognitive-behavioral therapies in its provision of a theory and model of emotions to patients. This strong psychoeducational component is arguably indispensable to the effective challenge of emotion myths.

CHAPTER FIVE

Mindfulness

The most prominent and widely used meditation technique in CBT is broadly known as "mindfulness training." Because of its empirically demonstrated effectiveness in helping patients work with difficult emotions (Baer, 2003; Hofmann, Sawyer, Witt, & Oh, 2010), mindfulness training is of particular interest for those therapists who seek to broaden the scope of CBT to enhance emotion regulation. Mindfulness relates to EST as a core capacity of awareness that is fundamental to the establishment and maintenance of an adaptive, flexible orientation to emotional experiencing. Mindfulness increases acceptance, a nonjudgmental and less guilt-ridden sense of emotion, and a recognition that emotions do not have to be controlled or suppressed but rather can be tolerated and experienced. Mindfulness training aims to foster a state of openness to experiencing emotions fully, in contact with the present moment, and without intense behavioral reactivity. Increasingly, prominent cognitive and behavioral approaches such as ACT (Hayes et al., 1999), mindfulness-based cognitive therapy (MBCT; Segal, Williams, & Teasdale, 2002), compassion-focused therapy (Gilbert, 2009), and DBT (Linehan, 1993a; see Chapter 4) have used mindfulness training as a central feature in their work with affect tolerance and emotion regulation.

Where does this increasingly popular notion of mindfulness begin? Although similar meditation practices probably existed as far back as 1000 BCE, what we think of as mindfulness training began 2,500 years ago, with the methods of the historical teacher who has come to be known as "the Buddha." Interestingly, the term "Buddha" simply means "one who woke up." According to the Buddha, training in *Sati* was very important. *Sati* was the original Pali (archaic Sanskrit) term that is now translated into English as "mindfulness." *Sati* is a particular and intentional state of mind that can be said to involve a blend of present-moment-focused attention, open awareness, and memory of oneself (Kabat-Zinn, 2009; R. Siegel, Germer, & Olendzki, 2009). *Samma-sati* (translated as "correct mindfulness") is one of the eight most basic tools that form the core of Buddhist mind training, known as "The Eightfold Path" (Rahula, 1958). Clearly, mindfulness training was a fundamental element of the original teachings of the Buddha.

As mindfulness meditation practices have entered the mainstream of CBT, a standard operational definition of mindfulness has emerged. According to Jon Kabat-Zinn, the developer of the mindfulness-based stress reduction (MBSR) method (Kabat-Zinn, 1994), mindfulness is "awareness that emerges through paying attention on purpose, in the present moment, and nonjudgmentally to the unfolding of experience moment by moment" (p. 4). This process involves the development of a special way of paying attention to our experiences that is rather different from our typical, everyday way of attending to our lives. Mindfulness represents a focused and flexible, moment-by-moment observation of the unfolding flow of thoughts, feelings, and bodily sensations that presents itself within our consciousness. From the perspective of a patient, aware observer, we come to experience thoughts *as* thoughts, emotions *as* emotions, and physical sensations *as* physical sensations. We are invited to suspend our judgment of these experiences and to diligently, yet gently, draw our awareness, again and again, to the flow of events in our consciousness.

One way of clarifying the distinction between mindfulness practice and our typical way of operating is to contrast a "doing mode" with a "being mode." When we are moving through our typical activities, pursuing goals, attempting to effect change on our environment, and pursuing objects in the world, we can be said to be acting in a "doing mode." Segal et al. (2002) note that this "doing mode" comes into action when our minds are not satisfied with the state of the reality we encounter. When we wish to have those things that we do not have or wish to push away that which we do not want, our minds enter this "doing mode." Some negative feeling or craving is triggered, and our mind comes into action, drawing upon our habitual patterns of thinking, feeling, and behaving to achieve some object or change in state. Often, this is not a problem. We are thirsty, so we seek something to drink. We see an obstacle on our path, and we walk around it.

Sometimes, though, the discrepancy between how things are and how we would like them to be is more difficult to address. Perhaps the action that is called for is vague or impossible. There may be an action we can take, but it isn't something we can do right now. In such cases, our "doing mode" does not really serve us.

Similarly, we are often troubled by our feelings or our thoughts. Naturally, our "doing mode" would suggest to us that we should take action. Often, that action amounts to pushing away these thoughts and attempting to avoid certain experiences. As we shall see, many researchers have suggested that attempts to treat our personal, internal experiences in this way can lead to more suffering (Hayes et al., 2001). When we attempt to suppress our feelings, thoughts, and mental events, they often are intensified and present themselves more frequently in our awareness (Wegner, Schneider, Carter, & White, 1987). In fact, the characteristics of this "doing mode" are often a lack of satisfaction, compulsive monitoring of one's state, hurriedness, self-criticism, and futile efforts to change what we cannot change. When we apply this "doing mode" to our emotions, we can struggle to rid ourselves of unpleasant feelings only to create an increasing wave of distress that grows in size and intensity relative to the strength and persistence of our struggle.

The mode of paying attention involved in mindfulness is sometimes referred to as a "being mode." When in this "being mode," we are not focused on the pursuit of goals or objects in the phenomenal world. When practicing mindful awareness, we are simply observing the stream of our consciousness, without judgment, description, or evaluation. In this way, we may make a deep contact with our present-moment existence. The experience of mindfulness is said to involve an enhanced awareness, clarity of perception, and a spirit of willing acceptance of present-moment reality, as it is. By cultivating such a perspective, we may more fully experience the richness of what it means to be alive.

The contemporary protégé Tibetan meditation master Yongyey Mingyur Rinpoche (2007) has described mindfulness as "the key, the *how* of Buddhist practice [that] lies in learning to simply rest in a bare awareness of thoughts, feelings and perceptions as they occur" (p. 24). Development of mindfulness cultivates an intentional mode of awareness that involves a paradoxical disidentification from the contents of one's conscious mind while gently allowing a nonjudgmental, full experience of one's present moment (Segal et al., 2002).

Several commentators have likened our typical state of mind to a sleepwalking mode of existence. The mental formations, projections of past experiences, generalized relationship expectancies, and emotional memories that we have cultivated so shape and affect our individual experience of reality as to weave a dreamlike and distorted experience of the act of being. As we have noted, the linguistic root of the word "buddha" (i.e., a fully enlightened being) means "one who has awoken." Hence, the psychospiritual ideal that has dominated Asian thought for millennia simply represents an awakening from the painful dream of experiencing life through the veil of literalized dysfunctional cognitions and patterns of emotional memories (Gilbert & Tirch, 2007). A number of studies have demonstrated the benefits of mindfulness training, including the treatment of depressive relapse, anxiety disorders, chronic pain, coping with illness, and many other psychological problems (Baer, 2003). Recent research on the neurobiology of mindfulness suggests that mindfulness training may enhance the functioning of emotional processing by enhancing the direct translation of bodily sensations into emotions, without overly relating these emotions to narrative memories. This process seems to involve potential augmentation of the function of the insula and the anterior cingulate cortex (Farb et al., 2007).

The techniques described in this chapter have been selected for their relative simplicity and their relevance to working with emotions. First, they are employed as foundational practices in a number of modes of mindfulness training. Second, they are relatively simple to teach and to learn in the context of ongoing CBT, given commitment and consistency on the part of the clinician and the patient. Finally, they all relate rather directly to the cultivation of enhanced emotion regulation capacities.

TECHNIQUE: BODY SCAN

Description

This technique is often referred to as the "body scan," as it has been labeled in MBSR training (Kabat-Zinn, 1990). Variations of this practice may be found in yoga, where it is referred to as *yoga nidra*. Beyond this, further examples of this practice may be found in exercises of global spiritual traditions, including Sufism, Esoteric Christianity, and Judaism. This technique consists of directing a mindful, nonjudgmental awareness throughout the body at a gradual and deliberate pace. The practitioner directs his or her attention to each part of the body in turn, bringing bare attention to whatever sensations are present at that moment. There is no effort to achieve a state of relaxation or, in fact, any alteration in state whatsoever.

Powerful emotions often manifest themselves in physical sensations. Teaching patients to be able to simply observe these physical sensations in a decentered way may provide some flexibility and leverage in the ultimate regulation of these emotions. Many patients' emotional schemas and fusion with emotion myths may lead to attempts at avoiding emotional processing or an overreliance on rationality. By making contact and fully experiencing these physical sensations in the body, patients make initial steps toward a more full and comprehensive mode of emotional processing (Segal et al., 2002).

Question to Pose/Intervention

This exercise may be taught in an individual or group format. After patients have learned this method, they may be invited to practice the body scan exercise daily. Typically, patients may be given an audio file, which contains a guided meditation, and a record form, which will allow them to monitor how frequently they engage in the homework and what their observations about the process are.

In order to guide patients through mindfulness training, the therapist must first take a few logistic concerns into account. Is the physical space adequate to allow for patients to lie on a yoga mat? Is the seating that is available conducive to a healthy sitting position? By maintaining his or her own mindfulness practice in the office, the therapist can build a sense of how conducive the environment is to such training. Also, the therapist might consider how much time he or she has to devote to mindfulness training in a given session. In the agenda-setting phase of a CBT session that incorporates a mindfulness intervention, it is often useful to discuss and plan with patients how much of the session will be devoted to the guided practice, allowing time for debriefing them and inquiring about their experience.

After patients engage in their first body scan exercise, they often are invited to share any observations they may have about the experience. It is important for the therapist to ask open-ended questions about such observations and to avoid any tendency to suggest the patients discuss the exercise in evaluative terms. The therapist may simply ask, "What was that like for you?" or "What observations might you wish to share about that first exercise?"

The therapist and his or her patients should define a clear aim for the guided practice. Typically, a daily 30- to 45-minute body scan practice is useful as a form of initial training in mindfulness. The patients may be given a guided exercise on an audio CD or mp3 file.

To promote homework compliance, patients are asked to complete a self-monitoring form. Patients record daily whether or not they practiced the body scan, as well as whether they used a guided recording or not, and note their daily observations regarding mindfulness practice.

Example[1]

The sections in *italics*, in this and other examples in this book, are meant to serve as a beginning script. The clinician is advised to follow this structure but to speak from his or her own experience, using his or her own words.

This exercise is usually conducted lying down or seated with the back straight, yet supple. It is probably best if you find a comfortable space, and lie there on a yoga mat, rug, or blanket. The setting should be at a comfortable temperature and in a place and time where you will be free from distraction or interruption. As you begin, let your eyes close and fall still. Allow yourself to gently direct your attention to the physical sensations you are experiencing in the present moment, bringing your attention to the presence of life in the body. For a moment, direct your attention to the sounds around you in the room. Next, broaden this sensory experience to take in the sounds just beyond the room. Then allow yourself to observe the sounds even farther away. With the next breath in, bring your attention back to the body and the experience of breathing.

---

[1] The following directions are adapted from several sources, notably the guided meditations of Jon Kabat-Zinn (1990). Some of the ideas and phrases are also adapted from the writings of Thich Nat Hanh (1992) and other clinical meditation sources.

Allow yourself to observe the flow of the breath, as it moves gently in and out of the body. There is no need to breathe in any special way; just allow the breath to find its own rhythm in time. As you breathe in, notice the physical sensations involved in the inhalation. When you release the breath, allow your attention to flow out with the exhalation. Each breath in will involve a gathering, a collecting of attention, and each out-breath will involve a process of letting go of that awareness. At this point, gently direct your attention to the physical sensations you are experiencing throughout the body at this moment. With each inhalation, allow your attention to gather at the contact points where your body meets the mat, chair, or cushion that supports you. As you exhale, notice the feeling of heaviness where your body is supported by the ground. There is no need to aim for any special state during this practice. There is no need to strive to relax or to "do" anything at all. Your aim in this work is simply to observe what you are experiencing moment by moment. Without judging, analyzing, or even describing your experience, you will now begin to direct your attention to the different parts of the body. As you gather attention at the level of physical sensation, allow yourself to suspend any evaluations and simply deploy a "bare attention" to whatever it is that you observe. With the next inhalation, allow your attention to move to the physical sensations in the abdomen. Notice the various sensations that accompany each in-breath and out-breath. After staying with this experience for a few seconds, bring your attention up from your abdomen, along the length of your left arm, and into the left hand. Allow your attention to spread, as if it were a warm presence radiating down the arm, all the while noticing the presence of life in the body. Merely observe the sensations in the hand. With each in-breath, allow yourself to imagine the breath flowing into the chest and abdomen and radiating down the left arm into the hand. Your attention will accompany this inhalation, as if you were "breathing in" an awareness of the physical sensations present in the hand. Without changing anything intentionally in the state of the hand, allow yourself to breathe into the sensations in each part of the hand for several seconds. With each exhalation, allow yourself to let go of that awareness. As you do this, allow yourself to notice the thumb ... the index finger ... the second finger ... the ring finger ... and the pinky. Next, breathe in a collected awareness of the sensations in the back of the hand ... the palm of the hand ... and the hand as a whole. When you feel that you have completed your gentle observation of the sensations in the left hand, allow your attention to radiate back up the left arm, noticing the presence of life in the lower arm, the bicep, the tricep, and all of the parts of the arm. With the next inhalation, allow your attention to gather again in the abdomen. Next, allow yourself to bring this attention to the sensations in the right arm and hand, in the same manner that you used with your left. At a comfortable pace, and with an attitude of gentle, nonjudgmental curiosity, direct your attention to each of the areas of the body in turn, breathing into the sensations in each foot (and each of the toes), each lower leg, shin, and calf, the pelvic region, the lower back and abdomen, the upper back and shoulders, the neck and contact point between the head and the spine, the muscles of the face, the forehead, and the scalp. Allow yourself to take this slowly and to engage in the exercise with a spirit of the client, accepting curiosity. When you observe discomfort or tension in any part of the body, again allow yourself to breathe into the sensations. As much as you can, attempt to stay with each sensation, merely observing it, being with it moment by moment. It is the nature of our minds to wander, and it is simply the most natural thing for our minds to do. As you engage in this practice, when you notice that your mind has drifted away from the focus on physical sensations, accept that this has happened, allow some room for this experience in your awareness, and gently draw your attention back to the physical sensations with the in-breath. After you have spent some time engaged in this practice, having brought a mindful awareness to the body over the course of several minutes (this practice can range from 15 to 45 or more minutes), gently allow your breath and attention to return to settle on the physical sensations in the abdomen. Now, with the next in-breath, allow your attention to focus on the sounds that surround you in the room. Next, bring the attention to the sounds outside of the room. Following this, allow your attention to gently settle on the sounds even farther away than that. Giving yourself a few moments to gather your attention and orientation to your presence on the mat, you can open your eyes, and resume your daily activities.

Homework

Patients may practice the body scan exercise daily. A recorded exercise of roughly 30 minutes should be sufficient to guide patients as they begin this work. It is useful to provide patients with a diary form (Form 5.1), so that they may better monitor and structure their practice.

Possible Problems

Mindfulness training will pose different challenges and potential problems for each person who engages in it. As we examine the range of techniques available, several of these possible problems may apply to more than one technique alone.

Although patients may intellectually grasp the notion of nonjudgmental awareness, they often cling to their judgments during the practice of mindfulness training. This is to be expected and is a part of the ongoing process of returning to an accepting stance. The questions that the therapist asks in sharing observations with patients are aimed at facilitating the development of an attitude of willingness. This may be something of a departure for many cognitive-behavioral therapists, who are often using the dialogue in therapy to facilitate cognitive restructuring.

As patients begin to discuss whether they have done the exercise "right" or have gotten it "wrong," it is the therapist's job to help them see past these judgments and discernments. The therapeutic dialogue may involve the therapist listening to the patients' evaluations of their experience and then proceeding to draw their awareness back to the ultimate aim of allowing the experience to be just as it is and to sit with that experience. It may be useful at such times to return to the contrast between the "doing" and the "being" modes. Thoughts may be viewed as objects in a stream of consciousness that can be disidentified through the process of observing or experiencing physical sensations in the present moment.

Patients often find themselves falling asleep during the body scan exercise because of the deep relaxation that frequently accompanies it. It is important for the therapist to normalize this response and to remind patients that, with practice, the body scan becomes much more an exercise in "falling awake" than in "falling asleep." Patients who have particular difficulty staying awake during this practice may opt to practice the body scan sitting up and/or with their eyes open.

Cross-Reference to Other Techniques

Other techniques that might be used in conjunction with the body scan include mindfulness of the breath, mindful awareness of movement, the making space exercise, mindfulness of sound,

3-minute breathing space, 3-minute coping breathing space, and mindful cooking, all of which are discussed in this chapter, as well as completion of the Emotionally Intelligent Thought Record (Form 8.2) and the "Stopping the War" Record (Form 6.4).

Form

Form 5.1: Daily Mindfulness Practice Record

TECHNIQUE: MINDFULNESS OF THE BREATH

Description

Awareness of the breath as a focus of attention is fundamental to most meditation methods the world over. This is particularly true of mindfulness training. Nevertheless, the way in which patients hold their attention in the mindfulness of the breath exercise is very different from many methods of relaxation and meditation. Typically, when we are enjoined to focus our attention, we might respond with an intense, one-pointed awareness, which we can only hold on to for just so long. Some methods of meditation, such as concentration meditation, seek to hone a "laser-like" focus on a single object. Mindfulness is a bit different. During the mindfulness of the breath exercise, patients use their breath as an "anchor" for their awareness. Yet the attention is "held lightly" on the breath.

Patients are taught to use this mindfulness of the breath exercise as a tool for developing a new perspective on their thoughts and feelings. At the point that this exercise will be implemented, patients should have already learned a definition of mindfulness and the aim of observing and decentering from the contents of consciousness. The body scan serves as an excellent introduction to these points, and it is often the case that patients will have already experienced mindfulness directly during the practice of the body scan exercise before they begin practicing mindfulness of the breath.

Question to Pose/Intervention

The therapist training patients in mindfulness of the breath usually does so by leading a guided meditation during the session. Often, this will take place in a group forum. This group mode of training is found in MBCT, MBSR, and other forms of mindfulness training. The guided exercise can also take place in an individual therapy session. As was the case with the body scan, when leading the guided mindfulness of the breath exercise, the therapist is not only speaking his or her way through the steps of the practice but is also taking part in the mindfulness meditation. This is a very important aspect of the practice. It is suggested that the therapist familiarize him- or herself with this exercise and then lead the meditation from memory rather than read a rote description of the technique from this or any other source. In this way, the therapist is modeling full participation in the present moment and is embodying a mindful perspective, as best he or she can.

The therapist can employ reflective listening and validating statements rather than a didactic style of instruction. The therapist is actually using this inquiry and discussion period to encourage patients' adoption of an accepting, kind curiosity about the nature of their experience. The following are examples of these questions: "What did you notice during that period of practice?" "In what way is this manner of paying attention different from our everyday mode of paying attention?" "What could this practice of paying attention to our breathing have to do with dealing with difficult emotions?" The heart of this practice resides in allowing whatever arrives in the moment to be just as it is, without any intervening judgment, analysis, or attempts to distort or change the experience. As such, it is important that patients' observations, discussions, and questions in this area be invited, allowed, reflected upon, and validated rather than subjected to a rational analysis.

Example[2]

The following directions will serve as a guide through this experience.

Find a place that is comfortable and quiet and that will be relatively free from distractions or interruptions. This is a meditation that is typically done in a seated position. You may choose to sit on a straight-back chair with your legs uncrossed, on a meditation cushion, or even on some pillows. For those not using a chair, if you are familiar with the postures involved in seated meditation, you may use such a posture. If these postures are unfamiliar, it is no problem at all; you can just sit cross-legged with the cushion or pillow beneath your buttocks. The main aim here is to keep your back in a straight yet relaxed posture. This will allow you to take a deep and full breath into the bottom of the lungs. In order to do this, it is a good idea to keep the knees lower than the hips, so that you are less likely to lean or slump forward. This might take a little getting used to, as we aren't always accustomed to sitting with an erect and self-supporting posture, but it is likely to feel quite natural with just a little practice. You might want to imagine your spine as a stack of poker chips or picture a slender thread gently pulling the top of your head to a dignified position, with the neck relatively free from tension. It is good to keep your feet on the floor when sitting in a chair. If you are on a cushion, allow your knees to rest on the floor. In this way, you will feel more grounded and connected to your support. As you begin, allow your eyes to close. Now, gently direct your attention to the sounds around you in the room. If it is quiet, or even silent, just notice the absence of sound, sensing the space around you. When you are ready, after several seconds, bring your attention to the sounds outside of the room. Next, direct your attention to the sounds even farther away than that. On your next inhalation, draw your attention inward to the physical sensations you experience just sitting in this relaxed posture. Just as you did in the mindfulness of the body exercise, allow yourself to collect your attention as you breathe in, observing whatever sensations emerge in your awareness. As you exhale, simply let go of that awareness as the breath leaves the body. Bring your attention to the presence of life in the lower abdomen. Notice whatever sensations are present as your pattern of inhalation and exhalation continues. Feel the sensations of the abdominal muscles as they expand and contract with the rhythm of your breathing. There is no special rhythm or method with which you should breathe. Allow the breath to find its own pace, essentially allowing it to "breathe itself." With a relaxed, yet attentive awareness, take notice of the changes in sensation as the cycle of the breath continues. As you do this, remain aware that

---

[2] The following directions are adapted from several sources, notably the guided meditations of Jon Kabat-Zinn (1990). Some of the ideas and phrases are also adapted from the writings of Thich Nat Hahn (1992) and other clinical meditation sources.

there is no need to change this experience in any way. Similarly, we are not aiming at creating some special state of relaxation or transcendence. We are merely allowing ourselves to truly be with our experience at this fundamental level, with an attitude of willingness and suspension of judgment, moment by moment. In time, the mind will wander. When this occurs, remind yourself that this is the nature of the mind, and that this is, indeed, part of the practice of mindfulness. Our mindfulness of the breath exercise involves a cycle of gently returning our attention to the breath, and it is not an experience to be struggled against in any way. When thoughts, images, emotions, or memories arise, we simply allow them to be where they are, making space for them in our awareness. There is no need to fight these mental events off or to cling to them. When we notice that our minds have wandered, we simply allow our attention to gently return to the flow of our breathing. During this entire process, we are intentionally adopting a gentle, compassionate perspective upon the flow of events in our consciousness. As a nonjudgmental and fully accepting observer, we are bringing this quality of kind and compliant watching to the river of our mind's activity. From time to time, it may be helpful to ground yourself in the present moment by feeling the physical sensations that you are experiencing. In doing this, you may connect with the sensations of the feet or knees on the ground, your buttocks on your chair or cushion, your spine, which is straight and supported, and the flow of the breath in and out of the body. You may continue this practice for about 20 minutes before completing it. In order to let the exercise go, you may again bring your mindful attention to the sounds around you in the room, the sounds that are just outside the room, and the sounds that are farther away even than that. When you are ready, open your eyes, gently rise, and continue with your daily activities.

Homework

The mindfulness of the breath exercise may be given as homework for daily practice. Having learned the form and structure of this exercise in session, patients may use a recorded guide to help them work through this practice on their own. After some time, they may choose to not use the recording and practice this in silence. However, it is recommended that patients begin by using a guided recording.

Possible Problems

Patients may complain that they encountered difficult emotions during their daily practice and that the mindfulness techniques "didn't work." This reveals a difference between a mindfulness-based approach and an approach that is focused more on symptom remission and control. During the practice of mindfulness, the patients' aim is to fully experience whatever may unfold before their mind, moment by moment, in a spirit of willingness, curiosity, and openness. This is very different from aiming to push away uncomfortable experiences or attempting to control the rise and fall of one's emotions.

When a patient comes to a session with a concern that mindfulness "isn't working" because of the presence of challenging emotions, the therapist may begin by validating the patient's emotional experience. In the spirit of empathy and nonjudgment, the therapist may proceed to use gentle inquiry to explore the patient's assumptions about what mindfulness would look like when it "is working" or "isn't working." The patient may actively learn that attempts at controlling and suppressing emotional experience may actually be amplifying and perpetuating psychological distress. The therapist can respond by employing both psychoeducation and reflective listening in this response. Reflective listening takes the form of paraphrasing and validating whatever the patient's experience of mindfulness practice has been. Psychoeducation will involve the therapist explaining the importance of willingness and bare observation in mindfulness and deemphasizing directly changing thoughts and feelings during the practice.

Cross-Reference to Other Techniques

The mindfulness of the breath exercise is related to the following practices: body scan, mindful awareness of movement, the making space exercise, mindfulness of sound, 3-minute breathing space, 3-minute coping breathing space, and mindful cooking as well as completion of the Emotionally Intelligent Thought Record and the "Stopping the War" Record.

Form

Form 5.1: Daily Mindfulness Practice Record

TECHNIQUE: MAKING SPACE: AN EXERCISE IN MINDFUL ACCEPTANCE OF THOUGHTS AND EMOTIONS

Description

The making space exercise is designed to help patients transition from a focus on the breath or the body to a direct awareness and acceptance of their inner experience. During this exercise, patients are encouraged to keep a gentler hold on the direction of their awareness but to be keenly aware of awareness itself. This aspect of mindfulness has been referred to as "choiceless awareness" (Segal et al., 2002) or "bare attention" (Thera, 2003). When practicing bare attention, whatever may arise in the flow of conscious awareness may be attended to mindfully, as if it were the breath or sensations in the body. In this way, patients "make space" for their experience.

It is important to remind patients that the aim of this practice is not to make "bad" feelings and thoughts "go away." Rather, it is an opportunity to recognize that, although we do not have a choice as to what arrives in our awareness, we do have an opportunity to choose how we pay attention. Also, we have the ability to choose where we place that attention. Perhaps we may even place our attention on the act of attending itself. In doing so, the making space exercise aims to bring patients into much closer contact with their attention as a dynamic living process.

Question to Pose/Intervention

Engaging in this practice allows one to ask, "Can I just sit with my experience, and adopt a stance of allowing, willingness, and bare observation?" By teaching this practice to our patients, we invite them to learn how to be "better" at accessing their feelings and thoughts rather than turning away from the negative to "feel better." From a certain point of view, this simple act of willingness and open attention is the crystallization of willingness.

The therapist is advised to suggest that their patients bring a compassionate, warm, and nonjudgmental attitude to the quality of their experiencing and self-regard throughout this exercise. This can be modeled and transmitted through the tone of voice and demeanor that the therapist manifests during the sessions of instruction that form the foundation of the patients' subsequent practice. If the therapist is able to mindfully be with his or her experience, he or she is far more likely to aid patients in finding their way to such an experience.

After an initial session of instruction and practice with the therapist, the patient can practice this exercise for a set period of time at home, spending roughly 20 to 30 minutes per day engaged in the exercise. The therapist and the patient can collaborate on exactly how long the patient may commit to practicing the making space meditation. This should be determined in advance, and the patient should be clear about the duration of each session, the course of his or her involvement with this exercise, and where and when he or she plans to practice. Although there is a guided meditation audio track on the CD accompanying this text, in time the patient may choose to let go of listening to this audio track and choose to begin to "just sit" with his or her awareness. In doing so, the patient is more closely following the traditional Buddhist meditation practice of *shikan-taza* ("just sitting"). More important, in being with silence and one's own awareness, the patient is coming into more intimate contact with the field of his or her own choiceless awareness, which is the ultimate aim of this exercise.

Example

As was the case with the mindfulness of the breath exercise, this practice usually takes place in a seated position. The initial instructions follow the same direction as the mindfulness of the breath exercise as well.

As you may see, your practice of mindful awareness of the breath may become the foundation for the cultivation of mindful attention in further exercises and throughout your day. As you begin, you may choose to sit in a straight-back chair with your legs uncrossed, on a meditation cushion, or even on some pillows. For those not using a chair, if you are familiar with the postures involved in seated meditation, you may use such a posture. If these postures are unfamiliar, it is no problem at all, you can just sit "Indian style" with the cushion or pillow beneath your buttocks. The main aim here is to keep your back in a straight yet relaxed posture. This will allow you to take a deep and full breath into the bottom of the lungs. In order to do this, it is a good idea to keep the knees lower than the hips, so that you are less likely to lean or slump forward. This might take a little getting used to, as we aren't always accustomed to sitting with an erect and self-supporting posture, but it is likely to feel quite natural with just a little practice. You might want to imagine your spine as a stack of poker chips or picture a slender thread gently pulling the top of your head to a dignified position, with the neck relatively free from tension. It is good to keep your feet on the floor when sitting in a chair. If you are on a cushion, allow your knees to rest on the floor. In this way, you will feel more grounded and connected to your support. As you begin, allow your eyes to close. Now, gently direct your attention to the sounds around you in the room. If it is quiet, or even silent, just notice the absence of sound, sensing the space around you. When you are ready, after several seconds, bring your attention to the sounds outside of the room. Next, direct your attention to the sounds even farther away than that. On the next inhalation, allow your attention to gently gather at the level of physical sensation. Observe the movement of the breath in the body, taking note of the physical sensa-

tions that accompany the flow of breath as it cycles through you. You may also wish to bring your attention to the places where you make contact with your support, feeling your feet on the ground, your buttocks in the chair, and your back feeling straight and supported. When you are ready, bring your awareness to the movement of the breath in the abdomen. Observe whatever sensations are present in the abdomen, allowing your attention to collect and gather on the inhalation and letting go of the awareness of particular sensations as you exhale. Allow this breath to flow in its own rhythm. Beyond this, allow yourself to settle into this awareness, abiding in a state of bare observation, suspending judgment, evaluation, or even description. As we have experienced in earlier practices, it is the nature of our minds to wander and drift away from the breath. When we notice this drift of attention, we may even briefly congratulate ourselves for having a moment of self-awareness and gently return our attention to the flow of the breath. How often in life do we allow ourselves to be immersed in these musings? How easy is it to identify with this stream of mental images, thoughts, and emotions? For a moment, you have noticed these mental events for what they are: objects in the stream of consciousness. As you do this, gently shepherd your awareness back to the sensations of the breath in the abdomen. After staying with this practice for a few minutes, allow your attention to refocus on the objects in your mind itself. As each new thought or image enters your mind, merely notice and observe it. You might even benefit from giving a simple label to each mental event as it rises and falls. For example, you may silently say to yourself, "Judging, I'm judging" or "Daydreaming, that was daydreaming." As such thoughts flow through your consciousness, bring a compassionate and nonjudgmental awareness to each of these mental events. Can we allow, accept, and be willing to stay with each of these mental occurrences? Let yourself simply "make space" in the wide field of your present-moment experience for any and every thought, emotion, or image. From time to time, distressing or upsetting ideas may arise. Simply allow yourself to stay with such experiences. As you inhale, allow your awareness to collect in this experience, making space for whatever arises. As you exhale, let go of this awareness. Pay close attention to the manner in which these thoughts emerge, rise, and ultimately fade from your awareness. No single thought is a permanent thought. We are not thinking the same exact thing as we were a decade ago, a year ago, a week ago, or even a moment ago. The flow of mental events continues. Allow yourself to be an observer of this stream, directing your attention to your mind itself.

From time to time, it may be helpful to ground yourself in the present moment by feeling the physical sensations that you are experiencing. In doing this, you may connect with the sensations of the feet or knees on the ground, your buttocks on your chair or cushion, your spine, which is straight and supported, and the flow of the breath in and out of the body. You may continue this practice for about 20 minutes before completing it. In order to let the exercise go, you may again bring your mindful attention to the sounds around you in the room, the sounds that are just outside the room, and the sounds that are farther away even than that. When you are ready, open your eyes, gently rise, and continue with your daily activities.

Homework

This is an exercise that some Buddhist meditation practitioners may practice for extended periods of time. In fact, many of the mindfulness practices presented in this text, and elsewhere in the third-generation CBT literature, are actually disciplines that may be pursued over a lifetime. However, applying these techniques to specific psychological problems such as emotion regulation does not necessitate a lifelong commitment to meditation training. Employing a more advanced mindfulness technique such as the making space exercise may be undertaken for a brief period (e.g., 2–3 weeks). During that time, the therapist and the patient may check in each week and review the observations, comments, and obstacles that presented over the course of the practice period. As the patient progresses in the therapy and mindfulness training, some exercises may seem apt for the development of a longer term practice. This is not mandatory, but may occur.

As with the body scan, a diary form is also included for patients' self-monitoring of homework compliance, observations, and questions.

Possible Problems

The first and most obvious problem that will present itself in the application of the making space exercise is what might be termed the "double-edged sword" phenomenon. Although mindfulness may appear concrete and simple, it may also seem abstract and complex, depending on how it is presented. It is important to remember that mindfulness training is less informational and more experiential.

When patients move from observation of physical sensations, which is overt and felt, to following the breath, they make a leap in the subtlety of attention and openness that they are pursuing. When patients then make the next leap from following the breath to intentionally engaging an accepting observation of thoughts and feelings themselves, they might risk falling into entanglement with abstract thinking or into distraction. Perhaps both of these obstacles are actually unavoidable traveling companions on the journey to a healthier relationship with emotions. The therapist can help patients return to the simplicity of the act of gently making space for whatever arises in awareness. Rather than overexplaining, the therapist is advised to use reflexive questions and validating statements to guide patients as they more deeply engage in the process of inquiry and compassionate curiosity that accompanies these students on the path to cultivating mindfulness. For example, the therapist might say, "It sounds like you are beginning to get wrapped up in some of the thoughts and feelings that you are experiencing during the exercise. Just as in earlier exercises, when you notice this happening, take a moment and give yourself credit for making that discovery. Then, simply and gently, see if you can just make space for whatever is, and bring attention back to the present moment with the next natural in-breath."

Cross-Reference to Other Techniques

The making space practice is related to all of the following: the body scan, mindfulness of the breath, mindful awareness of movement, mindfulness of sound, 3-minute breathing space, 3-minute coping breathing space, and mindful cooking as well as completion of the Emotionally Intelligent Thought Record and the "Stopping the War" Record.

Form

Form 5.1.: Daily Mindfulness Practice Record

TECHNIQUE: 3-MINUTE BREATHING SPACE

Description

We know that mindfulness exercises are not really just meant to be brief visits to an altered state of consciousness during a period of meditation (Tirch & Amodio, 2006). As we have seen, mindfulness training is aimed at the development of an ongoing change in the relationship between a person and his or her flow of experiencing. By bringing attention to the here and now, without judgment or immersion in logical analysis, a person may be able to experience things as they are, not just as the mind says things are. This is a platform on which adaptive decision making, self-care, and behavioral actions directed toward valued directions can take place (K. G. Wilson & DuFrene, 2009). Obviously, just practicing mindfulness on the meditation cushion, chair, or mat once a day is not likely to be sufficient. The aim of the mindfulness trainer may be for patients to begin to take mindfulness with them in each step of their day. The 3-minute breathing space exercise is meant to facilitate just that sort of generalization of mindfulness skills. Developed by Segal et al. (2002) in the context of MBCT, this exercise is meant to be "generalization practice." The exercise provides a structured, deliberate way in which patients may pause in the midst of the flow of their life stressors and bring themselves back to a mindful perspective.

Question to Pose/Intervention

This exercise is drawn from the MBCT group protocol (Segal et al., 2002). It is easily taught in a group format, but also may be employed in one-on-one instructional settings. Like the other mindfulness exercises included in this book, it is meant to be first taught directly to the patient in session by the therapist. Initially, the therapist might suggest that the patient practice the 3-minute breathing space exercise a few times a day at specifically planned points in time. For example, the patient might agree to engage in this exercise three times each day, just before each meal. In this way, the patient is provided with structure and regularity in his or her practice. After 1 or 2 weeks of such practice, the patient might be encouraged to apply the 3-minute breathing space several times a day, specifically when he or she has an intuitive sense that it would be advisable to return to a mindful and accepting perspective.

Example[3]

The 3-minute breathing space is best begun in a seated position. It is possible to engage with this practice while standing, but we will begin practicing while seated. This practice is designed to help you to breathe life into your mindfulness practice, by taking your practice off of the meditation cushion and applying it directly in the flow of your everyday life. To begin this brief application of mindful awareness, first bring part of your attention to the soles of the feet. Allow yourself to make any adjustments to your seated posture that may be necessary so that you might sit with a dignified, erect, yet relaxed demeanor. The back is straight. The sit bones are supported. You can feel yourself rooted to the earth at the contact points where your body

---

[3]This exercise is adapted from the MBCT protocol (Segal et al., 2002). Copyright 2002 by The Guilford Press. Adapted by permission.

meets your chair and the floor. Allow your eyes to close or, if you prefer, just allow the eyelids to relax as you cast your gaze gently at the floor before you. Next, bring attention to the flow of experience that unfolds before your mind. Observing thoughts, feelings, and physical sensations, allow yourself to notice, as much as you can, what is presenting itself in this very moment. We are now paying particular attention to those feelings, ideas, and sensations that may be experienced as unpleasant or upsetting. Rather than pushing these experiences away, we are allowing them to be just as they are. Taking a moment, allow yourself to simply acknowledge the presence of these experiences, making space for whatever emerges and flows through our field of inner observation.

Now, having allowed ourselves to sit in the presence of this moment, with whatever it brings, it is time for us to collect and focus our attention toward a single object. This focus can be gentle and open, but involves collecting our attention and focusing it on the flow of our breath. Observing the breath, we direct our attention to the movements of the body as the breath breathes itself. Breathing in, you know that you are breathing in. Breathing out, you know that you are breathing out. Take special notice of the bellows-like movement of the abdomen, as our body gently allows the very air to move through us, moment by moment. Taking a minute to stay with the flow of the breath, allow your attention to blend with the movement of breathing itself, as best you can.

Next, we bring our attention to a third step in this practice. Having gathered our attention on the flow of the breath, moment by moment, we are now allowing the scope of our awareness to widen to gradually encompass the entire body. Bringing our attention into the body as a whole as we inhale, it is as if we are breathing attention itself into the body, our sense of the body gently expanding as we inhale, taking notice of the interiority and spaciousness that arrives with the attention. As we exhale, we are completely letting go of that awareness. It is as if our whole body is breathing, softening around our experience. Staying with this experience for about a minute, we are allowing ourselves to make space within, as best we can, for whatever arrives.

As we let go of this exercise itself, we again bring part of our attention to the soles of the feet. Next, we bring part of our attention to the top of the head. And, again, we bring part of our attention to everything in between. Then, when you are ready, allow your eyes to open and let go of this exercise entirely.

Homework

Unlike some of the longer mindfulness training practices, the 3-minute breathing space might be applied as a specific, in-the-moment coping tool in a very direct way. This might result in a period of homework practice with a specific schedule or something much more unpredictable and responsive to the patient's environment. The therapist is advised to prepare the patient for this kind of adaptability and flexibility. In doing so, the patient may make a beginning in applying mindfulness directly to emotion regulation and affect tolerance in the flow of life.

Possible Problems

We can examine five potential roadblocks to cultivating mindfulness, which are sometimes known as the "Five Hindrances" (Kamalashila, 1992). The first of these hindrances involves the desire for sense experiences. The pull of appealing stimuli in our environment or even in our imagination can persistently draw us into a fused engagement with pleasurable or exciting thoughts, images, and experiences. This is a very natural tendency, but it is one that can provide persistent distraction during mindfulness training. The second of these hindrances is ill will, the mirror image of the first hindrance. Our habitual entanglement with our painful experiences, irritants in the sensory field such as coldness or itching, and anything generally unpleasant to us is a persistent and formidable distraction. In these first two hindrances, we can see how our attachment to having what we want to have and to getting rid of what we do not want both conspire to draw us out of direct engagement with the present moment and into an immersion in the verbal stories our minds continually weave.

The therapist can work with these two hindrances quite simply, by anticipating the pull of sense experiences and by discussing this with patients directly. The therapist should explain to patients that both pleasant and unpleasant inner experiences might arise during mindfulness training, and that both can be met with bare attention and a return of attention to observation of each individual moment.

The third hindrance to meditation practice is described as anxiety and restlessness. This represents the fidgetiness and psychomotor agitation that can emerge when we direct our intention to simply keep our physical bodies relatively still for a few minutes. In this hindrance, we can see the effect of the years of our learning history on the mind and body. The activation of our threat perception processes, neurophysiological arousal, or even simple worrying is bound through years of classical and instrumental conditioning to provoke a response. Mindfulness training gives us an opportunity to notice and to take action to change these habitual patterns. The therapist can elicit the patient's thoughts and feelings about how he or she would typically respond to feelings of agitation. Together, the patient and the therapist can practice directly staying in the presence of anxious agitation in session, remaining mindful throughout the process, with eyes open and in the midst of the discussion.

The fourth hindrance is known as sloth or torpor. It represents a low level of energy, a state of exhaustion, and a general slowness of responding. This hindrance may manifest itself as "lazy" avoidance, as procrastination, or as the anhedonic and vegetative symptoms that so often accompany depression. The mindfulness practitioner may simply be tired or have overeaten when sloth arises, but this may, indeed, be the result of depression or an aversion to fully experiencing some unprocessed emotions. Scheduling and commitment to practice even in the face of an urge to procrastinate, can be clearly prescribed by the therapist in response to this hindrance.

The fifth hindrance is described as doubt or indecision. Part of this might be related to a discomfort with uncertainty, which is characteristic of people with generalized anxiety disorder. This doubt may also involve self-doubt, arising from a negative belief about one's own capacities and strengths. Such negative self-evaluations are common among patients presenting for psychotherapy. Part of the aim of mindfulness training involves patients' gradual acknowledgment of such doubts as part of the flowing landscape of the mind. Patients apply mindful awareness to see thoughts as thoughts, emotions as emotions, and physical sensations as physical sensations, without surrendering the control of their behavior to the stream of emerging private events that continuously presents itself in the mind.

In the 3-minute breathing space, we can see an example of applied mindfulness in action. Accordingly, we can notice how each of the five hindrances present themselves naturalistically, as patients attempt to weave a mindful perspective into the fabric of their lives. Training a person in the use of the 3-minute breathing space provides an opportunity for the validation and normalization of obstacles as an inevitable part of a developing mindfulness practice. None of us are immune to the influence of these five hindrances. Indeed, each person who pursues a course of training in mindful awareness must gradually and repeatedly come face to face with such obstacles. It is exactly this tension, our persistent encounter with the contents of our consciousness, that trains us to bring a kind and engaged awareness to bear upon our experience in and of this present moment.

Cross-Reference to Other Techniques

The 3-minute breathing space is related to the following: the body scan, mindfulness of the breath, mindful awareness of the movement, the making space exercise, mindfulness of sound, 3-minute coping breathing space, and mindful cooking a swell as completion of the Emotionally Intelligent Thought Record and the "Stopping the War" Record.

Form

Form 5.1: Daily Mindfulness Practice Record[4]

TECHNIQUE: 3-MINUTE COPING BREATHING SPACE

Description

The foundation prepared by the practice of the body scan and mindfulness of the breath practice opens the way for subsequent formal exercises, which direct the attention to thoughts and feelings themselves, such as the making space exercise. Similarly, longer periods of formal practice may prepare patients to bring mindful awareness to bear on their experiences as they happen in their everyday lives. The next step in the generalization and application of mindfulness skills in MBCT involves deploying a mindful attentional stance during actual periods of distress. The 3-minute breathing space exercise provides patients with a sufficiently structured, yet "user-friendly," approach to employing mindfulness in a direct fashion, for the purposes of affect tolerance, dealing with distressing situations, and coping with things that may seem overwhelming.

When the 3-minute breathing space is used as a coping tool, patients are encouraged to apply the breathing space exercise at times when they are naturally responding, in the moment, to difficult emotions and thoughts that may arise in response to stress in the environment. As with the previous breathing space exercise, this breathing space practice also begins with a focus on sensations in the body that arrive with strong feelings or troubling thoughts. However, during the 3-minute coping breathing space, patients are encouraged to consciously adopt an extended sense of willingness and contact with the experience, as it is felt in the body in the present moment. This means that rather than a bare, distant observation, patients are "saying

---

[4]The flowing and "applied" nature of this mindfulness training technique might suggest that patients do not always need to be monitoring their implementation of the 3-minute breathing space.

yes" to their experience and establishing an intimate connection with the flow of their experience. Although this sort of nonjudgmental observation may seem like a form of distancing, in this case it paradoxically involves an immersion in direct experience that is qualitatively different from how sensation, emotion, and thought may be processed when patients are in their "automatic pilot" mode of everyday attention. The instructions for the 3-minute coping breathing space extend this concept of willingness and openness to experience and encourage patients to deliberately and consciously say to themselves that, whatever the feelings and thoughts that may arrive, "it's OK to feel this way" and "It's OK, whatever it is, it's OK. Let me feel it" (Segal et al., 2002).

Question to Pose/Intervention

When the therapist begins to train a patient in the direct application of the 3-minute coping breathing space to adaptive coping, he or she should be prepared for potential misunderstanding of the aim of the exercise. The tendency to engage in experiential avoidance is persistent and will continue to make itself known throughout the course of mindfulness training. In providing a 3-minute coping breathing space, the therapist is actively suggesting that the patient "do" something to affect his or her state under conditions of difficulty. This can easily be misinterpreted by the patient, because it might seem to suggest that the patient is using this mindfulness exercise to push away "bad" experiences. One way that a therapist may be able to better anticipate and address this central tendency is to mindfully attend to his or her own process while introducing and explaining the coping breathing space technique. By bringing some degree of cultivated mindful awareness to the therapeutic relationship during such an exchange, the therapist may be better able to model, instruct, and reinforce a softening around troubling private experiences. The therapist may choose to ask questions such as, "Can you just make space for and allow this experience as it unfolds before you in this moment?" Although such questions may not involve the direct first-order change of cognitive content that cognitive-behavioral therapists have become accustomed to over the past two decades, they do provide an alternative perspective, a decentering, and a potential refuge from attached immersion in unpleasant internal experiences.

Example[5]

This next exercise is meant to be applied when you are facing difficult feelings or emotions. When historically unpleasant emotions, bodily sensations, and thoughts emerge in our awareness, our first instinct may be to try to escape or suppress these experiences. For this exercise, this 3-minute-long practice of creating space through awareness of the breath and the body, we are going to practice a radical willingness to connect with our experience, just as it is, in this very moment. So, as we begin, bring part of your awareness to the soles of your feet. As much as you can, allow your attention to collect around your physical experience in this moment. If it is possible, allow yourself to sit down in a comfortable place. Allow yourself to make any adjustments to your seated posture that may be necessary so that you might sit with a dignified, erect,

---

[5]This exercise is adapted from the MBCT protocol (Segal et al., 2002). Copyright 2002 by The Guilford Press. Adapted by permission.

yet relaxed demeanor. The back is straight. You can feel yourself rooted to the earth at the con-
tact points where your body meets your chair and the floor. Allow your eyes to close or, if you
prefer, just allow the eyelids to relax as you cast your gaze gently at the floor before you. Next,
bring attention to the flow of experience that unfolds before your mind. Observing thoughts,
feelings, and physical sensations, allow yourself to notice, as much as you can, what is present-
ing itself in this very moment. We are now paying particular attention to those feelings, ideas,
and sensations that may be experienced as unpleasant or upsetting. Rather than pushing these
experiences away, we are allowing them to be just as they are. Taking a moment, allow yourself
to simply acknowledge the presence of these experiences, making space for whatever emerges
*and flows through your field of inner observation. Allow yourself to **describe and acknowledge***
the difficult experiences that may be arriving. For a moment, allow yourself to put these experi-
ences into words, noting them as mental events—for example, "I am having the thought that I
am unloved" or "I am feeling frustration and jealousy." In this way, we are again making space,
as best we can, for whatever arises, making intimate contact with this very moment, moment
by moment. Next, allow yourself to gently yet decidedly redirect your attention to the act of
breathing. Breathing in, we know that we are breathing in; breathing out, we know that we are
breathing out. For the next minute, allow your awareness to follow the breath as it enters the
body through the nostrils, moves through the core of the body, and leaves through our out-
breath, observing the depth and fullness of each breath, in this very moment. Watching as the
breath breathes itself, as it completes and begins a new cycle, we continue to simply make space
for our experience, just as it is.

During this next minute of our practice, allow your awareness to expand. With the next
available in-breath, allow your attention to encompass the body as a whole. In this moment,
we are paying particular attention to any sensations in the body that involve discomfort or
unnecessary tension. Rather than turning away from these experiences, you are blending your
attention with the flow of the breath. Allow yourself to "breathe into" this experience. With the
next natural out-breath, allow yourself to soften and open to these sensations. Breathing out,
you continue to make space for whatever arises in the flow of your experience. Say to yourself,
"This is OK. Whatever it is, it is OK to experience it. Let me feel this." Bring part of your aware-
ness to the muscles of the face. Without judging, notice how the expression and position of your
face and body are related to this unfolding stream of thinking and feeling.

As you prepare to let this exercise go, bring part of your attention to the soles of the feet.
Next, bring part of your attention to the top of the head. Now, notice again, for this moment,
everything in between, including thoughts, feelings, and bodily sensations. As you exhale, allow
your eyes to open, and consciously let go of this exercise. Take a moment to acknowledge your
capacity for choice and willingness. You have just decided to allow yourself these 3 minutes of
fully being with your experience, moment by moment. As best as you can, bring this openness
and mindful awareness with you throughout your day.

Homework

The 3-minute coping breathing space may be assigned as a homework exercise, but it is best
applied in a flexible and responsive way. This practice aims at deploying mindfulness and acceptance as a mode of "responding" rather than "reacting to" stressors in the environment. As such,
patients may wish to rehearse this exercise sufficiently, so that they feel comfortable engaging

with the exercise under conditions of some stress. From this point, patients may choose to wait until they are in active need of coping resources to actually begin this technique.

Possible Problems

Many of the potential problems that apply to other mindfulness techniques will also apply to the 3-minute coping breathing space. There are some unique points about this exercise as well, however. Patients might not actually apply this exercise in the presence of stress or difficult emotions. As we know, people often have habitual patterns of responding when faced with stress. Choosing to adopt a new approach *in vivo* can be daunting and elusive. In addition, the 3-minute coping breathing space is a method of responding that involves letting go of avoidance in the moment. Rather than choosing a coping method that takes them farther away from a challenging emotional response, patients are actually choosing to make space for and to approach disturbing feelings and thoughts. This requires a leap of willingness on their part. Having some grounding in prior mindfulness training can help facilitate this leap. It may also be useful for the therapist to openly discuss possible resistance and apprehension that patients may feel in deploying the 3-minute breathing space. The therapist and his or her patients may even choose to brainstorm potential obstacles to using the technique and find methods to address them. For example, patients can discuss situations in which they might feel reluctant to apply the technique, such as social situations or places that feel potentially embarrassing. The therapist and his or her patients might consider ways in which patients could briefly excuse themselves for a few minutes in order to center themselves and apply this technique as an active coping mechanism.

Cross-Reference to Other Techniques

The 3-minute coping breathing space is related to the following techniques: the body scan, mindfulness of the breath, mindful awareness of movement, the making space exercise, mindfulness of sound, 3-minute breathing space, and mindful cooking as well as completion of the Emotionally Intelligent Thought Record and the "Stopping the War" Record.

Form

Form 5.1: Daily Mindfulness Practice Record[6]

TECHNIQUE: MINDFUL AWARENESS OF MOVEMENT

Description

As the therapist and the patient endeavor to gradually transfer the facility for mindful awareness from the context of a meditation exercise to the context of everyday activity, mindful movement, specifically mindful walking, is a common exercise. This practice is part of classical Buddhist meditation traditions such as Zen, in which a similar, slow-moving walking exercise is know as

---

[6]The flowing and "applied" nature of this mindfulness training technique might suggest that patients do not always need to be monitoring their implementation of the 3-minute coping breathing space.

kinhin. In this exercise, the patient is learning to bring the quality of mindfulness, particularly the connection to physical sensation, moment by moment, into the act of moving through space and time as he or she walks. It is a deceptively simple exercise that can be experienced as very rich by practitioners. This exercise also has the benefit of being easily adaptable and practiced throughout the day, whenever the patient has the opportunity to put one foot in front of the other in a safe context.

Question to Pose/Intervention

"What physical sensations did you notice during the practice of mindful walking? What thoughts and feelings did you notice while you engaged in mindful movement? In what way was the quality of your attention different during this mindful walking experience compared with your everyday awareness? What did you notice about the speed of your walking? What did you notice about the rhythm of your walking? How might this practice help you to come into a more healthy relationship with your emotions?"

Example

As we have learned, mindfulness is more than just a technique that we use to address our problems. It is a natural, human state of being that can allow us to more fully experience the richness of the present moment. As such, our aim is to gradually carry this state of mindful acceptance into our everyday lives. We begin with specific practices lying or sitting, and then transition toward taking mindful actions. A good place to begin is with the simple act of walking. This practice of mindful awareness of walking can take place either inside or outside. Find a place where you may walk for some time with relatively little concern for onlookers or interruptions. You may choose a park, a city block, or even a path through the rooms of your home. Begin standing with your feet slightly less than shoulders-width apart. Keep your knees supple, while supporting your body weight fully. Your back should remain straight, with your arms hanging relaxed from your shoulders. As you gaze forward, allow your eyes to have a "wide-angle" focus, taking in your entire visual field. Your head should be resting nobly on the top of your spine, freeing the neck from the tension of muscle control. As you inhale, collect your attention at the base of your feet. Allow yourself to sense the connection between your feet and the ground. With each inhalation, allow your attention to observe the presence of life in the legs and the feet, feeling the distribution of your weight throughout the support of your body. As in earlier exercises, with each exhalation, let go of attachment to this awareness. After some time experiencing this, allow your weight to transfer to the right leg, taking note of all the richness of the sensations involved. Next, allow yourself to draw your attention to the left leg. You may experience a sensation of the leg lightening or "emptying" as you rely upon it less for support. Allow your attention to be divided between the legs, noticing the different sensations present throughout your lower body. When you are ready, allow the left foot to slightly rise from the floor. Notice the sensations in the muscles and tissue of the leg as it lifts and gently moves forward to take a first step. Gradually and deliberately, move the left leg forward, all the while gently observing the physical sensations that accompany this action. As you complete this first step, notice the sensations involved as you place the left foot back on the floor. Feel the weight transfer to this foot and leg, as your body uses it for support and its contact with the ground grows heavier and more present. As this occurs, notice whatever sensations emerge in the right leg and foot, as it lets go of the weight and support, growing lighter as the movement continues. As your weight is transferred to the left foot in a stable fashion, repeat this process with the right foot. Breathe into the sensation of the right foot leaving the floor. Observe the presence of life in the body as the right foot moves forward to take your next step. Again, notice the physical sensations as this right foot makes contact with the ground, and you complete this next step. As you do this, allow your motion to flow from one step to the next rather than complete these steps as discrete, robotic movements. Notice how your intention guides your body, drawing it forward slowly in space and time. Your movements may be similar to a Tai Chi Chuan practitioner, as they slowly yet smoothly move through their series of exercises. Continue to take these steps in this fashion, continuing along the path that you have chosen. As you do this, some of your attention remains connected to the flow of the breath and the spreading sensations throughout the body. As you walk, connect your attention to the presence of life throughout the body, noticing any sensations that present themselves with an attitude of kind and gentle acceptance. Your gaze will be held softly focused ahead of you, aware of the surroundings but also persistently aware of your presence in your body. As with our earlier practices, the mind will inevitably wander from the attention to the act of walking. Whenever this occurs, take note of where the mind is at that moment and kindly direct the attention back to the act of walking. It may be useful to use the sensation of your feet on the ground or the relaxed straightness of your spine as focal points to draw your attention back to the physical sensations that emerge moment by moment. The pace of your walk should be moderately slow but reasonably comfortable. You may wish to begin the exercise at a slow and gradual pace, almost as an "invitation" to your present-moment awareness. In time you may find yourself walking at a more "normal" pace. Note any tendency to speed up excessively as you would notice any distraction in your mindfulness practice, and gradually allow yourself to return your attention to the physical sensations of walking, anchoring your awareness through your in-breath and physical contact with the ground. This exercise can take place over a 15- to 20-minute span. After working with this exercise for a few days or weeks, you might choose to bring this quality of awareness to other activities, making the transition to applied mindful awareness. In this way, we might have the experience of connection with our observing self as we face our everyday lives.

Homework

This exercise may be assigned as structured homework, to be practiced at regular intervals. It also may be assigned as a relatively spontaneous exercise, to be engaged in during the course of the patient's everyday life.

Possible Problems

Obviously, the range of problems and obstacles that are present for the preceding exercises also apply to the practice of mindful movement. It is particularly important that the therapist practice and demonstrate mindful walking with patients in session. Small offices and the convention of remaining seated during the session might lead some therapists to be reluctant to do this, but it is very important. Patients might engage in mindful movement too rapidly or might claim that they understand the concept without actually having the experience. Also, the therapist and his or her patients may need to solve logistical problems, for example, determining locations and times for engaging in this activity. Privacy and space may be a concern. Patients might not feel comfortable publicly engaging in slow, unusual movements. Places in nature or safe, open spaces that are not too crowded might be suggested. Problem solving the logistics of mindful movement might seem banal or obvious to a therapist, but it can make the difference in whether or not patients comply with homework and overcome resistance to procedure. We advise the therapist to engage in this discussion with patients in as mindful, patient, and present a fashion as possible. In this way, the context of mindfulness that is established in the session can be transferred to the actual practice of mindful movement.

Cross-Reference to Other Techniques

Mindful awareness of movement is directly related to the following: mindfulness of the breath, the making space exercise, mindfulness of sound, 3-minute breathing space, 3-minute coping breathing space, and Mindful Cooking as well as completion of the Emotionally Intelligent Thought Record and the "Stopping The War" Record.

Form

Form 5.1: Daily Mindfulness Practice Record

TECHNIQUE: MINDFUL COOKING

Description

The quality of mindful attention can be brought to almost any activity. The characteristics of mindfulness, such as nonjudgment, contact with the present moment, and the ability to experience mental events as a process unfolding before an observer, may create a more vivid or connected experience throughout the chosen activity. Beyond this phenomenological dimension, consciously bringing mindful awareness to activities of daily living provides patients with myriad opportunities to practice enhancing their capacity for emotion regulation, as they engage in their necessary, and often habitual, behaviors. Cooking is an aspect of our lives that is often overlooked, as our culture propels us to a hurried existence, which often relies upon fast food or, at the very least, meals at home that are prepared in an expeditious fashion. To slow ourselves down and engage with the behaviors that are essential for our nurturance and physical being is to recognize with great care and attention the intimate connection we have with our environment. The following exercise provides a relatively simple example in the preparation of tea. Tea has a special place in Zen tradition: The tea ceremony has a long and revered history as an art form and mindfulness practice in Japan. Our example in this text extends the preparation of tea to the drinking of the tea. In doing so, this mindfulness practice guides patients through the process of transformation of food, through conceptualization, preparation, and consumption. Again, this exercise is meant as a form of "generalization practice" as well as a form of mindfulness training in itself.

Question to Pose/Intervention

"What did you notice about the preparation of tea that you would not have noticed before? What did you notice in terms of the five senses? What thoughts, emotions, and bodily experiences presented during this practice? How was this experience different from the way you might normally prepare or consume food or drink? How might this experience relate to cultivating a healthy relationship with your emotions?"

Example[7]

Our first mindful cooking exercise can involve any kind of food preparation, but it is best to begin with something very small, with explicit directions. The example we use here is the simple preparation of tea. Before you begin this exercise, make sure you are working in a clean space, preferably free from clutter. You may wish to have a chair or stool near the stove. You will need a pot to fill with water for boiling. You will also need a teacup or mug, a teabag or a tea leaf strainer, and maybe a saucer. Please be careful as you engage in the steps of this exercise, because you will be working with a stove and hot water. The potential danger in using fire and/ or an electric heating element as well as boiling water can be seen as a reminder that we are not seeking to "zone out" or go into some sort of trance when practicing mindful awareness. On the contrary, we are actually aiming more to "fall awake" and to be fully alert and present to what is happening in the field of our attention. Place the pot, the tea, and anything else you might need to make a pot of tea on the stove. If possible, take your seat on the stool or chair beside the stove. With your eyes open, bring part of your attention to whatever physical sensations present themselves to you in this moment. Begin to allow your awareness to follow the flow of your breathing. Observe the flow of the breath, as it moves in and out of the body. With a "light touch" in "the back of your mind," allow part of your awareness to follow the breath by silently saying "Breathing in, I know that I'm breathing in" as you inhale and "Breathing out, I know that I am breathing out" as you exhale. Continue this for a few cycles of breath. Next, bring part of your attention to the body. As you breathe in, allow yourself to "breathe attention" into the body as a whole. Keep your eyes open as you do this. Our aim at this point is to simply observe whatever is present, not to change anything, relax anything, or analyze anything at all. If relaxation arrives, that is perfectly acceptable. You can treat it like a trusted guest who has dropped by on a winter night.

Relaxation is welcome, but creating it isn't our aim. After a very few minutes, get up from the chair. As best as you can, keep alive some of the gathered mindful awareness that you have just tuned into, as you carefully fill the pot with water and place it on your stove. Feel the handle of the pot in your hand. What does it feel like? What is its texture? What is its temperature? How heavy is the pot, both before and after you have filled it with water? What sounds do you hear in front of you? Behind you? Above you? Can you hold part of your attention in the feet and feel the weight of the body as you do this? Allow yourself to turn on the heat and

---

[7]The following directions are adapted from several sources, notably the guided meditations of Jon Kabat-Zinn (1990). A portion of the tea preparation instruction is adapted from an exercise by Steven Hayes (Hayes & Smith, 2005). Some additional ideas and phrases are also adapted from the writings of Thich Nat Hanh (1992) and other clinical meditation sources.

boil the water. As you are waiting for the water to boil, what is going through your mind? As each new thought, image, or emotion enters your awareness, mindfully and patiently observe it, moment by moment. When does this thought begin? When does it end? Can you notice the space between your thoughts? What is the quality of this waiting? Soon you will notice the water is boiling. When it boils and you become aware that it is time to turn off the heat and pour the water into the tea, what do you notice in your body? How do you experience this motivation toward action in your physical being? In your thoughts? In your emotions? Remove the tea from the heat, turn off the stove, and then pour the hot water into your cup. Add the teabag or strainer. Watch the water as it begins to change. Notice the shade and color of the water as it darkens into tea. Observe the changes. In a few minutes the tea will be ready. Remove the teabag or strainer and place it aside. What do you now notice about the color of the tea? Bring your hands to the cup. Notice the warmth of the cup. Notice the texture of the surface of the cup. Notice how your body responds in this moment to touching the cup. How is this experience of a cup of tea different? Prepare to take a sip by bringing the cup to your lips. Notice any steam before your face. Blow across the surface of the tea and notice what happens. Smell the tea. Take a sip. What is the taste? What is the texture in your mouth? What is the temperature of the tea? What images come to mind as you sip the tea? Take a moment to recognize the stream of associations that present themselves before you in this simple act of having a cup of tea. When you are ready to leave this exercise, place the cup down, make a decision to let go of the formal practice of mindfully drinking a cup of tea, and allow yourself to exhale. As you exhale, let go of the exercise entirely. Now that the exercise is complete, give yourself credit for bringing a bit more presence into your everyday experience. See if you can carry some of this presence with you as you go about your day.

Homework

Unlike many of the previous exercises, the mindful cooking exercise is meant more as an example of how mindfulness can be brought into activities rather than a regular practice. After engaging in this practice as an example, patients may seek to apply their further mindfulness training to activities such as cooking, checking e-mail, and housekeeping, for example. Nevertheless, these activities do not necessarily need to be engaged in from a formal or guided perspective.

Possible Problems

As we present this exercise at this point in our text, you can probably infer the range of potential obstacles that patients may encounter as they engage in applied mindfulness. Please refer to the Possible Problems section of each technique included in this chapter if you are unclear about what challenges might lie ahead. One particular caveat is worth mentioning: Mindful cooking will require deliberate attention to safety when working with heat and kitchen tools. The therapist should remind patients of this. As we have seen, mindfulness involves "falling awake" rather than sinking into a trance, and cooking with an attention to the present moment should embody this principle, with attention to the necessary details of the activity.

Cross-Reference to Other Techniques

Mindful cooking is directly related to the following: mindfulness of the breath, mindful awareness of movement, the making space exercise, mindfulness of sound, 3-minute breathing space, and 3-minute coping breathing space as well as completion of the Emotionally Intelligent Thought Record and the "Stopping The War" Record.

Form

Form 5.1: Daily Mindfulness Practice Record

CONCLUSIONS

Mindfulness training has emerged as a very important and increasingly popular element of many variations of CBT. In order to implement mindfulness-based techniques effectively, the therapist should establish a very clear conceptual understanding of what mindfulness means. Mindfulness is a mode of paying attention in the present moment in a state of patient willingness. This attentional stance can be learned by a specific series of exercises and can lead to an augmentation of the patient's capacity in regulating his or her emotions.

In order to use mindfulness-based techniques, the therapist must ground him- or herself in an established mindfulness practice. Mindfulness training is far less about amassing information than it is about developing facility in an experiential technique. This involves the conscious deployment of attention and the activation of a range of functions throughout the central nervous system, breath, and body. In time, this mode of attention can be applied in the course of everyday activities and can be present throughout much of the patient's life.

Patients may see the practices involved in mindfulness training as mediation, and, in fact, much of what has been presented has been adapted from traditions that might be called "meditation" practice. However, the term "meditation," although somewhat accurate, may have cultural baggage and associations that are inaccurate or misleading for many therapists and patients. Mindfulness training can be presented as a simple method of training the mind in a flexible, acceptable, and adaptive mode of attention. This training can help patients to better manage stress, to reduce the impact of anxiety, and to tolerate difficult emotional states.

Mindfulness can serve as the metaphorical "mortar" between many of the other "bricks" provided in the techniques presented in this book. For example, adopting a mindful mode of attention may help patients to identify and distance themselves from maladaptive emotional schemas. Mindfulness might facilitate the growth of self-compassion or willingness to tolerate distress. As such, mindfulness is a compatible complement to much of our work in emotion regulation.

CHAPTER SIX

Acceptance and Willingness

Few of us would dispute that it is important to reject harmful or dangerous situations and to seek safety, survival, and even comfort. For example, if I see a bus coming straight at me, I get out of the way. When I notice that the food I am about to eat smells bad, I choose to throw it out rather than poison myself. Natural selection has ensured that we have inherited a tendency to avoid things that are bad for us. However, the tendency to avoid the unpleasant can become overgeneralized and rigid, resulting in difficulties when we are faced with events or aspects of life that we cannot change or avoid (Hayes, Luoma, Bond, Masuda, & Lillis, 2006).

Attempts to avoid unpleasant thoughts and emotions can sometimes cause us to experience them more frequently or more intensely (Purdon & Clark, 1999; Wegner et al., 1987; Wenzlaff & Wegner, 2000). We might strive to push away unwanted feelings and ideas, only to find them popping up again and again. When we experience emotionally challenging thoughts and feelings, we sometimes respond to them as though they were literally true or real (Hayes et al., 2001). For example, if I have the thought, "Nobody would ever want to spend time with me," I might literalize this and experience it as though it were a fact. Accordingly, my behavioral options might become narrower, as I isolate and limit the possibilities in my life. This chain of events can unfold such that experiential avoidance stands in the way of living a meaningful and purposeful life.

Experiential acceptance, often described as "willingness," offers an alternative way of relating to private experiences. Acceptance-based processes "involve taking an intentionally open, receptive, and nonjudgmental posture with respect to various aspects of experience" (K. G. Wilson & DuFrene, 2009, p. 46). This willingness to make direct contact with difficult experiences is not undertaken as an end in itself. Willingness represents a choice to fully experience even the most difficult internal events, in the service of a pursuit of our valued directions in life.

In this context, acceptance or willingness does not mean endorsing or seeking out unpleasant experiences. We do not suggest that a person should force him- or herself to enjoy, desire, or embrace the pain and struggle of life. When we ground ourselves in reality, we are forced to admit that life involves a certain degree of pain and suffering. This inherent suffering can arrive in the form of difficult private experiences or even as unwanted real-world events that are beyond our ability to change or control. Willingness does not mean "giving up" in the face of these sources of pain. By adopting an attitude of radical acceptance, a person is recognizing the reality of his or her situation and the inevitability of feeling some sadness and pain in life (Linehan, 1993a).

A variety of therapies have emerged in the last 10 years that emphasize the cultivation of acceptance. Acceptance-based processes are a central feature in ACT (Hayes et al., 1999) and DBT (Linehan, 1993a; see Chapter 4). Other therapies, such as metacognitive therapy (Wells, 2009) and MBCT (Segal et al., 2002), also emphasize accepting and observing mental events for what they are. Older forms of cognitive-behavioral therapy (CBT) have also maintained an emphasis on accepting difficult feelings in the pursuit of important goals. For example, exposure techniques all involve the patient willingly experiencing challenging states of anxiety in order to overcome phobias and other forms of anxiety (Barlow, 2002; Marks, 1987). Cognitive therapy (CT) also encourages the patient to cease thought suppression and to move toward difficult emotions, particularly in the treatment of anxiety disorders (Clark & Beck, 2009).

There are some differences, however, in how and why acceptance is pursued. Third-generation CBT methods tend to use experiential and mindfulness-based methods in the gradual cultivation of willingness rather than traditional, straightforward behavioral exposure. Similarly, although CT or metacognitive therapy might address willingness by actively restructuring a patient's beliefs about the advantages of acceptance, ACT or DBT practitioners would be more likely to engage the patient in exercises that encourage willingness to emerge in the presence of challenging private events. Within the ACT paradigm, willingness is not pursued in the service of symptom reduction or in the service of directly changing thoughts and feelings. The aim of willingness for the ACT therapist is, ultimately, for the patient "to feel all of the feelings that come up for you more completely, even the 'bad' feelings, so that you can live your life more completely" (Hayes & Smith, 2005, p. 45).

The techniques described in this chapter involve the patient gradually coming to understand the value of adopting a stance of willingness or radical acceptance in living a full life as well as in adopting more effective emotion regulation strategies. These techniques have an obvious connection to mindfulness practices. Both mindfulness and acceptance involve a shift in perspective concerning the contents of one's consciousness (see Chapter 5). Accordingly, some of the techniques presented here involve a deliberate and purposeful deliteralization of internal events. Acceptance and mindfulness can also both be seen as involving an inherent compassion for oneself. There are qualities of "noncondemning" and self-validation that emerge when we are willing to stay with our experience moment by moment. These qualities are intimately connected to the emergence of a compassionate mind.

EST is related to the ACT model of psychological functioning and psychotherapy processes (Hayes et al., 1999; K. G. Wilson & Dufrene, 2009) in that its aim is to cultivate a psychologically flexible, adaptive, and responsive broadening of the patient's behavioral repertoire in the presence of distressing emotional experiences. EST also endorses pursuing therapeutic movement in the core processes involved in psychological flexibility in the current ACT model, these being contact with the present moment; willingness to experience private experiences fully; defusion, or deliteralization of cognitive content; the capacity to experience the self as an observer; authorship of valued directions; and committed action in the pursuit of valued aims (K. G. Wilson & DuFrene, 2009). For these reasons, techniques, concepts, and processes that have emerged from the ACT tradition are amenable to integration with an EST approach to emotion regulation.

TECHNIQUE: INTRODUCING WHAT WE MEAN BY "ACCEPTANCE"

Description

There are many psychotherapeutic inroads that a clinician may use to begin work with acceptance. Some involve experiential exercises and some are more informational. The word "acceptance" has a few meanings in the English language. Also, many of our patients are firmly entrenched in strategies that involve experiential avoidance. As a result, a psychotherapist who plans to use methods based in acceptance and willingness may need to begin by simply teaching patients what acceptance means in this context.

There are several steps involved in the process of developing willingness. These include helping patients to be aware of the many ways they use avoidance or control-based strategies, exploring and questioning how useful or workable these strategies have been for them, and validating patients' experience of frustration or sadness in the face of strategies that have not yet released them from their struggle (Luoma et al., 2007).

Question to Pose/Intervention

"How long have you been experiencing difficult or painful emotions? Can you remember a time before you were facing any of the difficult private experiences that you are facing today? What are you struggling against? What have you had to give up because of your struggle? Who taught you that you could make 'bad' feelings just go away by fighting against them? How have you tried to get rid of your feelings? How has that worked out for you? Can you remember a time when you just let yourself feel a feeling for what it was? Do you ever remember taking a step back from thoughts that were entangling you? What was it like to stop fighting against your experience and just observe your mind as it did what minds do? What do you think it would be like to drop your struggle against your experience and pour your energy into pursuing the valued directions that matter most to you in your life?"

Example

Patient: It's kind of like I've been depressed for as long as I can remember. It feels as though this sense that I'm just not good enough has been with me forever.

Therapist: It certainly does sound like you've been carrying this for a long time. Can you remember a time before you felt so inadequate?

Patient: I think probably when I was about 4 or 5—just before I went to school. I think that back then I didn't really have any sense of whether or not I was good enough.

Therapist: So for the last three decades or so you've been telling yourself that you're not good enough. You have had this persistent sense, this sad feeling, that there was just something wrong with you?

Patient: Yes. It is always with me, I think.

Therapist: Have you tried to fight this thought, this feeling? I mean, how have you tried to deal with this idea popping into your mind?

Patient: I wish I didn't feel this way, but I do. Oh, I've fought it in lots of ways. I drove myself to be a straight-A student, even when it meant that I kept away from having a life. I would keep myself isolated at school or at work so that I wouldn't face the rejection. I've read all sorts of self-help books. I've been on Zoloft since God knows when. Sometimes, when I'm home alone and can't sleep, I can put away a bottle of wine and just cry myself to sleep.

Therapist: That really sounds like an exhausting struggle. How have these methods worked so far?

Patient: Clearly, they haven't. Nothing stops it.

Therapist: Yes, you've told me how persistent this is, this sense that "I'm not good enough." It must be really frustrating to face these thoughts and feelings that just won't stop.

Patient: Sometimes I just can't stand it.

Therapist: I'm sure there are lots of other ways that you've tried to struggle against this sense that you just aren't good enough, and as we go, I want to notice them so that we can see just how hard you've been working to stop having this thought "I'm not good enough."

Patient: OK.

Therapist: What do you think would happen if you gave up this struggle?

Patient: You mean just stay depressed? That sounds awful.

Therapist: That's not what I mean exactly. I know that overcoming depression is important to you. I mean, what if you stopped struggling against the idea that your mind is going to keep causing this thought, "I'm not good enough," to pop into your head? What might happen if you allowed yourself to be willing to hear your mind tell you that thought, as you put your energy and heart into pursuing a life that really mattered to you?

Patient: I'm not sure what that would be like. Why would I do that?

Therapist: Well, for a very long time, your mind has learned to respond with these words "I'm not good enough" when you deal with things in your environment. You've tried so many things to stop having that thought, to avoid it, to control it, but it pops up again and again. That is how thinking and feeling work sometimes: The more we try to push certain experiences away, the more they show up again and again.

Patient: Yes, I think I know what you're talking about.

Therapist: So, if we found out that you could really engage deeply with the things in your life that bring you joy and meaning, but the price of that engagement would be your hearing your mind tell you that you "weren't good enough," might you be willing to accept those words as events in your mind and go about the business of living your life?

Patient: Well, yes, I suppose ... if it meant I could get my life back ... maybe have a life really for the first time ever, then I would be willing. How do I do that?

Homework

There are many ways that willingness and acceptance can be practiced for homework. We might begin by assigning a simple, daily self-monitoring task so that patients might notice when they are and are not adopting a stance of willingness to experience just what arrives in the present moment, without needless defense. This exercise, using Form 6.1, is adapted from a number of similar ACT self-monitoring forms, particularly the Willingness, Depression, and Vitality Diary (Robinson & Strosahl, 2008). This assignment involves patients committing to spend a week deliberately engaging as fully as they can in behaviors that are meaningful to them, that are rewarding in some intrinsic way, and that may even build their sense of mastery in life, a form of behavioral activation (Martell, Addis, & Jacobson, 2001). They are also committing to willingly accept and observe whatever thoughts and feelings arrive as they go through the week. Each day, patients rate their experience across three dimensions, using a 1–10 scale. The first dimension is the degree of willingness that is experienced throughout the day. The second dimension is the amount of distress that is experienced while willingly engaging in valued behaviors. The third, and final, dimension is the degree of engagement experienced each day. For our purposes, engagement represents a blend of how rewarding patients found their daily activities, how purposeful and rich in meaning they found their daily lives, and how much their daily activities enhanced their sense of personal mastery.

Possible Problems

Many patients have come to therapy because they are experiencing particularly difficult states of anxiety and depression. There may be some initial resistance to adopting an attitude that accepts emotional experiences just as they are, without overt efforts at creating new mood states. In order to address this, the therapist can take time to explore with their patients the costs and benefits of experiential avoidance. One way this can be done is by exploring patients' entire history of attempts at using avoidance as a coping strategy. Typically, both patients and their therapist will discover that years of experiential avoidance actually brought about more harm than good. This exercise may be useful for the therapist to do for him- or herself to establish a direct sense of how experiential avoidance affects people's lives.

Although mindfulness and acceptance-based therapies are not pursuing direct change of thoughts and feelings, numerous studies have demonstrated that such methods actually can result in a reduction of the symptoms of anxiety and mood disorders (Bond & Bunce, 2000; Forman, Herbert, Moitra, Yeomans, & Geller, 2007; Hayes et al., 2004; Zettle & Hayes, 1987). It can be useful to discuss this effect of willingness with the patient. However, willingness to experience an emotion just so it will go way is not "real" willingness. Real willingness requires a commitment to open oneself to whatever emerges in the field of one's consciousness, fully and without unnecessary defense.

Cross-Reference to Other Techniques

Introducing what we mean by "acceptance" is directly related to techniques involving defusion, mindfulness, and the Emotionally Intelligent Thought Record.

Form

Form 6.1: Willingness Journal

TECHNIQUE: DEFUSION

Description

"Defusion" is a term drawn from the ACT literature that represents a process of "making contact with verbal products as they are, not as what they say they are" (K. G. Wilson & DuFrene, 2009, p. 51). The behavioral term "verbal products" here refers to thoughts and mental events as private verbal behaviors. In practicing defusion, a patient notices his or her thoughts and feelings as mental events rather than as literalized truths or objects in an external reality. Although traditional CT utilizes a decentering approach so that the patient differentiates thoughts, feelings, and facts, the ACT therapist approaches defusion using different techniques.

The dominance of linguistic processing mechanisms over direct human conscious experience can result in a disconnection from moment-to-moment experience and a reification and concretization of imaginary constructs, verbal representations, and transient emotional experiences (Hayes et al., 1999, 2001). As a result, people may all too often spend their time responding to internal events as though they were profoundly threatening or saddening events in the outside world. This literalization of mental representations has been referred to as "cognitive fusion" (Hayes et al., 1999). Thought–action fusion, which involves the belief that thoughts reflect reality or will lead to feared outcomes, has also been proposed in traditional cognitive models of obsessions (Rachman, 1997).

Defusion techniques seek to allow the patient to broaden his or her range of possible behavioral responses in the presence of difficult thoughts and feelings. This shift in the way a mental event exerts an influence on behavior is sometimes referred to as a *transformation of function*. In addressing defusion, the therapist assists the patient in experiencing a greater degree of psychological flexibility. The following examples provide a few simple exercises designed to promote defusion, helping the patient to experience his or her challenging private events without being controlled by them.

Question to Pose/Intervention

"Can you have a thought without having to buy into that thought? Do you need to believe everything that you think? Can you notice the process of thinking as it unfolds before you in the moment rather than identifying with the contents of your thoughts? Can you look *at* your thinking rather than *from* your thoughts?"

Example

The following example is an excerpt from a session that involves the therapist using "milk, milk, milk"—a classic example of defusion that is described in the original ACT text (Hayes et al., 1999).

Therapist: Now, today we've been talking quite a bit about how we might choose to look at our thoughts in a new way, a way in which we are less attached or wrapped up in the content of our thoughts.

Patient: Yes, I think I get what you've been describing, pretty much.

Therapist: I would like us to take a moment to explore this with an exercise right here in the session. Would that be all right?

Patient: Is it a meditation exercise?

Therapist: Not really, this is more of an experiment to see if you can get a taste of this shift in perspective.

Patient: OK, I'm up for it.

Therapist: Very well. If you would, please think of the word *milk* for a few moments. Take as long as you need, and then let me know what comes to mind.

Patient: All right, I'm thinking of milk and I'm thinking of ice cream, which is sort of made from milk. I'm thinking of putting it in my coffee. Oh, I'm thinking of pouring it into cereal, too.

Therapist: That all makes sense, doesn't it? OK. Does anything else come to mind?

Patient: Well, I guess I can imagine what it tastes like. I drink milk sometimes just by itself, a cold glass of milk.

Therapist: So, as you think of the word *milk*, these images, these memories start to show up in your mind?

Patient: Yes, of course.

Therapist: Of course, yes. So, during this next part of the exercise, I would like you to repeat this word, *milk*, over and over again, out loud, and at a rapid pace. Please close your eyes and do this with me when I ask you to, all right?

Patient: OK.

Therapist: Ready, and … begin … [At this point, both the therapist and the patient begin to repeat the word *milk* over and over again. The therapist gradually takes the lead in setting the pace, and they begin to rapidly say "milk, milk, milk …" at an increasing rate. Soon the words seem to trip slightly over themselves and the pace of the words makes them a bit difficult to follow. The volume has increased slightly. This continues until the therapist calmly asks the patient to stop. It has taken about 40 seconds. This cessation of the repetition is followed by a brief silence.] So, now, might you please say the word *milk* just one more time.

Patient: Milk.

Therapist: And when you say this word now, what is different about the experience?

Patient: The word started to sound funny when we were saying it. It didn't seem to mean anything. The ideas that were popping into my head before aren't really there now.

Therapist: Isn't that something? Just a few minutes ago, the word immediately pulled up all of these images and related things, and after less than a minute of repetition, the experience of the word is very different.

Patient: That is weird, but it is different.

Therapist: Next, if it is acceptable, I'd like to try this same technique with a thought that has caused you some trouble or distress this past week. Would that be all right?

Patient: Sure, let's see what happens.

Homework

Defusion is less of a specific psychotherapy technique and more of a central process involved in establishing psychological flexibility, according to the ACT model (K. G. Wilson & DuFrene, 2009). (A similar technique was introduced by Freeston et al., 1997, as a form of thought exposure for obsessive–compulsive disorder.) There are a wide variety of possible defusion exercises that might be assigned as homework; these techniques often use metaphor or visualization of thoughts in a new context as a homework practice. Three examples that can be assigned as homework are included in Form 6.2, with descriptions of the metaphors and techniques employed. The techniques in this form are adapted from a number of ACT sources (Hayes & Smith, 2005; Hayes et al., 1999) and can also be found in various Internet sources (e.g., *www.contextualpsychology.org*).

Possible Problems

In some cases, *defusion* may also be confused with *cognitive restructuring*. Both defusion and cognitive restructuring involve noticing automatic thoughts as they emerge and employ shifting awareness so that thoughts can be examined further. In the case of cognitive restructuring, the aim becomes a direct change of the *content* of the thought, which takes place through logical analysis of the thought's utility and validity. Defusion does not engage with content in the same way. In using a defusion technique, the therapist is not necessarily aiming for any direct change of the thought's content. Defusion aims to allow the patient to observe his or her private events and to relate to them as mental phenomena rather than facts in order to disentangle the patient from the behavioral control that these thoughts exert over him or her. In doing so, the patient may move toward greater flexibility, with the opportunity to take back his or her life. Of course, cognitive content may change along the way, but this change may be construed as "second-order" change and as just a part of a larger process.

The therapist should notice when the discussion with the patient starts to turn toward cognitive disputation rather than defusion. At such times, the therapist can directly discuss the difference between disputing the logic of a thought and recognizing a thought as "just a thought" and not reality. The therapist might engage in a functional analysis of the thought, examining how buying into a particular thought affects the patient. Also, the therapist might directly distinguish between questioning the "helpfulness" of a thought and questioning its "truth."

Cross-Reference to Other Techniques

Defusion is itself a part of mindful awareness, so it is obviously related to the variety of mindfulness techniques illustrated in this text. Defusion is also clearly related to introducing what we mean by "acceptance" and to using metaphors to cultivate willingness and defusion, discussed next.

Form

Form 6.2: Defusion Practices for Everyday Living

TECHNIQUE: USING METAPHORS TO CULTIVATE WILLINGNESS AND DEFUSION

Description

The use of metaphors is a central component of an ACT-consistent approach to therapy. Although a number of therapies, including traditional CBT, may employ metaphors to illustrate a psycho-educational point or to facilitate a shift in perspective, a therapist using ACT-based methods is likely to use metaphors more often and for rather different reasons, as explained next.

ACT is based on a behavioral theory of language and cognition—relational frame theory (RFT; Hayes et al., 2001)—that proposes a behavioral account of the use of metaphor. This theory can seem somewhat complex to many psychologists outside the behavior analytic tradition. However, it is not necessary to establish a deep understanding of the details of RFT to employ ACT-consistent moves in therapy. Even a brief look at the RFT perspective on metaphors can help the clinician either in using one of the many established metaphors in the ACT canon or in generating his or her own metaphors.

In ACT metaphors employ figurative language in a way that can teach new responses to disturbing emotional contexts (Hayes et al., 1999). The metaphor is not meant just to transfer knowledge: It is meant to establish a new relationship between events in the patient's mind with a resulting change in behavior. This change in the effect of a private event on a patient's behavior can be described as a transformation in stimulus functions (I. Stewart, Barnes-Holmes, Hayes, & Lipkens, 2001). In order for an ACT-consistent metaphor to accomplish this goal effectively, it should meet the following criteria: The metaphor is based on everyday commonsense elements; it "evokes a rich sensory pattern" (p. 81); it describes a series of events, interactions, or relationships that are representative and symbolic of elements of the patient's life that are likely to come up between sessions; and it may have several interpretations if the patient is facing a broad problem and fewer possible interpretations if he or she is facing a specific, focused problem.

When a patient is cultivating willingness, metaphors may assist in generating psychological flexibility. The "Monsters on the Bus" exercise in the Example section is a classic ACT metaphor that, among other things, emphasizes and illustrates the potential benefits of practicing acceptance in the service of a life well lived (Hayes et al., 1999).

Question to Pose/Intervention

"I would like to illustrate this idea with a brief story. Would that be all right? How can you relate the story that we have been looking at to the stories that emerge in your life? If you knew that the difficult thoughts and emotions that are showing up in this situation were a necessary part of what it takes for you to live a vital, meaningful, and rewarding life, would you be willing to experience them, to carry them with you on your journey?"

Example: The "Monsters on the Bus" Metaphor[1]

Let's imagine that you find yourself in the role of a bus driver. You have your uniform, your shiny dashboard, your comfortable seat, and a powerful bus at your command. This bus that

---

[1]This exercise is adapted from Hayes, Strosahl, and Wilson (1999). Copyright 1999 by The Guilford Press. Adapted by permission.

you are driving is very important. It represents your life. All of your experiences, all of your challenges and strengths, have brought you to this role, as the driver of your bus, your life. You have decided on a destination for this bus. It is a destination that you have chosen. This destination represents the valued directions that you are willing to pursue in your life. Getting to this destination is deeply significant to you. It matters that you get there. Every inch that you travel toward this valued aim means that you have, indeed, been taking your life in the right direction for you, in this moment. As you are driving, it is necessary that you keep to your course and follow the correct path toward your valued aim.

    Like any bus driver, you are obliged to stop along the way and pick up passengers. The trouble with this particular journey is that some of these passengers are truly difficult to deal with. These passengers are actually monsters. Each one represents a difficult thought or feeling that you have had to contend with over the course of your life. Some monsters might be self-criticism. Others are feelings of panic and dread. Others represent frantic worries about what will come. Whatever has troubled you and distracted you from the rich possibilities of life is hopping on your bus in the shape of one of these monsters.

    These monsters are unruly and they are rude. As you're driving, they are shouting insults at you and shooting spitballs. You can hear their calls as you drive. "You're a loser!" they shout. "Why don't you just give up? It's hopeless!" is heard ringing through the bus. One even shouts, "Stop the bus! This will never work!" You think about stopping the bus to scold and discipline these monsters. But if you did that, you would no longer be moving in the direction that matters to you. Perhaps you should pull over to the side of the road and throw these monsters off the bus. Again, this would mean you having to stop moving in the direction of your values. Maybe if you made a left turn and tried a different route the monsters would become quiet. But this too is a detour from living your life in a way that takes you toward realizing your freely chosen, valued aims.

    All of a sudden you realize that while you have been preoccupied with devising strategies and arguments for dealing with the nagging monsters on the bus, you have already missed a couple of turns and have lost some time on your journey. You now understand that in order to get to where you want to go, and to continue moving in the direction that you have chosen in life, you need to continue driving and allow these monsters to continue their catcalls, teasing, and nagging all the while. You can make the choice to take your life in the right direction, while just making space for all of the noise that the monsters generate. You can't kick them off, and you can't make them stop. But you can make the choice to keep living your life in a way that is meaningful and rewarding to you, to keep driving the bus, even when the monsters yammer away as you go.

Homework

The use of metaphors to illustrate the value of willingness and acceptance, as well as other processes, is not designed as a formal homework exercise. That being said, however, many patients may relate their experience between sessions to the metaphors they have learned in session. For example, a patient who struggles with significant social anxiety, yet who must also attend team meetings at work, might offer the observation, "Today, I was really freaking out in the meeting, but it was just like the 'monsters on the bus.' I kept doing what I knew was needed, even though the anxiety was coming and going." Gradually, the metaphors are increasingly related to both life experiences and the active processes that take place in the therapy sessions. As a result, the patient develops a capacity for a shift in perspective and the potential for an emergent psychological flexibility. Thus, the "homework" in the use of metaphors to cultivate willingness involves the patient applying these metaphors (see Form 6.3) when stressors emerge to facilitate acceptance and defusion. The therapist may check in with the patient in each session to learn how he or she applied the metaphors that were used.

Possible Problems

A patient may be very willing to entertain the use of metaphors and to go on imaginary journeys with the therapist in order to illustrate a point or facilitate an experience. However, if the therapist launches into a metaphor in a tangential or sudden way, he or she may lose the connection with the patient in the moment. Similarly, the metaphors can be delivered in a pedantic or professorial way that the patient might experience as invalidating. In order to best employ metaphors in session, the therapist is advised to briefly ask for the patient's permission and collaboration in the exercise. For example, the therapist might say, "I would like to use a short story to take a closer look at what we are discussing. Would that be all right?" In order to facilitate an attuned, empathic psychotherapeutic alliance throughout the use of a metaphor, the therapist might aim to match the patient's affect and pacing.

The patient may grow impatient if metaphors take too long to explain or if the therapist is using a metaphor at a time when the patient is experiencing an urgent need to discuss another topic. Agenda setting and collaboration early in the session can be used to make time for the patient to bring up the agenda items he or she feels are important and also to allow time for the therapist to introduce metaphors and other techniques. In the best-case scenario, both the therapist and the client are entering into this metaphor together, connected to the present moment and open to the transformation of stimulus functions that may emerge from the use of figurative language, perspective shifting, and defusion.

Cross-Reference to Other Techniques

Work with metaphors has an obvious connection to defusion, mindfulness techniques, and introducing what we mean by "acceptance." Techniques for cultivating self-compassion, like metta meditation and imagining the compassionate self, are related to metaphors also.

Form

Form 6.3: The Monsters on the Bus

TECHNIQUE: "STOPPING THE WAR"

Description

The following exercise is based on a meditation found in Jack Kornfield's *A Path with Heart* (1993). This exercise might be considered as a mindfulness practice, but it is included among our acceptance and willingness techniques. It is included in this section because it aims to assist patients in letting go of the conflicts and struggles that they maintain in their day-to-day lives. This exercise involves making a choice to "stop the war" against our emotional experiences. Interestingly, this exercise is also a form of metaphor in that it uses the symbol of a "war" or "battle" to represent the inner struggles against the flow of our experiencing that can hook us into attachment or fusion with our private events.

Question to Pose/Intervention

This exercise may be introduced after the patient has used mindfulness practice in session and, preferably, the concept of willingness. While guiding the patient through this meditation, it is important to speak the words at a slow and even pace, taking pauses and allowing brief silence. This assists the patient in a state of mindfulness and acceptance within him- or herself.

Example[2]

Take a few moments to allow yourself to become comfortable where you're sitting. Make any small adjustments to your position and posture that you may need, as you begin this exercise, so that you might be at ease. Adopt a posture that is secure and grounded. Allow your eyes to close. Without deliberately changing the pace of your breathing, begin to gently bring attention to the flow of the breath in and out of the body. Bring part of the attention to the soles of the feet. Next, bring part of the attention to the top of the head—now, to everything in between. Returning attention to the breathing, simply follow the breath: as you are breathing in knowing that you are breathing in, and as you are breathing out knowing that you are breathing out.

Begin to notice the sensations that are present in your body. If there are feelings of tension, pressure, or discomfort, bring your attention to these as well. As much as you can, bring an attitude of willingness to these experiences. As you breathe in, breathe attention especially into those areas of the body that present you with discomfort, tension, or resistance. Can you make space for these experiences? Bring part of your attention to the feeling of resistance, to the struggle that you are experiencing around these sensations. Notice the tension that is involved in fighting these experiences, moment by moment. When meeting each of these sensations, throughout the body, open yourself to the experience. Let go of the fight. Bring gentle attention to your breath. Let yourself be exactly as you are in this moment.

As you exhale, let go of the attention to physical sensations entirely. With the next available natural in-breath, bring your attention to your thoughts and emotions. What thoughts are flowing through your mind? What feelings are moving in your heart? Bring an open, receiving attention especially to those thoughts and emotions that you would typically struggle against. As much as you can, in this moment, allow yourself to soften around these thoughts and feelings. Can you make space for these events in the mind and heart? Can you let go of this war within yourself, if even just for this very moment?

Return your attention to the flow of the breath, to your feet on the ground, to your seat in the chair, and to your back feeling straight and supported. As you breathe in, bring attention to the struggles in your life. What battles are you continuing to fight? See if you can feel the presence of these battles. If you struggle with your body, bring awareness to that. If you struggle

---

[2]The following meditation is based on the "Stopping the War Within" exercise by Jack Kornfield (1993).

against your emotions, notice it in this moment. If there are thoughts that intrude, thoughts that you wage war against, bring a gentle awareness to this struggle. For a moment, allow yourself to feel the weight of these struggles, these battles. How long have these armies within you been fighting?

Softening around even this experience, allow yourself to bring an open, compassionate attention to the struggles. Let go of these battles. As you exhale, for a moment allow yourself to feel a complete willingness to be exactly who you are, right here and right now. In this moment, allow yourself to accept the totality of all that life has brought to you and all that you have brought to life. Isn't it time to stop the war that you have been waging within yourself? Allow yourself again to choose to let this war go. With courage and commitment, allow yourself to fully accept who you are, right here and right now.

Bring part of the attention to the soles of the feet. Next, bring part of the attention to the top of the head. Now, to everything in between. Returning attention to the breathing, simply follow the breath: as you are breathing in knowing that you are breathing in, and as you are breathing out knowing that you are breathing out.

When you are ready, open your eyes and allow yourself to let go of this exercise and resume your day.

Homework

This exercise can be assigned as a daily meditation to be practiced between sessions. This assignment may take place over a week or more. After patients have developed a regular mindfulness practice, they may choose to make this meditation a central aspect of their practice. This is not a goal to aim for, and it is not necessarily the "best" meditation for this purpose. This exercise may also be used in session to help patients make contact with willingness, without it being assigned as homework at all. Form 6.4 ("Stopping the War" Record) can be used by patients to record their daily practice of this exercise.

Possible Problems

Experiential exercises like "Stopping the War" are very different from what many patients might expect to encounter in a psychotherapy session. Some may view this sort of technique as exotic, alien, or even part of a religious tradition that they oppose. The therapist may invite the patient to take part in the exercise as an experiment that will be undertaken in the session together. The therapist may elicit the patient's negative automatic thoughts and assumptions about "meditation" exercises in session.

Also, the therapist may discover that the patient harbors automatic thoughts regarding being judged by the therapist while undertaking the exercise or fears of embarrassment when engaging in this visualization. The therapist may use a double-standard technique in such cases, asking the patient, for example, "What would you say to a beloved friend if she told you that she was too frightened to engage in this exercise, even in her therapist's office?" Also, the advantages and disadvantages of engaging in the exercise might be explored.

Even when a therapist asks for permission, matches the patient's pace and affective tone, and engages in a collaborative stance, the patient may not be willing to undertake the exercise. This presents an opportunity for the therapist to model acceptance, flexibility, and compassion.

After listening to the patient's mixed feelings or objections, it may be advisable to flexibly adopt a different method or engage a different process in order to help the patient meet his or her aims in therapy.

Cross-Reference to Other Techniques

This technique is related to mindfulness techniques, defusion techniques, introducing what we mean by "Acceptance," and using metaphors to cultivate willingness and defusion.

Form

Form 6.4: "Stopping the War" Record

CONCLUSIONS

When we discuss acceptance and willingness in emotion regulation, we are not talking solely about techniques but an emphasis on processes that are involved in psychotherapeutic change. Training patients to cultivate a willingness to remain in the presence of difficult emotional experiences can permit them to habituate to this displeasure and to discover new behavioral options. Habituation, in this sense, is not operationalized solely as a decrease in symptoms and signs of anxiety in the presence of a feared stimulus. In terms of acceptance-based interventions, habituation represents a broadening behavioral repertoire when faced with unpleasant or unwanted emotional responses. This opening of possibilities can allow patients opportunities to more deeply engage with the valued aims and directions that they pursue. The intrinsic rewards that come from such behavior can help them to engage in a virtuous circle of progress and movement in life. Several of the dimensions described in this book interrelate in this process. For example, mindful awareness of the present moment, self-compassion, and a willingness to experience mental events fully, while not allowing ourselves to be controlled by the contents of our thoughts and feelings, all are involved in an ongoing flow of emotion regulation that can take place in the context of a life well lived. Similarly, acceptance and defusion can enable patients to stand back from their emerging automatic thoughts, encouraging a stronger awareness of emotional schemas and an enhanced ability to question negative thinking.

CHAPTER SEVEN

Compassionate Mind Training

As we have discussed, mindfulness, acceptance, and compassion are interrelated. Practicing mindful awareness and a willingness to contact the present moment "just as it is" involves an emergent form of self-kindness and self-validation. Accordingly, mental training designed to intentionally foster a "compassionate mind" (Gilbert, 2007) has become a growing trend in third-generation mindfulness and acceptance-based cognitive and behavioral therapies. This emphasis on compassion within CBT is part of a greater integration of compassion-focused methods and Buddhist influences within psychotherapy in general (Germer, Seigel, & Fulton, 2005). Paul Gilbert (2009) has drawn upon Buddhist influences, evolutionary psychology, and affective neuroscience to develop a comprehensive form of CBT known as compassion-focused therapy (CFT). In this chapter, we outline several techniques, drawn from CFT and Buddhist practices, that emphasize compassionate mind training.

Obviously, many therapies discuss the value of warmth and empathy in the psychotherapeutic relationship (Gilbert & Leahy, 2007; Greenberg & Paivio, 1997; Rogers, 1965). However, CFT and other compassion-focused approaches are characterized by an emphasis on patients' specific "compassionate mind training." Compassion-focused approaches hypothesize the cultivation of compassion to be a central process in emotion regulation and psychotherapy, particularly when dealing with patients who struggle with feelings of shame and who exhibit self-critical thinking (Gilbert, 2007; Gilbert & Irons, 2005).

Gilbert (2007) describes compassion as a "multi-faceted process" that has evolved from "the care-giver mentality" found in human parental care and child rearing. As such, compassion involves a number of emotional, cognitive, and motivational elements: care for the welfare of others, sympathy, distress tolerance, empathy, nonjudgmental awareness, distress sensitivity, and the ability to create opportunities for growth and change with warmth (Gilbert, 2007). Gilbert (2009) asserts that "its essence is a basic kindness, with deep awareness of the suffering of oneself and of other living things, coupled with the wish and effort to relieve it."

The underlying theory for CFT links "psychotherapeutic processes with evolved psychological systems, especially those associated with social behavior" (Gilbert, 2007). Drawing from evolutionary affective neuroscience (Depue & Morrone-Strupinsky, 2005), the CFT model describes three primary affect regulation systems that operate in humans (Gilbert, 2009). The first of the three emotion regulation systems is referred to as the "incentive/resource-focused" system, which involves the range of human behaviors that contribute to pursuing aims, consuming, and achieving (Gilbert, 2007, 2009). The incentive/resource system likely involves dopaminergic systems to a greater degree than do other emotion regulation systems. The second emotion regulation system involves a highly sensitive "threat focus." Faced with the persistent presence of threats, such as predators, disease, and natural disasters, our ancestors evolved to possess a "better safe than sorry" process for quickly detecting threats in the environment and responding rapidly. The threat-focused system involves older evolutionary structures in the brain, such as the amygdala and the limbic system, involving the serotonergic systems (Gilbert, 2009), activating the defensive behavioral response, such as the classic "fight, flight, or freeze" response. In contrast, the third emotion regulation system is referred to as a contentment safeness and connection-based system. It is reflected in "affiliative-focused" behaviors, such as nurturance, validation, and empathy, involving the oxytocin and opiate systems (Gilbert, 2007). Humans have evolved to naturally respond to kindness and warmth through a down-regulation of the anxiety systems and a felt sense of "soothing." This involves a genetically predisposed capacity for humans to feel "safeness" and to feel soothed in the presence of stable, warm, empathic interactions with others (Gilbert, 2009). This affiliative-focused "safeness system" involves nonverbal behaviors that may resemble the stable, caring context that engaged and effective parents may establish with their child (Bowlby, 1968; Fonagy, 2002; Fonagy & Target, 2007; Sloman, Gilbert, & Hasey, 2003). One of the aims of CFT is training patients in accessing and employing this system of self-soothing through the felt experience of compassion.

In a similar conceptualization of compassion, Wang (2005) hypothesizes that human compassion emerges from an evolutionarily determined "species-preservative" neurophysiological system. This system has evolved in a relatively recent evolutionary time frame compared with the older "self-preservative" system. This species-preservative system is based on an "inclusive sense of self and promotes awareness of our interconnectedness to others" (Wang, 2005). Considerable evidence on a wide range of animals, especially primates, supports the view that compassion, empathy, altruism, and other forms of kindness are widespread (DeWaal, 2009). Ancestral humans who practiced compassion, group protectiveness, sharing of food, and care for the young or sick were more likely to survive than those characterized by indifference to one another's welfare (D. S. Wilson & Wilson, 2007).

Relative to some other animals, human infants and children may seem defenseless, requiring, as they do, a great deal of care and protection in their early life. As a result, particular brain structures and other elements of the nervous and hormonal systems have evolved that promote behaviors that involve protection of and care for others. Wang's review of the relevant literature suggests that the prefrontal cortex, cingulate cortex, and the ventral vagal complex are involved on a structural level, in the activation of this species-preservative system (Wang, 2005). These structures are all involved in the development of healthy attachment bonds and may also be involved in the cultivation of mindfulness (D. Siegel, 2007).

In a related approach, Neff has integrated contemporary social psychology with fundamental elements of Buddhist philosophy to develop a theory of "self-compassion" that is distinct from both "self-esteem" and compassion for others (Neff, 2003). According to Neff, self-compassion involves three primary elements: self-kindness, an awareness of our common humanity, and mindful awareness. Higher levels of reported self-compassion have been found to be correlated with lower levels of depression and anxiety (Neff, 2003; Neff, Hseih, & Dejitthirat, 2005; Neff, Rude, & Kirkpatrick, 2007). These relationships have been found to persist, even after controlling for the effect of self-criticism. Neff and colleagues' research has demonstrated positive correlations among self-compassion and a range of positive psychological dimensions (Neff, Rude, et al., 2007). These factors include, but are not limited to, life satisfaction, feelings of social connectedness (Neff, Kirkpatrick, & Rude, 2007), and personal initiative and positive affect (Neff, Rude, et al., 2007).

Grounded in an evolutionary perspective, EST construes the healthy functioning of a self-soothing capacity based on the experience of attuned attachment relationships to be a central process in adaptive human emotion regulation. Indeed, the nature of healthy adaptive emotional schemas suggests that an accepting, validating, and open-hearted relationship with oneself may lead to a healthier emotional life. As such, cultivating self-compassion can be an essential element of an emotional schema-based approach.

TECHNIQUE: THE "LOVINGKINDNESS" MEDITATION

Description

The term "lovingkindness" is a translation of the word *metta*, which in the ancient Pali language represented a deeply caring sense of goodwill and concern for the welfare of all beings. This form of goodwill involved no attachment to the objects of care. At its most fundamental level, metta represented a form of aspiration toward universal love and kindness. Traditionally, it was believed that regularly practicing metta meditation would result in a cessation of hostility and aggression in the practitioner. It was thought that this would lead to a greater degree of spiritual and personal health, including helping the meditator overcome problems like insomnia or nightmares. These ideas are reflected in recent neuroimaging research of long-term practitioners of compassion meditation (Lutz, Brefczynski-Lewis, Johnstone, & Davidson, 2008), which shows that advanced compassion-focused meditators responded to aversive stimuli with an increased activation of brain regions involved in empathy, love, and positive emotions, such as the anterior cingulate cortex and insula. This supports Gilbert's (2009) assertion that compassionate mind training can result in a shift in mode of emotion regulation from a threat-based, anxious, or aggressive response system to an affiliative, compassion-oriented soothing system.

In the lovingkindness meditation, we are presented with a unique example of a prescientific intervention, designed specifically to foster more adaptive emotion regulation and address anxiety and aggression, that is now being supported by the empirical evidence. The practice is very simple and involves the meditator visualizing him- or herself as innocent and deserving of compassion and care. When this image is formed, the meditator then begins to recite a phrase that aspires to self-compassion, such as "May I be filled with lovingkindness, may I be peaceful and at ease, may I be well." Accompanying this visualization and recitation, the person engaged in this training also aims to foster a direct sensory experience of compassion and love by focusing on sensations in the body that are related to such emotions. This is practiced regularly for about 30 minutes, over a long period of time, traditionally. After self-compassion is generated, this exercise can be used to cultivate compassion for others, even those toward whom one might have anger or ill will. In this way, as the patient remains engaged with this meditative practice as much as he or she can, the patient is gradually habituating to the experience of compassion and increasing his or her ability to flexibly remain in the presence of the difficult feelings that may arise when he or she directs compassionate attention inward.

Question to Pose/Intervention

The intervention itself follows the basic format of the mindfulness practices that are explained in detail earlier in this text. The therapist will guide the patient through the steps of this exercise, which the patient can later follow either from memory, from having approximately memorized the instructions in the patient handout, or from following a recorded guided lovingkindness meditation. There are several examples of guided lovingkindness meditations available. It may also be advisable for the therapist to record the guided meditation as it takes place in session and to give the patient a copy of this recording. Like mindfulness practices, this meditation should take place in a quiet, safe place, with the patient seated on a meditation cushion or a straight-backed chair or lying flat on the floor.

Example[1]

Lovingkindness is a quality that can help us to abide with difficult experiences rather than struggle against that which we cannot change. This quality of warm, compassionate regard for the self and others is also associated with the cultivation of a sense of well-being that can translate into positive actions taken in the service of a meaningful and rewarding life. The meditation we are about to embark upon may be viewed as one of the most ancient and enduring "mental health" practices in human history. For over 2,500 years, people have sat silently, drawing their attention to the cultivation of love and appreciation for themselves and all living beings in this way. As you take your seat to begin this meditation, take a moment to realize that you share an aspiration with centuries of fellow travelers as you embark upon your own private journey toward compassion. Set aside about 20 minutes to engage in this exercise at first; later on you may want to devote a little more time to it or let it go entirely. Unlike some other meditation exercises, this exercise involves a focus on specific emotions and specific images. At first, this kind of exercise might elicit feelings different from those you are aiming to explore. It may even bring about some frustration. All of this is OK. As best as you can, allow yourself to be kind and patient with yourself. You are exploring ideas and practices that may be very new and different to you. The kindness and patience that you can direct toward yourself in the face of frustration can provide yet another opportunity to practice and deepen your capacity for self-compassion.

As you begin, take a seat on a straight-backed chair or meditation cushion. Just as you would in a mindfulness meditation exercise, allow yourself to bring your attention to the flow of the breath. Make any small adjustments that you might need to make in order to be as comfortable as possible. As the exercise proceeds, if you need to adjust your posture from time to time, that is OK. Bring part of your attention to the flow of your breath. As much as you can, without judgment, just observe the breath as you breathe in and out. Gather your awareness of the physical act of breathing, and simply follow the flow of the breath, moment by moment.

Form an image of yourself in your mind. Imagine that you are seated in the same posture that you now sit in. You may wish to picture yourself as a child. You are innocent and worthy of love and compassion in this image. If you do not wish to imagine yourself as a child for this exercise, simply imagine yourself as you are now, but held in a kind, loving appreciation. Recognize, just for a moment, that all beings wish to be happy and free from pain. All people have an inborn

---

[1]The following exercise is adapted from many sources on metta meditation, including the writings of Jack Kornfield (1993) and Jon Kabat-Zinn (1990).

motivation to feel loved and be held in kindness and acceptance. Realize that it is all right for you to wish to be happy and free from suffering. As you do this, begin to silently repeat the following phrase: "May I be filled with lovingkindness. May I be well. May I be peaceful and at ease. May I be happy." Hold the image of yourself in your mind as you repeat this. Allow the rhythm of repetition to flow with your breath. Allow yourself to engage in this exercise gently but with a spirit of immovability. Allow your "heart" to open to the meaning of these words. As you continue though this exercise, let yourself blend the feeling of being loved and held in unconditional kindness with the flow of the words themselves. Whenever your mind has wandered, which is an inevitable behavior of the mind, gently direct your mind back to the phrase, the image, and the feeling of loving. "May I be filled with lovingkindness. May I be well. May I be peaceful and at ease. May I be happy." It is natural that distractions will come and go. Practice a warm acceptance of yourself as you proceed through this exercise and allow yourself to gently return your attention to the repetition as many times as is necessary. When the time that you have allowed for this exercise has past, simply let the phrase go. As you exhale, let the image of yourself and the deliberate focus on feelings of warmth and compassion go as well. Allow yourself to simply be with the flow of your breath: breathing in knowing that you are breathing in, and breathing out knowing that you are breathing out. As you exhale, allow your eyes to open, and let go of this exercise.

Homework

The lovingkindness meditation may be practiced regularly as a form of homework and a method of pursuing ongoing compassionate mind training. This exercise might take as little as 10 to 15 minutes per day, but can be practiced for periods of up to an hour or more in one sitting. It is more worthwhile for patients to maintain a regular practice each day than to engage in one or two periods of longer, more intense meditation without establishing a reliable, repeatable practice. Patients may practice with a recorded guide at first and may also practice by remembering and following the written directions provided here. It is helpful to monitor patients' daily practice and any observations that may arise around the practice. Patients can complete Form 7.1 to help them further explore the practice of lovingkindness.

Possible Problems

Many patients may find it difficult to direct compassion toward themselves. Developmental experiences such as abuse, trauma, or neglect may lead them to associate the experience of compassionate acceptance with shame, danger, or other unpleasant emotions. Several steps may be useful in assisting patients to approach self-compassion, when the very idea of compassion evokes anxiety.

A developmental analysis and shared case conceptualization may be helpful in these situations. The therapist may begin this process with psychoeducation, reviewing the idea that humans learn to relate certain environmental events to an activation of their threat detection systems. The therapist can explain that often people will develop safety behaviors or avoidance in response to this activation of threat detection.

The therapist and the patient can review the history of developmental events and relationships that contributed to the patient's fear of compassion. Together, they can isolate avoidance and safety behaviors that have developed in response to this history.

The therapist may employ a functional analysis of the responses in session. New responses can be planned and rehearsed in session, with a great deal of emphasis placed upon the therapist validating these emotional responses and teaching self-validation to arising difficult emotions. First, the patient may be taught to consciously employ a mindful orientation to these experiences in order to observe and defuse from shame-based and self-attacking cognitions. From this point, the lovingkindness meditation may be practiced for a short duration during session, with a debriefing following. The therapist and the patient can then rehearse noticing thoughts and emotions, affect labeling, and responding with self-compassionate self-talk in session.

Cross-Reference to Other Techniques

The lovingkindness exercise is clearly related to the range of mindfulness-based exercises that are presented. The mindfulness of the breath exercise, in particular, can serve as an introduction to the initial stages of the lovingkindness meditation. The compassionate mind training exercises that follow in this chapter are modern adaptations and developments in compassion training, all of which have some relationship to the practice of metta meditation found in the lovingkindness practice.

Form

Form 7.1: Questions to Ask Yourself after Completing Your First Week of Engaging in Lovingkindness Exercise

TECHNIQUE: IMAGINING THE COMPASSIONATE SELF

Description

CFT aims to train patients in developing multiple aspects of compassion, including compassionate attention, compassionate thinking, and compassionate behavior (Gilbert, 2009). Imagery-based techniques feature prominently among those employed in this approach. Although such visualization methods are not a formal extension of Buddhist training, we can see the roots of compassionate imagery in various Buddhist traditions. Tibetan and Japanese Vajrayana Buddhist schools embrace a variety of techniques for using the imagination to identify with various symbolic images of mythological characters. Each of these characters represents an aspect of healthy perspective, wisdom, compassion, or effective action. The purpose of these techniques is to experientially connect with qualities that are conducive to liberation from suffering. For example, a meditator might form an image of a *bodhisattva* of compassion in her mind and imagine her breath moving in and out with the rhythm of that person's breathing. The details and colors of the mythological character's clothing and countenance might be vividly imagined. In such visualizations, the meditator may even adopt the posture and hand gestures of the imaginary figure, and may attempt to access a deeply felt emotional experience of compassion during the meditation period.

The exercises found in CFT do not necessarily invoke religious or spiritual iconography. In fact, part of the inspiration for the compassionate self exercise was drawn from an adaptation of acting exercises to mental health interventions, so that clinicians might contact and better relate to the affective states of their patients (Gilbert, 2009). The compassionate self exercise is meant to enable patients to engage in a multisystem form of role play in which they can guide themselves toward an experiential knowledge of self-compassion.

Self-compassion and emotional self-validation are meant to facilitate a shift from a threat-focused emotional processing system to the activation of a felt sense of safeness that emerges in the soothing, affiliation-focused emotion regulation system. This is accomplished by using the imagination. Just as imagining sexual imagery might activate our sexual response, imagining compassionate imagery can activate our compassion response. This compassion response involves our affiliative soothing processes (Gilbert, 2009). In this way, the practice of imagining the compassionate self is a direct method of pursuing emotion regulation. The example below has been based on CFT (Gilbert, 2009) for use in emotion regulation, and is modified for EST purposes.

Question to Pose/Intervention

"What would your ideal, compassionate self look like? What are the qualities that you would associate with a compassionate person? How might you hold your posture if you were as wise, emotionally strong, and kind as you could possibly be? What would it feel like to be forgiving and relaxed? What would the expression on your face be like if you could remain loving and calm, even in the face of stressful challenges?"

Example

As we begin, allow part of your awareness to settle upon the flow of the breath in and out of the body. Allow your eyes to close. Feel free to make any adjustments that may be necessary for you to become comfortable where you are sitting. Over the course of this exercise, you may find it useful to make such small adjustments from time to time. This is perfectly natural and completely acceptable as you engage in our exercise. Again, bring part of the attention to the flow of the breath. There is no need to adjust the rhythm of your breathing or to create any specific pattern or state. Simply allow the breath to breathe itself. Breathing in, know that you are breathing in. Breathing out, know that you are breathing out. Bringing attention to the soles of your feet, feel your connection to the ground. Feel yourself seated in the chair, with your back straight and supported. Taking a few moments more, allow yourself to breathe attention into the body as a whole. Next, bring part of your attention to the sounds that are in the room. [Pause for a few seconds.] Now bring part of your attention to the sounds that are just outside of the room. [Pause for a few seconds more.] After a few moments, bring attention to the sounds that are farther away even than that. Next, bring part of your attention to your eyes—these eyes that you have looked out from for as long as you remember. Taking a few moments, allow yourself to realize how many different stories you have told yourself about the person who looks out from these eyes. There are so many different aspects of who we are, each vying for attention and control of our behavior, moment by moment. With the next natural in-breath, breathe attention into your whole body. As you let go with the next natural out-breath, again bring attention, with the eyes closed to your imagination. In this moment, allow the most compassionate, warm, and caring aspects of your self to be present. Using your imagination in these next moments, begin to construct an image of your compassionate self. Allow your facial expression to begin to reflect the kindness and intuitive wisdom that we all possess. You can do this by allowing your lips to gently curve into a half smile. In doing so, in this moment, you are adopting an expression of compassion. Allow your mind to steadily and gradually compose an image of your compassionate self. We will be giving this image particular qualities. This image will possess wisdom.

This image will possess strength. This image will be noncondemning. This image will radiate warmth. During this exercise, in this very moment, you have the freedom to allow your imagination free reign. This image of the compassionate self doesn't need to look like "you" as you imagine yourself to appear in your day-to-day life. The image of your compassionate self may resemble someone from your past or a fictional or mythological character, or it may involve a combination of aspects that are meaningful to you. From time to time, as in mindfulness exercises, the attention may wander away from this image. As best as you can when you notice your mind has wandered, gently and kindly bring your attention back as you breathe in. How do you want your compassionate self's image to appear to you? Is it a version of you? Is it an image of a person? Is it an image of a force of nature like a wave? Is this a female or male image? What does this compassionate self sound like? Imagine that you are looking out from behind the eyes of this compassionate self. In this moment you are a deeply warm, loving, strong, and compassionate being. Recognize the calmness and wisdom that you possess. Take a moment to feel the physical sensations that accompany the arising of a compassionate mind. Recognize the strength and healing quality of a vast and deep kindness. Recognize that this warmth and kindness, this powerful compassion exists within you as an abundant reservoir of strength. Stay with this image for a few moments. For as long as you need to, allow yourself to recognize and feel that you are, indeed, capable of great kindness. With the next natural in-breath, bring bare attention to the flow of the breath into the body. As you breathe out, allow yourself to let go of this image of the compassionate self. Breathing in, you know that you are breathing in. Breathing out, you know that you are breathing out. Bring part of your attention to the soles of the feet. Next, bring part of your attention to the top of the head. And now bring part of your attention to everything in between. Next, bring part of your attention to the sounds that are in the room. [Pause for few seconds.] Now bring part of your attention to the sounds that are just outside of the room. [Pause for a few seconds more.] After a few moments, bring attention to the sounds that are farther away even than that. With your next available out-breath, allow yourself to let go of this exercise completely. Take a few moments, and when you're ready to allow your eyes to open, gently allow yourself to settle into your everyday awareness, and perhaps allow yourself to take some of this compassion with you throughout the day. (Based on and modified from exercises in Gilbert, 2009.)

Homework

This exercise can be practiced in a structured, meditative fashion at particular intervals of the day or week. Patients might decide to set aside a specific amount of time to engage in this exercise in such cases. Alternatively, they can practice this as they move through their daily activities, whenever an opportunity presents itself. In this way, patients may gradually generalize their accessing a compassionate mind, and may be better able to contact a compassionate and self-validating perspective. Patients can also complete Form 7.2 to help them further explore their compassionate selves.

Possible Problems

For some patients, engaging in self-compassion exercises may evoke a sense of self-consciousness or even associations of shame and self-recrimination. This may be due to elements of their interpersonal learning history or difficult relationships in their family of origin that relate to abuse, neglect, or other sources of abandonment and shame. As such, the therapist introducing such techniques is advised to consistently maintain a slow pace in such work, emphasizing emotional validation. Socratic questioning and guided exploration of the emotions and thoughts that arise throughout the process of compassionate mind training may be a necessary component of the therapy process. For example, a patient may report that she feels "embarrassed" when constructing an image of a compassionate self. The therapist may begin by validating that emotional response, explaining that a new and different sort of exercise such as this could naturally trigger emotions such as embarrassment or shyness. The therapist may then proceed to inquire about what automatic thoughts are arriving in the moment in session. If the patient were to report self-critical or shame-based thoughts, such as "I'm going to make a fool of myself" or "I can't do this," the therapist may choose to review alternative, compassionate ways of thinking. For instance, the patient may tell herself, "I feel a little embarrassed, but I'm in a safe situation, and I can spare a few moments to see what self-compassion feels like."

When patients engage in generalization training, such as the informal application of the compassionate self exercise, it is important that they reserve part of their attention for what they are actually doing in their day-to-day lives. The therapist should review with his or her patients situations in which it would be safe and functional for them to devote part of their attention to a compassionate mind or mindfulness-based practice. For example, it might be perfectly acceptable to vacuum a guest room floor while holding an imaginary vision of the compassionate self. Allowing a significant portion of the attention to drift to compassionate imagery while driving through midday city traffic might pose far more problems.

Cross-Reference to Other Techniques

The imaging the compassionate self exercise has a direct relationship to the lovingkindness and compassionate letter-writing exercises. This exercise begins with a grounding in mindfulness and relates to the mindfulness of the breath exercise. The imagining the compassionate self exercise can be used as a form of generalization practice and has a clear relationship to the 3-minute coping breathing space and mindful cooking exercises as well.

Form

Form 7.2: Questions to Ask Yourself after Completing Your First Week of Imagining the Compassionate Self

TECHNIQUE: COMPASSIONATE LETTER WRITING

Description

Several forms of psychotherapy employ techniques that involve the patient writing letters and narratives (Pennebaker & Seagal, 1999; Smyth & Pennebaker, 2008). These exercises can assume a variety of forms and purposes, including writing a letter to the source of a schema (Leahy, 2003b; Young et al., 2003), writing an unsent letter to a person to express suppressed emotions (Mahoney, 2003), and other forms of narrative exposure using expressive writing. This exercise uses the simple act of writing a letter to train the patient in accessing and enacting a more compassionate and mindful perspective. This practice of compassionate letter writing has been adapted from a similar exercise in CFT (Gilbert, 2009, 2010) and an exercise developed by Neff (Gilbert, 2009; Neff, 2003).

Compassionate letter writing can be engaged in as a form of homework or can take place during the session. Patients are asked to write a letter to themselves from their compassionate mind, reflecting self-kindness, a sense of our common humanity, and mindfulness (Neff, 2009). Gilbert (2009) suggests that engaging in compassionate letter writing can down-regulate the threat-focused emotional system, and can reduce anxiety and judgment-based emotions and automatic thoughts.

Form 7.3 is a homework-based version of compassionate letter writing and contains detailed instructions. It is designed as a do-it-yourself exercise; however, it is advisable that a therapist review and introduce this exercise in a careful fashion, even if it is being employed as a homework technique.

Question to Pose/Intervention

"Can you imagine a kind and wise friend, who holds you in unconditional compassion, love, and acceptance? What would such a friend tell you when you begin to slide into shame and self-attacking? Can you remind yourself that all of us have regrets, fears, and struggles? Can you step back from the flow of your thoughts and emotions to recognize that your suffering connects you to the rest of humanity, knowing that all human beings feel pain, guilt, and regret? If a loving friend was making helpful suggestions about how you could take action to live a meaningful and healthy life, what would be the tone and feeling quality of those suggestions? Would a wise, resilient, and caring friend seek to tear you down or to hold you up so that you might flourish and live?"

Example[2]

As we begin this exercise, allow yourself to take a moment and mindfully bring attention to the flow of the breath. Without any particular aim, observe the rhythm and flow of your breathing in and out of the body. Bring part of your attention to your feet on the floor, to your buttocks in the chair, to your spine feeling straight and supported, and to the top of the head. Allow yourself to notice whatever physical sensations present themselves in this moment. Breathing in, you know that you are breathing in. Breathing out, you know that you are breathing out. In front of you, there is a pencil and some paper. We have enough time to engage in this exercise at whatever pace feels right for you, and it is probably best if we approach this without any hurry. This is time for you to connect with and to speak from a wise, kind, and noncondemning aspect of yourself. There is no need for us to rush.

You might remember our practice of imagining and experiencing your compassionate self. If it is helpful for you, you might choose to form this image in your mind as you begin. Imagine yourself as kind, as emotionally strong and resilient, and as a loving and accepting presence. This is the voice that you will be bringing to your letter writing today. You will be writing from

---

[2]The following exercise is adapted from compassionate letter-writing exercises developed by Gilbert (2009) and Neff (2003).

this understanding, self-accepting, broad perspective. In this way, we are contacting a wisdom that you were born with and giving it a voice.

As you begin, remember the simple act of self-validation. There are many good reasons for the distress you are currently experiencing. Your brain and mind have evolved and emerged through millions of years of life progressing on this planet. You were not designed to deal with the particular pressures and complexities of our current social environment. Your learning history has presented you with strong challenges and situations that have caused you pain. Can you open yourself to a compassionate understanding that your struggle is a natural part of life and that it is not your fault?

Take a moment to step back and observe the flow of thoughts and feelings that emerge moment by moment. Hold this process of unfolding mental events before you, and recognize the impermanence of the contents of your mind.

As much as you can, connect with the basic kindness and care that you would bring to a beloved friend. You might have regrets or might have engaged in behaviors that you feel guilty about. You may have goals that you have yet to attain. You may have great anger toward yourself and may engage in self-attacking speech. If you were writing this letter to a truly beloved friend, a person whom you held in great kindness, what would you want to say? What would you write in your letter? Wouldn't you validate your friend's suffering? Wouldn't you reach out to let him or her know that whatever he or she has done, this friend is still worthy of love and kindness? Wouldn't you try to help your friend find ways to take action, to move his or her life to a greater state of well-being and meaningfulness?

As you write, think about what compassionate actions you could take to help better your current situation. What kind of compassionate attention might you bring to your life right now? How can you be as understanding and patient as you can with yourself?

In the next few minutes, allow yourself to compose a compassionate letter that gives a voice to your compassionate self. We will read it together and reflect on the exercise when you are done.

Homework

This letter-writing exercise (Form 7.3) can be engaged in during session or assigned as homework. If used as homework, the therapist should explain the exercise in detail and begin the process in session. The form provides a self-administered version of the exercise instructions. There are advantages to engaging in this exercise as homework. Because it may take more time than one session can allow, assigning the letter writing as homework may give the patient sufficient time to deeply engage in the exercise without rushing.

Possible Problems

Many patients may have had experiences in their personal histories that contribute to a fear or aversion toward self-compassion or positive self-regard. They may have experienced childhood abuse, severe rejection or shaming, traumatic memories, or distant and invalidating parental behaviors. Consequently, activating a compassionate voice may be difficult or may elicit fears of being punished. The therapist may inquire about the memories that get in the way of self-compassion or the beliefs that lead to resisting this experience. For example, the patient might say, "I don't really deserve this. I am bad." Further inquiry might lead to examining the experiences that gave rise to this belief and whether the patient would treat a child with derogation and shaming. The therapist may ask, "What would have been different for you if you had been able to direct compassion and kindness toward yourself?"

Many patients might associate self-compassion with self-indulgence. They may believe that harsh self-criticism is necessary to drive themselves toward greater achievements (Neff, 2003). The therapist might address this with a functional analysis of these assumptions, with cognitive restructuring techniques or even a defusion-based intervention. Psychoeducation may also be useful in such cases. Indeed, self-compassion has been found to correlate with greater personal initiative and life satisfaction (Neff, 2003; Neff, Rude, et al., 2007). According to Neff (2009), "Self compassionate individuals are motivated to achieve, but this goal is not driven by the desire to bolster one's self-image. Rather, it is driven by the compassionate desire to maximize one's potential and well-being" (p. 8).

Cross-Reference to Other Techniques

As we have noted, mindfulness is frequently considered an element of, or precursor to, self-compassion (Gilbert, 2009; Neff, 2009). Thus, the mindfulness of the breath as well as mindfulness-based generalization exercises may help prepare the patient to engage in the compassionate letter-writing exercise. This exercise is a part of the same compassionate mind training process that is found in the lovingkindness, compassionate other, and imagining the compassionate self exercises. In addition, self-validation and other validation techniques may also be helpful.

Form

Form 7.3: Self-Compassionate Letter Writing

CONCLUSIONS

Compassionate mind training is based on the knowledge that human beings have evolved to respond to kindness and affiliation, and that compassion directly activates a soothing capacity in humans. Although some of these techniques are variations on prescientific practices, the evidence from affective neuroscience, social psychology, and evolutionary theory suggests that training in self-compassion can augment the patient's capacity for emotion regulation. CFT presents the clinician with a specific model involving three modes of emotion regulation: threat detection, incentive/resource focused, and affiliation focused. This model is a clarification and simplification of the range of affect regulation theories that are currently in discussion, many of which are addressed in this text. Compassion-focused techniques are compatible with the range of emotion regulation methods provided here, and the blend of mindfulness, willingness, and self-compassion can serve as a foundation for ongoing work in emotion regulation, regardless of the specific therapeutic modality that is being employed.

CHAPTER EIGHT

Enhancing Emotional Processing

Emotion-focused therapy (EFT; Greenberg, 2002) is a short-term, evidence-based therapy that has emerged from the tradition of humanistic psychotherapy. Based on theories of emotion and attachment, EFT proposes that the psychotherapeutic relationship itself serves an emotion regulation function, as an "affect-regulating bond" (Greenberg, 2007). Processes that are hypothesized to be involved in this relationship resonate with elements of other approaches outlined thus far, including acceptance, empathy, focus on the present moment, and the activation of inherent, human affiliative soothing systems. The concept of an emotional schema is also in accord with Greenberg's EFT perspective on emotion (Leahy, 2003b). Greenberg's entire premise involves cultivating emotional intelligence and a broadening set of emotion regulation techniques in response to challenging emotional experiences through the therapeutic relationship. This is entirely resonant with the aims of EST, in that EST responds to specific sets of meta-experiential beliefs and strategies about how one might relate to an emotion. Beyond this, both EST and EFT recognize the adaptive function of emotional experiencing as information processing. For example, EFT theory holds that an emotion contains its related cognitive content and that activating an emotion might lead to a clearer understanding of that content (Greenberg, 2002).

In EFT, the therapeutic relationship is construed as the central process wherein psychotherapeutic change becomes possible. According to Greenberg and Watson (2005), the therapeutic relationship operates in two principal ways. Primarily, the relationship directly results in emotion regulation through the function of a soothing dyad. The patient may generalize and internalize the experiences that arise within this dyad, resulting in a greater capacity to self-soothe. Secondarily, the therapeutic relationship also serves as a context within which the patient may experience emotional deepening, and it may enhance specific skills necessary for effective emotion regulation.

The EFT therapist works in a highly collaborative manner, oscillating between guiding the patient's emotional experiencing and following the emotional directions that the patient moves toward (Greenberg, 2002). Techniques commonly place the therapist in the role of "emotion coach" (Gottman, 1997), gradually facilitating the patient's increasing capacity for emotion regulation and the tolerance of difficult affective states.

Cognition is seen as a component of overall emotional processing in EFT, but it is not viewed as the sole regulatory role (Greenberg, 2002). Within this paradigm, emotions may influence cognition just as cognition may influence emotions. Emotions themselves may even be used to regulate other emotions. In EFT, "appraisal and emotion are seen as occurring simultaneously to generate emotional meanings" (Greenberg, 2007). Indeed, Greenberg and Safran (1987) propose that emotion is a "high level synthesis of affect, motivation and behavior" (Greenberg, 2002, p. 10). This conceptualization of integrated and interdependent cognitive-affective functioning can be understood as a form of emotional intelligence. As a result, emotion coaching might be viewed as training in the development of emotional intelligence and an enhancement of adaptive emotional processing.

The concept of emotional intelligence (EI) has been defined as an individual's ability to relate to emotions across several dimensions (Greenberg, 2002; Mathews, Zeidner, & Roberts, 2002; Mayer & Salovey, 1997), including identifying emotions, expressing emotions, appraising emotions, understanding emotions, generating emotional feelings, regulating emotions in self and others, and using emotion knowledge. This concept was widely popularized by Daniel Goleman's best-selling book *Emotional Intelligence*, although Goleman credits Mayer and Salovey as pioneering the conceptualization of EI (Goleman, 1995). The Mayer and Salovey model asserts that EI consists of a system of intelligence that relates to the processing of emotions (Mayer, Salovey, & Caruso, 2000). This model suggests that EI functions in ways that are analogous to the functions of general intelligence, leading to methods of EI assessment, theories of EI development, and an expanding body of EI research (Mathews et al., 2002). Ciarrochi, Mayer, and colleagues have put forward an applied, clinical definition of EI, which is relevant to emotion regulation techniques (Ciarrochi, Forgas, & Mayer, 2006; Ciarrochi & Mayer, 2007) From this perspective, EI represents "the extent to which one is able to engage in value-consistent behavior in the context of difficult emotions or emotionally charged thoughts" (Ciarrochi & Bailey, 2009, p. 154).

The techniques that follow in this chapter are partially derived from EFT and aim toward patients' enhancement of their emotional processing. By strengthening EI, patients may become better able to understand their emotional experiencing and may relate to their emotions in a more flexible and adaptive way.

TECHNIQUE: ENHANCING EMOTIONAL AWARENESS

Description

If patients are going to begin to work with, and perhaps transform, their emotional processing, practicing and enhancing their ability to notice and selectively attend to their emotions is an important first step. As we have seen, mindfulness practices may serve as a useful introduction to decentering from and observing internal experiences. In addition to cultivating mindful awareness, it may be useful for patients to practice their ability to observe, describe, and explore their experience of emotions.

EFT suggests several ways that patients may begin to practice attending to their emotional experiencing (Eliot, Watson, Goldman, & Greenberg, 2003; Greenberg, 2002). Patients may begin to attend to physical sensations and to question where in the body they are experiencing an emotion. For example, "When I feel anxious I notice that my shoulders tense and my teeth seem to grind together." They may label the emotion, identify the thoughts that are related to the emotional experience, and examine its function in their lives (Greenberg, 2002). EFT also distinguishes between primary emotions and secondary emotions. Primary emotions represent direct emotional responses to stimuli in the world, while secondary emotions represent emotions about other emotions. Distinguishing these elements of emotional processing are important parts of EFT emotion coaching.

Two forms included in this book provide ways for patients to rehearse enhancing emotional awareness: Form 2.3, the Emotion Log (Greenberg, 2002), and Form 8.1, which contains a series of EFT-based questions for patients to answer for themselves (Greenberg & Watson, 2005). The specifics of the implementation of these forms are discussed later in the Homework section.

To help bring structure, reliability, and repeatability to patients' practice of enhancing emotional awareness, the EFT therapist routinely uses an Emotion Log (Greenberg, 2002). This tool provides a simple way for patients to identify the situations and emotions that arise daily. The therapist can ask his or her patients to allow some of their attention to be directed toward their emotions each day. Patients should learn to attend to internal physical cues in order to notice their emotions. External cues are also important, and patients may learn to enhance their attention to emotional experiencing in certain situations that typically provoke an emotional response. When they become aware of their emotions, patients can use the Emotion Log to simply note what emotions present each day.

Form 8.1, Questions to Ask Yourself to Enhance Your Emotional Awareness, is a direct, step-by-step outline of questions and responses that are aimed at enhancing emotional experiencing. It presents a series of daily life questions that patients ask themselves. Patients record their responses to these questions and then review them with the therapist in session. These questions highlight a number of aspects of emotional processing that might not be typically associated with emotions for many patients. For example, a patient is asked about the physical experiences associated with emotions, the label he gives to emotions, and his thoughts that accompany the emotions. Also, the patient is asked if he is experiencing mixed emotions and, if so, to identify the emotions that are being experienced. The patient is asked to identify personal needs that these emotions are related to as well as behavioral urges that are involved in the emotional experience. In this way, the range of aspects of emotional processing that comprise dimensions of EI can be rehearsed and potentially strengthened through training.

Question to Pose/Intervention

"Using the five senses (vision, hearing, smell, taste, and touch), what can you notice around you in your environment? Turning your awareness inward, what physical sensations do you notice in the body in this moment? Where in your body are you experiencing sensations that you relate to your emotions just now? If you were to give a label—the name of a feeling—to your emotion, what would it be? What thoughts are going through your mind that you associate with this emotion? What needs or wants do you associate with this emotional state? What urges toward action arrive with this emotion? Is this a clearly defined emotion, or are you experiencing a mix of emotions? If so, what are the labels for the emotions you are feeling?"

Example

The following example involves a patient who complained about her inability to focus at work. Although this was her stated presenting problem, she appeared quite sad and frightened by her father's ongoing treatment for lung cancer. The patient rarely wanted her response to her father's treatment to be on the therapy agenda.

Patient: This week it has just been very difficult to focus at work and get anything done because I've been so stressed out.

Therapist: Stressed out?

Patient: Yeah, I guess I've sort of had my father's illness on my mind all week, and it makes it hard to get anything done. I'm very worried about whether or not I'll meet my deadlines. My boss is really demanding, and I just don't know what is wrong with me that I can't buck up and get the job done.

Therapist: It makes a lot of sense that your father would be on your mind, doesn't it? I know that he is facing some difficult, truly challenging medical treatments. I know, particularly from our discussion last week, that you are very concerned.

Patient: I just wish this whole thing didn't get in the way of work.

Therapist: Yes, I get that. Our emotions do show up on their own schedule, and when they arrive they sometimes ask a lot of us. What are you feeling right now?

Patient: Right now?

Therapist: Yes. How might you describe what you are feeling in this very moment?

Patient: I'm not sure. Sometimes I don't know what I feel. I just get stressed out and don't want to feel anything at all.

Therapist: I suppose it's natural to try to shut out or keep away feelings that are difficult to be with. Sometimes, I think, we do this without even knowing. Let's see if we can tune in a bit to your emotional experience in this moment. Would that be all right?

Patient: Yes, it's just that I'm not sure how to do that.

Therapist: That's OK. We can walk through the steps together. So, in this moment, what do you notice around you in your environment, using all of your five senses?

Patient: Well, I can hear the cars going by outside. I can feel my weight on the chair. When I look around, I can see the light and shadows in the room. Is this the sort of thing you mean?

Therapist: Yes, that's exactly what I mean. Now bringing your attention inward, what physical sensations do you notice in the body?

Patient: I guess I can feel a little tension in my throat. Now that you mention it, I can notice a little pressure on my temples. In fact, I kind of feel like I might cry.

Therapist: So these are sensations that you can connect with some emotion?

Patient: Yes.

Therapist: How would you label the emotion you are feeling in this moment?

Patient: When I stop and let myself feel it, I'm just so sad. I'm sorry.

Therapist: It's OK to be sad. I know that this is a very difficult time for you, with everything that you are facing. This sadness, when it arrives, what thoughts go through your mind? Is it all right for us to talk about those thoughts for a few moments?

Patient: Yes, of course. I guess I just really don't want to have to see my father go through these treatments. He is so strong and so positive, and it is just so devastating for him. I don't want this.

Therapist: Of course you don't. Your emotions, your response to this, are very natural and are very human.

Homework

Patients may work with either of the forms included in this section. The Emotion Log (Form 2.3) is more fundamental and less time consuming and may be particularly useful as an introduction to working with emotional awareness. Because this exercise focuses on noticing and labeling emotions, it may be particularly effective for patients with alexithymia.

The Questions to Ask Yourself to Enhance Your Emotional Awareness form (Form 8.1) involves a more thorough process and will take a bit more time to complete. This exercise may be assigned as homework to patients who have been introduced to working with emotional awareness in session and may serve as a follow-up to the Emotion Log.

Both of these homework exercises should be introduced in session, with therapist and patient working through the form together at least once as an example. The homework exercises may be assigned for a week or more so that the patient may have sufficient time to practice, apply, and generalize the skills involved in these forms.

Possible Problems

The forms and concepts discussed in this section may seem very simple and basic to clinicians and others who have spent some time exploring their emotional responses. Patients who present with a history of trauma or who have a developmental history that includes an emotionally invalidating family environment may have a habitual pattern of avoiding emotional experiencing (Wagner & Linehan, 2006; Walser & Hayes, 2006). Furthermore, affect avoidance is an aspect of experiential avoidance, which has been hypothesized to be a core process involved in many forms of psychopathology (Hayes et al., 1996). Focusing on and identifying emotions can provoke a great deal of anxiety and may also trigger efforts at avoidance or resistance.

Techniques for enhancing emotional experiences are like a set of Russian nesting dolls. Inside each of the questions asked there remains a world of other questions and associations. For example, when asking a patient "What needs do you associate with this emotion?," the therapist may discover a variety of automatic thoughts, emotional schemas, maladaptive assumptions, and patterns of emotional avoidance. As a result, the therapist will need to strike a careful balance in applying guided discovery to address the whole emotional experience and in shaping a new emotional response pattern in the patient. The therapist should normalize the patient's emotional experience, validate his or her emotional processing, and guide him or her to question the nature of the emotion and its related cognitions.

Cross-Reference to Other Techniques

Strategies for enhancing emotional awareness relate to a number of different techniques, particularly the mindfulness-based techniques. Mindfulness training can prepare the patient with decentering skills, which will be useful in enhancing emotional awareness. The making space meditation is particularly useful as a preparatory exercise for working with emotions. The 3-minute breathing space exercise also may be useful for opening up a field of awareness in which the patient can closely examine his or her emotional responses. Emotional schema-based techniques (examining beliefs of the danger, shame, guilt, incomprehensibility, uniqueness, need for control) can be helpful in examining the beliefs and strategies that are invoked when emotions are accessed. In addition, the Emotionally Intelligent Thought Record (described next) can also be useful in enhancing emotional awareness.

Forms

Form 2.3: Emotion Log

Form 8.1: Questions to Ask Yourself to Enhance Your Emotional Awareness

TECHNIQUE: THE EMOTIONALLY INTELLIGENT THOUGHT RECORD

Description

Beck's Dysfunctional Thought Record has become a central technique in cognitive therapy. This thought record provides a structured format for patients to engage in cognitive restructuring, identifying the situation that gives rise to an emotion, labeling and rating the degree of emotion, identifying the automatic thoughts and degree of belief in the thought, providing alternative or rational responses (and the degree of belief), and then rating the resultant emotion. For example, a patient who tells himself, "I can't stand feeling anxiety," may use restructuring techniques to identify an alternative thought, such as "I am strong enough to handle this, after all."

Having the patient complete the dysfunctional thought record is a useful technique, but when working with someone with emotion regulation and affect tolerance problems, the therapist may be seeking to target processes other than change of the content of cognitions. As we have been suggesting, a range of processes can be used in working with emotions, such as mindful contact with the present moment, radical acceptance, labeling and clarification of emotions, commitment to valued aims, behavioral experiments, emotional schema techniques, cognitive defusion, and relaxation training. This may seem like a lot for a therapist and patient to juggle together.

The aim of the Emotionally Intelligent Thought Record is to have patients ask themselves a number of questions that address a variety of these processes involved in a comprehensive approach to working with emotions. The Emotionally Intelligent Thought Record is designed to be used with patients who have already been introduced to concepts such as mindfulness and acceptance. Rather than seeking cognitive change exclusively, the series of questions outlined in this technique aims to bring patients' awareness to their present-moment experience in a way that will develop a greater capacity to remain in the presence of difficult experiences, while taking action in pursuit of a life well lived. Like the Dysfunctional Thought Record, the Emotionally Intelligent Thought Record seeks to provide a clear, workable format for homework practice in the hope of the development and generalization of particular skills.

The Emotionally Intelligent Thought Record is conceptualized from a particular perspective on thinking and feeling. This thought record is meant to be used from the assumption that internal events (such as thoughts and emotions) are not so much static constructs as they are a part of an ongoing flow of action, taking place in this moment. The Emotionally Intelligent Thought Record aims to bring the patient's attention to his or her moment-to-moment experiencing outside of the direct presence of the therapist, generalizing this experience through a daily homework exercise. From a certain point of view, the Emotionally Intelligent Thought Record is an exercise in applied mindfulness. Through its use, the patient practices decentration from distressing events in the mind, gradually bringing him- or herself into a different relationship with internal experiences that seems to drive his or her suffering. The questions presented in the next section and the clinical example clarify the specifics of the intervention.

Question to Pose/Intervention

The questions that form the structure of the Emotionally Intelligent Thought Record relate to fundamental experiential exercises from third-generation cognitive and behavioral therapies as well as the format of the Dysfunctional Thought Record. The work sheet itself begins with a brief instruction so that patients may be reminded of their therapist's instructions in session. Like the traditional Dysfunctional Thought Record, the Emotionally Intelligent Thought Record begins by asking patients to notice and establish the situation they find themselves in during their experience of disturbing emotions.

During the subsequent period of self-observation and inquiry, patients are meant to be practicing the application of "radical acceptance," whereby they adopt an observing stance regarding their experience. In doing so, the patients are examining and experiencing their reality not in the way they fear, believe, or insist it to be, but just as it is, in the moment, moment by moment.

Each successive set of questions invites patients to view their experience from this mindful, defused perspective, while examining their physical, emotional, cognitive, and behavioral responses.

Although this exercise is not explicitly aimed at cognitive restructuring, it does inevitably involve change in the form and function of patients' cognitions. If any change in thought content is witnessed, the therapist would be advised to help this change in thought to move toward a balanced, accepting, and empowered perspective rather than emphasizing an exclusively "rational" approach.

Processes that may be involved in this exercise include perspective taking, affect labeling, decentering, cultivating mindfulness, promoting cognitive defusion, exposure to affect, cognitive restructuring, and commitment to the behavioral pursuit of valued aims.

The therapist may ask the following questions in session, while referencing the Emotionally Intelligent Thought Record:

- *Step 1:* "What is going on around you, in your environment, right now? Where are you? Who is with you? What are you doing? What are you noticing in the environment that is affecting you?"

- *Step 2:* "Sometimes our response to something in our environment can be felt in the body, like 'butterflies in the stomach,' for example. Bringing our attention, as best as we can, to these sensations can be helpful. Developing awareness and sensitivity to these experiences can take practice, so if you don't notice anything in particular, just allow yourself that experience, while taking a moment or two to give yourself some time to observe whatever may be present. In this situation, what physical sensations do you notice yourself experiencing in your body? Where in your body do you feel such sensations? What are the qualities of such sensations?"

- *Step 3:* "Labeling our emotions using 'feeling words' can be helpful. What 'feeling word' would best describe and 'label' this emotion that you are feeling in this moment? How intensely would you say you are feeling this emotion? If you were to rate this emotion on a scale of 0–100, with 100 being the most intense feeling you could have and 0 being no presence of this feeling at all, what would that rating be?"

- *Step 4:* "What thoughts are going through your mind in this situation? Ask yourself, 'What is going through my mind right now? What is my mind telling me?' What is 'popping into your head' in this situation? What does this situation say about you? What does this situation suggest about your future? As best as you can, notice the flow of thoughts that unfold in your mind in this situation. What are some of the thoughts that are arriving?"

- *Step 5:* "We have learned to try to get rid of, or get away from, things that seem threatening or unpleasant. This makes a lot of sense. But attempts to suppress or eliminate distressing thoughts and feelings sometimes makes them that much stronger. So, for a moment, take this opportunity to learn to stay with your experience, just as it is. Following the flow of your breath in this moment, as much as you can, make space for whatever unfolds before your mind."

- *Step 6:* "Now that you have noticed, and allowed yourself to more fully experience, the sensations, emotions, and thoughts that have shown up in this situation, how might you best respond in this moment? Adopting a mindful, 'emotionally intelligent' attitude, you can recognize that these thoughts and feelings are events in the mind, and not reality itself. Working with your therapist, you can learn many ways to respond to distressing thoughts and feelings. Here are a few questions to ask yourself that you can practice over the course of the coming week:

    o 'What are the costs and benefits to me of believing these thoughts?'
    o 'How might I act if I really believed this?'
    o 'How might I act if I didn't believe this?'
    o 'What might I say to a friend who was facing this situation?'
    o 'What needs are involved in this event, and how can I best take care of myself now?'
    o 'Can I mindfully observe these events in my mind, choose a course of action, and act in a way that will serve my aims?'"

- *Step 7:* "Ask yourself the following questions:

    o 'How can I best pursue my own aims and values in this situation?'
    o 'Is there a problem here that I need to solve in order to live my life in a meaningful and valued way?'

    o 'How can I interact with others in this situation in an effective way that suits my aims and values?'

    o 'Does this situation call for a behavioral response? Does any action need to be taken?'

    o 'Is doing nothing an option?'

    o 'How can I take care of myself best in this situation?' "

Example

Therapist: You've described several situations this past week when your fear of vomit was very troubling. It seemed to be on your mind a lot during your children's playdates, didn't it?

Patient: It really did. A lot of the children at the nursery school have been sick with the flu lately, and I just couldn't stop worrying that one of the kids would come home with a stomach virus. It really freaked me out.

Therapist: And if one of them did come home with a stomach virus, what did you fear might happen?

Patient: Well, I was afraid they would throw up, of course. Then I would have to deal with it, which would freak me out, and I just don't know if I could handle it.

Therapist: I know that this thought, "I don't know if I could handle it," has shown up along with a lot of anxiety in the past.

Patient: It sure has, but I think it's *true*. What kind of a mother can't deal with her own children throwing up?

Therapist: So when this thought shows up, it brings friends and it means business, doesn't it? So now it seems that you're having the thought that you are somehow defective as a mother.

Patient: Of course I am! Why would we even be having this discussion if I weren't.

Therapist: You know, a lot seems to be coming up for you in this very moment, so I would like to use this part of our session as an opportunity to practice a new way of working with these thoughts and feelings.

Patient: What do you mean?

Therapist: As part of our agenda for the session today, you might remember that we discussed introducing a new self-therapy practice exercise. Why don't we take a look at that self-therapy exercise right now and rehearse it together in this session. Would that be all right?

Patient: Sure. I am looking for just about anything to take this feeling away today.

Therapist: Well, I'm not so sure we are aiming to "take any feelings away" just now. In fact, part of our work is going to be allowing some of these feelings and thoughts to stay here, in the room, as we work together. Do you remember our earlier mindfulness work?

Patient: Yes, sure. I'm still practicing the "mindfulness of the breath" exercise each morning. Just for 15 minutes, though. Are you going to be asking me to just "accept" these feelings?

Therapist: You are right, accepting feelings is part of it, but there is more that we can do. Sometimes acceptance is passive, just letting things take their course. But sometimes acceptance can be very active. It can involve seeing things clearly as they are, while deeply engaging with what matters most to us in our lives.

Patient: Yes, I remember that, and it's been a little bit helpful when I pick up the kids.

Therapist: So, this "willingness to feel things more fully" *has* been helpful?

Patient: I said a little bit! (*laughing*) but ... yeah, it has been helping.

Therapist: All right, so here we are, in this office, at 2:00 in the afternoon, and we are discussing your fear of your children vomiting.

Patient: Yes, and I hate even thinking about it.

Therapist: That makes sense. So, could you briefly describe the situation you are in that is activating these thoughts and fears about vomit, please?

Patient: I'm sitting with my therapist, and we are talking about my fear of vomit. It's two in the afternoon, and later I will have to pick up my kids from nursery school.

Therapist: So, as we've seen, sometimes the first place to look, in order to bring our awareness more fully to our experience, is to check in with what sensations are showing up in the body.

Patient: Like in the "body scan" exercise?

Therapist: Like that, yes. This time, though, we are checking in on our experience in "real time" so that we can train our awareness to really "be with" our experience in this moment, as we live our lives. So, bringing your attention, as best as you can, to the presence of sensation in the body in this moment, what physical sensations do you notice yourself experiencing in your body?

Patient: I feel like my breath is short, like there is pressure on my chest.

Therapist: Good. You were able to notice that fairly rapidly. Now, without trying to change or alter that experience, would you be willing to just allow yourself to stay with this feeling of shortness of breath, and this feeling of pressure on your chest, as we proceed with this exercise?

Patient: Yes, I can do that. It's not like it's going to go away anyway! (*Laughs.*)

Therapist: (*laughing with the patient*) That's a pretty keen observation there. Now, taking a moment to truly make space for and allow this experience, what "feeling word" would best describe and "label" this emotion that you are feeling in this moment?

Patient: Feeling word? You mean like a name of an emotion?

Therapist: Yes, that's it exactly.

Patient: Well, then it would be "anxiety." This definitely feels like "anxiety," or maybe you could also even call this "fear.

Therapist: Good, you were able to label that experience quite clearly, weren't you?

Homework

The steps of the Emotionally Intelligent Thought Record (Forms 8.2 and 8.3) are best introduced in the session as an interactive process. Rather than simply handing Form 8.2 or 8.3 to the patient and going through the steps, the therapist is better advised to learn and practice these steps and questions in advance and to gradually work through the questions that are included in the form during the session. The purpose of the work sheet is to notice, distance, label, allow, and alter one's relationship to difficult experiences as one moves toward effective action. Often metaphors of practicing a new skill may be helpful. For example, the therapist may offer the following observation: "When we learn a new skill, repetition and 'overlearning' are sometimes helpful. So this work sheet can provide you with a structure to practice engaging with your experience in a new way. If you were learning how to play the violin, you might practice scales or exercises. If you were learning how to play golf, you might go to the driving range. You might want to think of the Emotionally Intelligent Thought Record like those exercises: a simple process that you can repeat often, so that you learn something new and important."

Possible Problems

The Emotionally Intelligent Thought Record is an exercise that may become fundamental to a way of working with patients, but it is not a "simple" tool for simplistic therapy. The use of this technique assumes that the therapist and the patient have begun working with the concepts of acceptance and willingness. Also, some prior training in the cultivation of mindfulness is highly recommended. An active, vital, empathic, and collaborative therapeutic relationship is also foundational to the effective use of this technique.

Patients who have intense difficulty with affect tolerance may show some initial resistance to certain aspects of this technique. First, bringing awareness to physical sensations can actually intensify the experience of anxiety at first. This is a normal, and perhaps necessary, step, but it needs to be addressed in a compassionate yet directive way by the therapist. In using the Emotionally Intelligent Thought Record, the therapist is, in effect, guiding his or her patients to remain in the presence of internal events that they may have a kind of "phobic" response to. This may reflect some underlying emotional schematic process, alexithymia, or a general tendency toward experiential avoidance. Whatever the driving force behind this tendency, the therapist's aim in such cases is to create an accepting, safe, empathic, and collaborative context, within which patients can come to observe troubling sensations as they rise and fall.

Second, patients may be unwilling to allow their experience to unfold, just as it is, in the moment. This can be viewed as an *in vivo* example of the tendency toward experiential avoidance that may be driving much of the struggles that patients present. Although this resistance may be seen as a "potential problem," it really is a manifestation of the greater problem itself. The Emotionally Intelligent Thought Record provides a structure for patients to gradually address this tendency to avoid and to move past this avoidance to effectively engage with their experience. Part of the therapist's aim is to strike a balance between a gentle and gradual shaping of effective engagement on the part of the patients and the consistent maintenance of a structured approach that does not collude with their attempts at avoidance.

Third, patients who strongly believe, "buy into," or demonstrate cognitive fusion with troubling thoughts may have a hard time stepping out of the trap of debating the "truth" of such thoughts. This can lead the well-intentioned therapist to become further entangled with his or her patients' cognitive content, falling into the "rabbit hole" of arguing with thoughts and increasing the amount of control that these thoughts may have over behavior. Cognitive restructuring techniques have demonstrated efficacy in certain applications and are an aspect of the

Emotionally Intelligent Thought Record. However, this technique emphasizes the adoption of a very different relationship with thinking and feeling than is often held by patients in CBT. Using decentration and disidentification, patients are invited to engage with and question their thoughts with almost a "sense of play." By changing the relationship or vantage point they have with their flow of thinking and feeling, the act of cognitive reappraisal can be aimed at addressing not only the structure of negative automatic thoughts but their function. The degree to which troubling patterns of thinking exert control of behavior and impinge on patients' ability to live a meaningful and rewarding life is a more central aim of the Emotionally Intelligent Thought Record than merely moving toward rational thinking.

Thus far, we have discussed patient-oriented problems in implementing this technique. There are, in addition, problems in using the Emotionally Intelligent Thought Record that may begin with the therapist. In order to use this technique effectively, several therapist- and therapy-related factors must be present. The therapist using mindfulness and willingness-based techniques is strongly advised to have developed and maintained a personal practice of mindfulness training for him- or herself. This element of therapist training and preparation has been emphasized in a range of third-generation CBT therapies (Roemer & Orsillo, 2009; Segal et al., 2002). Additionally, the Emotionally Intelligent Thought Record is meant to be a part of a thoughtful approach to therapy, which involves a fully developed case conceptualization. Both therapist and patient are best served by a course of therapy that involves the therapist having a clear and cogent understanding of the patient's patterns of experiential avoidance, symptom presentation, maintaining and mitigating factors involved in the expression of symptoms, and learning history and as clear an understanding as possible of the patient's emotional schemas. Further, an understanding of the patient's valued aims and his or her degree of commitment to these aims would also be helpful. Without this broader understanding, importing this technique into a free-standing traditional mode of CBT would be less than optimal.

Cross-Reference to Other Techniques

The Emotionally Intelligent Thought Record relates to enhancing emotional awareness, mindfulness techniques, affect labeling, identifying emotional schemas, and many other techniques presented in this text. This daily thought record is meant to summarize and provide generalization practice for the entire human act of emotion regulation, involving, as it must, mindful awareness, acceptance, self-compassion, values-consistent behaviors, cognitive restructuring, and an emotionally intelligent awareness of emotional schemas.

Forms

Forms 8.2 and 8.3 present two variations on the Emotionally Intelligent Thought Record. The first is a great deal longer and provides a comprehensive description of each of the questions. This long version is meant to be used during the first 1 or 2 weeks of working with the Emotionally Intelligent Thought Record, gently and comprehensively walking patients through the questions that their therapist might ask in session. This provides an opportunity for patients to rehearse and generalize the work they have been engaging in during sessions. Once the client has demonstrated an understanding of the steps involved, they may switch to the short form (8.3), which provides brief versions of each question, with less explanation of the steps undertaken.

Form 8.2: Emotionally Intelligent Thought Record (Long Form)

Form 8.3: Emotionally Intelligent Thought Record (Short Form)

CONCLUSIONS

These techniques, drawn from EFT and integrative CBT, focus patients' efforts directly on the enhancement of their emotional processing. The methods described are based on the concept of the therapeutic relationship serving as an intrinsically affect regulating bond (Greenberg, 2007). Within this context, various processes described throughout this text may be at work, such as mindful awareness, self-compassion, cultivating willingness, and change in emotional schemas. The forms and exercises presented here can be used to focus patients' emotion regulation training specifically on various elements of restructuring or working with emotional schemas.

Each of the practices described in the techniques in this chapter clearly prioritizes enhancing emotional processing in a step-by-step manner. These tools are provided in a manner that does not lock therapists into a particular way of conceptualizing a case and that is not bound to a particular theoretical modality. Therapists should apply their own clinical judgment regarding integrating these techniques, and their work in enhancing emotional intelligence, into the case formulation and treatment plan that they have developed for each patient.

CHAPTER NINE

Cognitive Restructuring

As we indicated in Chapter 1 emotional regulation can include any intervention that affects the intensity and discomfort of emotional experience and the degree of impairment. Thus, cognitive therapy can be viewed as a set of interventions relevant to emotion regulation. Indeed, Beck's (1976) seminal book *Cognitive Therapy and the Emotional Disorders* reflects the recognition that cognitive processes may lead to, maintain, or exacerbate emotional experience. There has been considerable debate about whether cognitive styles or processes are a vulnerability factor in depression and anxiety. For example, once depression is in remission, formerly depressed patients are no different from never-depressed controls in endorsing automatic thoughts or dysfunctional attitudes (Miranda & Persons, 1988). This raises the question of whether cognitive distortions or biases are simply part of depression—a kind of "epiphenomenon"—and not a predisposing factor. However, other research demonstrates that cognitive biases or distortions are latent vulnerabilities—they are mood dependent. When primed through affect induction, these cognitive distortions become manifest for previously depressed patients currently in remission (Ingram, Miranda, & Segal, 1998; Miranda, Gross, Persons, & Hahn, 1998). Other research demonstrates long-term vulnerability of explanatory style to future depressive and manic episodes (Alloy, Abramson, Safford, & Gibb, 2006; Alloy, Reilly-Harrington, Fresco, Whitehouse, & Zechmeister, 1999). Moreover, the "cognitive style" of rumination is also a predictor of future depressive episodes (Nolen-Hoeksema, 2000; Roelofs, et al., 2009). Consistent with Gross's outline of emotion regulation, cognitive restructuring is an effective "antecedent" emotion regulation strategy (Gross, 1998a, 1998b; Gross & Thompson, 2007). By modifying the interpretation of events, the individual can effectively reduce the emotional impact. This is also consistent with EST in that concepts of durability, danger, incomprehensibility, and lack of control can be modified by regulating emotion through reinterpretation of potentially stressful events. In this chapter, we examine how cognitive restructuring can be used in emotion regulation.

Although there is a dispute as to whether cognitive restructuring is an essential component of mood change, there is considerable evidence that it can be helpful. Use of cognitive therapy techniques focusing directly on symptoms predicts improvement in therapy (Roelofs et al., 2009). The importance of the mediating role of cognitions in change is supported by the findings that sudden gains in therapy are preceded by changes in thinking, that patients with sudden gains (whose cognitions have changed) maintain these gains 2 years later, and that changes in cognitive content mediate improvement in panic symptoms for patients in CBT (DeRubeis &

Feeley, 1990; Tang & DeRubeis, 1999). However, other evidence questions the mediating role of cognitive change in sudden gains in social phobia (Tang, DeRubeis, Hollon, Amsterdam, & Shelton, 2007). Nonetheless, there is considerable evidence for the efficacy of cognitive therapy in the treatment of depression and in all of the anxiety disorders (Hofmann, Schulz, Meuret, Suvak, & Moscovitch, 2006).

A wide variety of techniques can be used to help the patient restructure dysfunctional thoughts. A compendium of almost 100 of the techniques is available in Leahy's (2003a) *Cognitive Therapy Techniques: A Practitioner's Guide* as well as Bennett-Levy et al.'s (2004) *Oxford Guide to Behavioural Experiments in Cognitive Therapy*. In this chapter, we have chosen several techniques that can be easily used by patients in their self-help homework, but the clinician interested in helping patients cope with difficult mood regulation issues may wish to consult these additional sources for further details.

TECHNIQUE: DISTINGUISHING THOUGHTS FROM FEELINGS

Description

Many patients who have intense feelings have difficulty recognizing that a feeling is not the same thing as reality and not the same thing as a thought. This is especially evident in "emotional reasoning" where the patient may tell her- or himself, "I just feel awful. Life is just terrible." Here the patient has a feeling ("awful") along with a thought ("life is terrible") that can be distinguished from the facts ("What is the evidence that life is terrible?"). In cognitive therapy, it is essential for the patient to get some distance from thoughts and feelings in order to evaluate them. This decentering can begin in the first session, where the therapist assists the patient in recognizing how thoughts may lead to feelings (and to behavior) and that alternative thoughts are also possible, thereby leading to different feelings and different behaviors.

Question to Pose/Intervention

"Imagine that you are walking along a street at night and it's dark and there is no one around. You now hear two men coming from behind you, walking fast toward you. You have the thought 'These guys are going to attack me.' What kinds of feelings would you have? What would do?" The patient might indicate that he would feel afraid and might try to run. The therapist can then proceed with the following: "But imagine that you thought, 'These are two people from the conference I was at.' What might you feel and do then?" The patient might indicate that he would feel relaxed or even curious to meet them and would simply continue on his walk.

Example

Therapist: One of the things that we find important is to distinguish between a thought and a feeling. A feeling is an emotion, such that you say you feel sad, anxious, afraid, happy, curious, hopeless, or angry. We don't dispute that you have a feeling—it would not make sense for me to say that you don't feel sad when you have told me that you feel sad. Feelings are simply true because you simply tell me that you have a feeling. What feelings are you having recently?

Patient: I feel sad and a little hopeless.

Therapist: OK. And I can see that you also recognize that your feeling can have a range of intensity; for example, you mentioned a little hopeless. So it's possible to feel more hopeless, less hopeless, or very hopeless. We will want to keep that in mind that your feeling varies in intensity. Now let's look at the thoughts that might make someone feel sad. These thoughts might be, "I will never get what I need" or "I will always be unhappy." Or there might be thoughts like, "I can't do anything right." Those are thoughts that might lead to the feeling of sadness or hopelessness.

Patient: Yeah, I've sometimes had those thoughts, too.

Therapist: Now a thought is not the same thing as a feeling. We can take a thought such as, "I never do anything right" and test it out against the facts. Let's take the thought, "It's raining outside." How would I test that out?

Patient: You would go outside and see if you get wet.

Therapist: Right. We would collect the facts. And it might or might not be raining. So, when you say you have the feeling of sadness and it might be related to the thought, "I can't do anything right," we could test out whether the facts support your thought. We can see if there is anything that you have done right. And then we would know how accurate your thought is.

Patient: Yeah, but I really do feel sad.

Therapist: That's absolutely right that you feel this way. But what if the thoughts that you had turned out not to be as absolute as your feeling? What if you believed that you did a lot of things right?

Patient: I guess I would feel a lot better.

Therapist: That's what we will have to look at. We'll have to see if your thoughts hold up against the facts. So, we have established a couple of things. First, thoughts and feeling are different. Second, we can test out whether thoughts are true. And, third, thoughts and facts are different. We also know that your thoughts can change and that might change the way you feel. So we have some work ahead of us.

Homework

The patient can be assigned Form 9.1 (Distinguishing Thoughts from Feelings), which lists the feelings that he has and the thoughts that accompany the feelings. The form also provides a short description of the "situation," that is, what is going on that triggers these feelings. In addition, the therapist can ask the patient to indicate on a scale from 0 to 100 the degree to which he has the feeling and the degree to which he feels confident in believing the thought.

Possible Problems

Some patients with a sense of anxious urgency may claim that they cannot use these techniques because they are too anxious. The therapist can stress that the use of these techniques is precisely for the purpose of reducing the sense of urgency and anxiety. However, more simple stress reduction techniques such as deep muscle relaxation or breathing exercises may be useful in preparing for the use of cognitive restructuring and the reduction of time urgency. In some cases, the patient may say, "I can't think of doing these things when I am upset. It doesn't occur to me." The therapist can ask the patient to write down three or four reminders of specific techniques to use so that the patient can "trigger" cognitive therapy techniques rather than time urgency. These reminders can be placed in prominent places that are likely to be associated with time urgency.

Some patients claim that they do not have any thoughts, just feelings. For example, the patient might say, "I just feel depressed. I'm not thinking anything." The therapist can assist the patient in identifying thoughts by suggesting some possible thoughts that other patients have had: "Sometimes when people are depressed they think [nothing will work out, I'm a loser, I can't do anything, I don't enjoy anything]" and follow up by inquiring whether any of these or other thoughts sound familiar. Another possibility is to have the patient identify the situations that trigger the depressed feeling and then examine what he or she might be thinking. The patient can write down these thoughts and attempt to monitor his or her thinking during the week to see whether any seem familiar. Some patients are assisted in identifying thoughts if the therapist can get them to focus on specific details (visual, auditory, olfactory, touch) associated with the feeling, thereby eliciting the contextual cues of the emotion.

Cross-Reference to Other Techniques

Inducing imagery to activate thoughts and feelings can be helpful. Also, patients can often distinguish thoughts from feelings by examining the list of cognitive distortions in the checklist below.

Form

Form 9.1: Distinguishing Thoughts from Feelings

TECHNIQUE: CATEGORIZING NEGATIVE THOUGHTS

Description

The cognitive model proposes that negative thoughts can be categorized in terms of the kinds of biases and inferential errors that underpin the way the patient is thinking. For example, the patient who is upset because she believes a friend thinks she is a loser may be engaged in "mind reading" and the patient who predicts, "I will always be alone," is using fortune telling. It is possible that these thoughts could turn out to be accurate, but the first step is to see whether there is a pattern to the style of thinking.

Question to Pose/Intervention

"A lot of times we find that we are having the same kinds of negative thoughts that make us upset. Now these thoughts could be true or false and we won't know until we collect the facts to find out. But it may be that you could be using certain ways of thinking that habitually upset you. We have a list of common biases in thinking that people have who get depressed and anxious, and it might be helpful to go through this list to see if you recognize yourself in using these thoughts." The therapist then presents the patient with Form 9.2 (Categories of Automatic Thoughts) and explains each one. The therapist can then ask the patient whether he or she often uses any of these specific ways of thinking and inquires how it makes him or her feel.

Example

Therapist: All of us get upset at times but sometimes we can get really upset and find that this is related to some things that we are thinking at the time. Right now we don't know how accurate your thoughts can be—perhaps they are true. But we haven't really examined that at this point. I have a listing of some ways of thinking that we find often goes along with feeling depressed and anxious. And I'd like to go through this list with you to see whether you might recognize some ways that you are thinking. (*Presents Form 9.2.*)

Patient: Well, I can see right off that I do mind reading. I was thinking that you thought I was boring.

Therapist: OK. That's an excellent example of a style of thinking that could upset you. How did it make you feel to think that?

Patient: Well, I felt sad and anxious, and I worried that you might not want me as a patient.

Therapist: Do you think you do a lot of mind reading with other people, too?

Patient: Yes. I do it with Becky a lot, and I think that she doesn't find me attractive and thinks I'm a drag.

Therapist: How about this one, "fortune-telling"? Do you do this, too?

Patient: I keep worrying that Becky is going to leave me or that she'll find someone more interesting.

Therapist: And how does this fortune-telling make you feel?

Patient: It makes me feel afraid, like I can't really count on her and then I think I'll be alone forever.

Therapist: The thought about being alone forever is another fortune-telling thought, isn't it?

Patient: I guess I'm doing these things a lot.

Therapist: We might want to see whether there are certain ways of thinking that you are in the habit of using and if this is related to your sadness, anxiety, and hopelessness.

Homework

The patient can be given Form 9.2 (Categories of Automatic Thoughts), which lists the specific categories. Then the patient can be asked to summarize, using Form 9.3 (Four-Column Thought Form), whether there is a pattern of certain kinds of thoughts that come up frequently and certain situations that elicit these thoughts.

Possible Problems

Some patients believe that they are unable to categorize a thought because it appears to fall into more than one category. For example, "Tom will think I'm a loser" is an example of both fortune telling and mind reading. This does not really pose any problem because thoughts can belong to more than one category. Another problem is that implicit in a thought, for some patients, is the evaluation of the thought. For example, the automatic thought above might "contain" an implicit evaluation that it would be catastrophic if Tom thought he was a loser. This can be distinguished as another underlying thought that can also be categorized. Finally, some patients are reluctant to categorize their thoughts because they believe that their thoughts are true. This is a valid concern, and the therapist should indicate that categorization does not mean that the thought is invalid, only that it is an example of one way of thinking. These thoughts can then be examined by considering the facts or logic.

Cross-Reference to Other Techniques

Other techniques that are relevant include using imagery to elicit thoughts and feelings, distinguishing a thought from a feeling, and examining the implications and assumptions of the thought.

Forms

Form 9.2: Categories of Automatic Thoughts
Form 9.3: Four-Column Thought Form

TECHNIQUE: WEIGHING THE COSTS AND BENEFITS

Description

Patients are often of a mixed mind regarding their negative thoughts. Some may believe that their negative predictions and interpretations help protect them, prepare them for the worst, avoid surprise and regret, or motivate them to achieve goals or that these thoughts are simply realistic. Indeed, there may be a grain of truth in each of these beliefs in the advantage of negative thinking. Sometimes it is useful to anticipate possible negatives to avoid being blindsided, and sometimes negative predictions allow us to plan to overcome obstacles or to avoid them in the first place. Simply urging people to think positively is not helpful and may, in cases of patients with low self-esteem, actually backfire. However, beliefs have consequences, and in order to modify a belief the patient needs to have some investment in the idea that such cognitive restructuring can be helpful. Thus, the therapist engages the patient in a dialogue about the costs and benefits of negative beliefs.

Question to Pose/Intervention

"Some beliefs have consequences for how we feel, what we do, and how we relate to people. We will be looking at a lot of the thoughts that you have and we will test them out against the facts.

But before we can do that we need to examine your mixed motivation about these beliefs. For example, you might think that some of these beliefs are helpful to you or that you need to have these beliefs for certain reasons. Examining the costs and benefits of these beliefs doesn't mean that they are wrong or right—It simply helps us look at what you might be gaining or losing from thinking certain things."

Example

Therapist: What are you thinking about when you are feeling so sad?

Patient: I just think I'm a loser.

Therapist: That must be a difficult thought to have. Sometimes we think that our thoughts will help us, even if they are negative and painful to have. Can you think of any advantages that you might get out of thinking that you are a loser?

Patient: Well, maybe if I criticize myself I'll get more motivated. I'll drive myself harder. But I can't think of any other advantages.

Therapist: How about the disadvantages of that thought?

Patient: It makes me depressed, hopeless, and it makes me feel that I will be alone forever.

Therapist: OK. So if you had to weigh the advantages and disadvantages of the thought that you are a loser—and divide up 100 points—is it 50:50, 60:40, 40:60?

Patient: I'd say that the disadvantages far outweigh the advantages. I don't know how you can really put numbers on this, but I'd say it's 10 for the advantages and 90 for the disadvantages.

Therapist: OK. So the disadvantages outweigh the advantages. What would change, then, if you believed this thought a lot less?

Patient: I'd feel a lot better—more hopeful and less depressed about myself.

Therapist: And do you really think that criticizing yourself has been that motivating?

Patient: Sometimes it can be—but most of the time I feel worse.

Therapist: Do you get more or less done when you feel worse?

Patient: Probably less done. I procrastinate and think about how bad things are.

Therapist: So, you might think that this self-criticism motivates you but sometimes it takes away your motivation.

Homework

Using Form 9.4 (Examining the Advantages and Disadvantages of Thoughts), patients can identify several negative thoughts that are associated with difficult emotions and identify the advantages and disadvantages.

Possible Problems

Some patients may deny that there is any advantage to a negative thought. Such patients may want to appear rational or may be so overwhelmed with the negativity of the thought and emotion that it is hard to imagine gaining anything from the thought. The therapist can encourage these patients to examine possible advantages: "Perhaps right now, at a rational and calm moment, there don't appear to be any advantages but usually there are some hidden away in your mind. What could anyone hope to gain from these negative thoughts?" If this does not work, the therapist can suggest some possible advantages: "Maybe criticizing yourself motivates you or seems realistic."

Cross-Reference to Other Techniques

Some patients may claim that there are no advantages to their thought; it just makes them miserable. The therapist might suggest that sometimes the advantages are hard to see, but that there may be some. The therapist can also suggest some possible advantages, "Is it possible that this thought keeps you prepared? That you won't be surprised?" Of course, it may be that there are no advantages that can be identified. Other patients may claim that the thought is advantageous. In this case, the therapist can examine what the patient is choosing as the consequence: "If you believe that you have to be perfect, are you then willing to pay the price of worry and self-criticism?"

Form

Form 9.4: Examining the Advantages and Disadvantages of Thoughts

TECHNIQUE: EXAMINING THE EVIDENCE

Description

The patient's belief in a thought may be modified by examining the evidence supporting or refuting the thought. The nature of an automatic thought is that it is automatic and often goes unexamined by the patient. Its credibility is often based on its emotional charge, and the patient who is depressed or anxious often has a biased selection of information and discount information that is countervailing. Moreover, the quality of the evidence should be considered. For example, the anxious patient may be using his or her emotions as evidence or may be focusing on one small detail or event and ignoring other information that would balance against his or her belief. In addition, the logical connection between the "evidence" and the thought can also be examined.

Question to Pose/Intervention

"A lot of the thoughts that we have can make us feel anxious and depressed. Sometime they are valid thoughts but other times we may be looking at events in a way that we don't use all the information that might be available. Let's look at this thought that is upsetting you and let's examine whether the evidence or facts support the degree to which you believe the thought. Draw a line down the center of the page, and on the left side let's list all the evidence in favor of this thought and on the right side all the evidence against the thought. In listing the evidence, you don't have to believe the evidence 100%. I would just like to examine all the possible ways of evaluating this thought so we can see if we can have a different perspective."

Example

Therapist: I can see that you are thinking that you will never be happy again. That's a really powerful thought that must be upsetting you quite a bit. How much do you believe that thought, using a scale from 0 to 100%?

Patient: I guess I would have to say about 95%.

Therapist: So, it's a thought that seems almost absolutely true to you at this moment. And when you have this thought at 95%, how sad and hopeless do you feel, using a scale from 0 to 100%?

Patient: About the same. About 95% for both. Sometimes I feel 100% hopeless.

Therapist: OK. So it's a thought that makes you feel sad and hopeless and, I imagine, if we changed the degree to which you believed that thought your feelings might also change. Does that make sense?

Patient: Yeah. But I really believe it's true. I've been depressed for the past 2 months.

Therapist: That's hard to be depressed like that. Sometimes, though, our thoughts may be partly true, but not as absolute as they feel. Let's take a look at the evidence that you are using—the facts—that make you think and feel this way. And let's see if there is any evidence against this thought. I would like you to draw a line down the center of the page here, and on the left side list evidence in favor of this thought and on the right side evidence against the thought. Let's start with the evidence that you have that you will never be happy.

Patient: Well, I am feeling depressed now and I've felt depressed for 2 months. I've had problems with depression before. I don't have a relationship right now.

Therapist: OK. I can see where that would make you feel sad. Now, let's see if there is any reason to believe that you might be happy again at some time.

Patient: It's hard to imagine that right now. But I guess I have been happy in the past. There are some things at work that I like to do.

Therapist: Let's look at some things that you have done in the past month that have given you some pleasure or a sense of accomplishing things.

Patient: It always seems like such drudgery. But I do get some pleasure out of running, although I haven't been doing that much exercise for the last few weeks. I enjoyed dinner with my friend Bill. He's a good friend, really cares. I enjoyed the special on television about the National Parks.

Therapist: OK. Let's write those down as evidence that you can experience some happiness some of the time. If you were not depressed, what would be some things that have made you feel good in your life?

Patient: Learning new things makes me feel good. It's good to grow. And I have enjoyed traveling—I had a great trip to Brazil last year. Watching football, especially with my friends.

Therapist: OK. We can add those things to your list. When you look at the evidence that you will be unhappy forever, it seems to be based on how you have been feeling in the last 2 months, which have been very hard for you. What do you make of the fact that you have felt happy before?

Patient: I have felt better. But it just feels so bad now.

Therapist: Sometimes we judge the future by the way we feel at the present moment. But it also makes sense to step back from the way you feel and look at your capacity to feel good before the recent crisis in your life. And, come to think of it, you also have times right now when you feel good. What do you make of that?

Patient: I guess I am focusing a lot on the current situation.

Therapist: Well, we do that when we are upset, don't we? But I am also thinking that you might even begin assigning some of these pleasurable things to yourself to see if it affects your mood. You might assign exercise, seeing friends, watching the game, learning new things, even planning some travel just to see if it helps a little bit.

Patient: That might help. I just feel so down so much now.

Therapist: Yeah. It's a hard time. But this sense of hopelessness seems to be based on just that—feeling down right now. If you looked at the evidence that you have been happy before, that there are things that you are doing—and could do more of—that make you feel better and that you have gotten over depressions before, what do you think about the idea that you will never be happy again?

Patient: I guess I don't believe it as much. Maybe there's hope.

Therapist: So, if you had to rate the degree to which you believe you will never be happy, using the scale from 0 to 100%, what would you give it?

Patient: Maybe 50%. But I still believe it to some degree.

Therapist: I would expect that a strong belief would hold on for a while. But in 10 minutes it's changed from 95% to 50%. Does that make you feel differently?

Patient: I guess I feel more hopeful. Maybe I can change.

Homework

The therapist can assign Form 9.5 (Examining the Evidence for a Thought) with the accompanying instructions:

> "Every day you may have some negative thoughts about yourself, your experience, or the future. You may be worried about bad things happening or label yourself in ways that are upsetting to you. Use the Examining the Evidence for a Thought form every day to list the evidence for and against your thoughts. Ask yourself if the evidence in favor of your negative thought is based on your emotions rather than the facts. See if you have a tendency to overlook or discount or minimize evidence against your negative thoughts. Then weigh the evidence and write out your conclusion about your negative thought."

Possible Problems

Some patients use their emotions as evidence of the validity of their thought: "I must be a loser because I feel so depressed." This emotional reasoning can be identified as the kinds of evidence that the patient is using and then examined in terms of the quality of the evidence: "If I felt exhilarated and thought I was God, does that make me God?" Another problem is that some patients believe that simply believing a thought very strongly confers validity to the thought: "There must be something to it if I believe it so strongly." The therapist can ask if there are strong beliefs that were once held about religion, politics, conventional conduct, or Santa Claus that are no longer believed.

Cross-Reference to Other Techniques

Other useful techniques include vertical descent, weighing the costs and benefits, and challenging the logical structure of thoughts.

Form

Form 9.5: Examining the Evidence for a Thought

TECHNIQUE: DEFENSE ATTORNEY

Description

Sometimes patients recognize that there may be arguments or evidence against their negative thoughts, but they lack the motivation and direction to challenge those thoughts. They may believe that they cannot challenge or evaluate the thoughts unless they already believe that the thoughts are irrational or extreme—they get stuck in an emotional vicious cycle: "I can't challenge the thought because I already believe it." The cognitive therapist can assist patients in gaining distance from the emotional charge of a thought by considering the thought as a participant in a trial. With this technique, patients take the role of defending themselves against the negative thought by becoming an "attorney" whose job is to defend the client, in this case the patients themselves.

Question to Pose/Intervention

"Sometimes when we feel down it's hard to stand outside of our thoughts and feelings and take a different perspective. But let's imagine that your negative thoughts were part of the prosecution in a trial—trying to find you guilty. They have been labeling you in all kinds of terrible ways (e.g., lazy, stupid, hopeless, condemned to sadness forever). We are going to use a technique called Defense Attorney where you play the role of a very skilled, highly motivated lawyer who defends *you* against these negative thoughts. Like all good lawyers, you don't have to believe everything your client says or does—you just have to defend him. So, your job, counselor, is to defend yourself. We can start with my playing the defense attorney and shift later with you playing the defense attorney. When I play the defense attorney, you will be the prosecutor."

Example

Therapist: (*citing the prior description*) I am going to play the defense attorney and you play the prosecutor. So, I'd like you to charge me with all of the complaints in your negative thoughts, such as, "He is a loser, a failure, will never be happy again." Just go at it and I will defend my client—you.

Patient: (*as prosecutor*) Let's see. Your client is just stupid and lazy.

Therapist: Do you have any evidence to support these charges?

Patient: Well, his relationship with Anna didn't work out.

Therapist: That seems irrelevant to the charge. Almost everyone has a relationship that doesn't work out, including Anna. Would the prosecutor want us to conclude that the entire world is stupid and lazy? Is Anna stupid and lazy?

Patient: (*as prosecutor*) He just screws up in everything he does.

Therapist: The facts do not support this outrageous and illogical claim. My client graduated from college, he holds a job where he is appreciated and rewarded, he has friends, he is a good son to his parents and a good friend to people who need him. This charge is absurd and is not consistent with the evidence.

Patient: Well, he could do better.

Therapist: So could the prosecutor. But he continues to dig a deeper hole for himself. Your honor, I would like to submit that my client has grounds for a charge of slander against the prosecutor for making public statements that are malicious and obviously untrue and that are intended to cause harm to my client and his reputation.

Patient: (*laughing*) I guess I get the point.

Therapist: It seems that your negative thoughts can't stand up to a strong defense.

Patient: That seems true. But I don't defend myself.

Therapist: Imagine a trial where the only person allowed to speak was the prosecutor. What would that look like?

Patient: Totally unfair.

Therapist: Perhaps that is how you are treating yourself.

Homework

The therapist can assign Form 9.6 (Defense Attorney Form) and Form 9.7 (What Would the Jury Think?). The patient can be asked to imagine that he is taking the job of defending himself against his worst critic, the prosecutor. He now has to use all of his intelligence, cunning, and experience to disprove the charges against him. He should attack the evidence and the logic and point out the unfairness of the charges that are made. Finally, he should examine how a fair-minded jury would evaluate this "trial" and then examine how he may be charging himself with accusations that do not withstand a defense.

Possible Problems

Some patients view the vigorous challenge of defense attorney as invalidating or condescending. We find it helpful to introduce this technique by anticipating this concern: "When we challenge a negative thought, we are not invalidating your feelings or your right to think the way you choose. But if the thought is causing you pain, it might be worth seeing if it can stand up to facts and logic. Please let me know, when we use this technique, if you are feeling better or worse." It is helpful to have the patient switch roles from defendant to prosecutor and back to defendant to practice both sides.

Cross-Reference to Other Techniques

Other relevant techniques include categorizing the automatic thought distortion, weighing the advantages and disadvantages, and weighing the evidence. The double-standard technique can often be used with this technique.

Forms

Form 9.6: Defense Attorney Form
Form 9.7: What Would the Jury Think?

TECHNIQUE: WHAT ADVICE WOULD YOU GIVE A FRIEND?

Description

People who are anxious or depressed are usually kinder toward and more tolerant with other people than they are toward themselves. Asking the patient what advice he or she would give a friend allows the patient to stand back from his or her negative thinking and see things more objectively. This is sometimes known as the "double-standard technique." Moreover, activating the relationship of "friend" may help dispel tendencies to be overly critical. The patient is put into the role of "helping" rather than criticizing and may recognize that he or she would be less critical and more supportive with a friend (or a complete stranger) than with him- or herself. Furthermore, the patient's more gentle and supportive treatment of others can lead to the question of why the patient would have a double standard. This often leads to a recognition that the patient is holding him- or herself to a more critical standard than others precisely because he or she is depressed, thereby completing a vicious cycle of feeling depressed or anxious because the patient gives in to self-criticism because he or she feels depressed and anxious. This technique can be used as either a direct question ("What advice would you give a friend?") or in a role play, with the patient playing the role of a helping friend and the therapist playing the role of the patient in need.

Question to Pose/Intervention

"Sometimes we are gentler and more supportive to others than we are to ourselves. Imagine that you had a good friend who was having the very same problem you are having. What advice would you give him?" Alternatively: "Let's imagine that I am your good friend and I am having the problems that you are having. Let's do a role play and I will describe my thoughts and feelings and I want to see how you would be supportive to me." Finally: "I noticed that you are more supportive to a friend than you are to yourself. Why is that? What would it be like if you were as kind to yourself as you are to others?"

Example

Therapist: I noticed that you were very critical of yourself, labeling yourself as a loser and as stupid. Sometimes we can see things differently if we imagine ourselves giving advice to a friend with a similar problem. If your friend were going through things like you are, what advice would you give her to be more supportive?

Patient: I would tell her that she has a lot going for her. I'd tell her that she is smart, she went to college, she has a good job, and her friends really respect her. I'd try to be supportive of her because I know how hard it is.

Therapist: That does sound supportive and caring. But it doesn't sound like the way you treat yourself. Do you see the difference?

Patient: Yeah. I am constantly criticizing myself. I don't stand up for myself.

Therapist: I can see that. What is the reason for that?

Patient: I guess it's because I am depressed. Nothing seems right.

Therapist: Would you think that your best friend deserves your support most of all when she is depressed?

Patient: I guess that makes sense.

Therapist: What do you think it would be like if you treated yourself as your best friend over the next few weeks?

Patient: I guess I would feel better.

Homework

The patient can complete two forms: Advice I Would Give My Best Friend (Form 9.8) and Why It's Hard for Me to Take Good Advice (Form 9.9). In the first form, the patient indicates (as in the role play) the advice she would give a good friend with a similar problem. This helps distance her from her negative thoughts and helps her recognize the extremity and unfairness of these thoughts. It also activates a caring and compassionate mind-set. The second form focuses on the resistance or reasons not to take the good advice and asks the patient to challenge these negative thoughts. For example, the patient may say, "I don't take the advice because I am depressed," and the constructive response to this is, "I need support when I am depressed. If I took this advice I might become less depressed." Other reasons to resist good advice include, "I don't deserve it" or "I don't believe it." Constructive responses include, "I am a human being and I deserve to be treated fairly—just like other people would be treated." When the patient says, "But I don't believe the constructive response," the therapist can indicate that "thinking about another way of seeing things is the first step in changing a belief." Or the therapist can inquire about the reasons for not believing the constructive response (see prior discussion).

Possible Problems

This technique often leads the patient to claim that she is easier on other people than on herself. This objection to the technique is helpful because it identifies underlying schemas of demanding standards, undeservingness, special person, or defectiveness and helps identify the beliefs about how one can best cope. For example, the patient may believe that she needs to criticize herself because she is "basically lazy" and criticism acts as a motivator. Or the patient may object that she should not treat herself as well as she treats others because she is defective. These schematic beliefs can be examined using the techniques in this chapter.

Cross-Reference to Other Techniques

All of the techniques in this chapter are relevant.

Forms

Form 9.8: Advice I Would Give My Best Friend
Form 9.9: Why It's Hard for Me to Take Good Advice

TECHNIQUE: DECATASTROPHIZING

Description

Most intense emotional responses are the result of viewing events as awful, catastrophic, or overwhelming. One of Ellis's prime targets in therapy was the patient's belief that events were "awful" (Ellis, 1962). While recognizing that many events are objectively difficult or even life threatening, the cognitive therapist attempts to put things in perspective in order to avoid over-reaction. For example, the patient who thinks, "It's awful that my friend canceled our dinner date," will overreact with intense emotion as if her life is threatened. Taking the catastrophe out of events involves a number of strategies. This includes identifying the tendency to catastrophize, for example, monitoring thoughts such as "That's awful," "I can't stand it," "It's terrible," or "I can't believe this is happening." These emotionally escalating thoughts can be examined in terms of costs and benefits of catastrophic thinking. It's essential that the patient come to recognize that the bias toward catastrophizing results in self-defeating dysregulation of mood. Next, the therapist can examine the evidence for and against the view that events are catastrophic, use the continuum technique to place events in the perspective of other less "bad" or more "bad" events, shift to a problem-solving mode, and extend time to place current frustrations in the context of a longer and more meaningful life.

It is important to help the patient recognize that negative events can be "truly negative" and that decatastrophizing does not need to be invalidating, minimizing, or dismissive. We have suggested that the therapist introduce this concept of invalidation in the context of placing things in perspective in order to anticipate this issue.

Question to Pose/Intervention

"It seems that you are thinking and feeling that what is happening is really awful or terrible. Sometimes when we are upset we think that we are being overwhelmed by events that we cannot tolerate, that are overwhelming. That may be part of anxiety and depression for us. It might be helpful to see if we can put these events into perspective for you to determine whether they might be less awful for you and possibly more manageable. This does not mean that your feelings are invalidated or that what is happening is OK or not important. It just means that we might be able to see things in a perspective where they are still negative but not as awful for you."

Example

Therapist: It sounds like you are feeling really upset about the breakup, and it's understandable that you would feel bad right now. I am wondering what this breakup is making you think.

Patient: I just think my life is awful. It's terrible that here I am at 27 years old with no relationship and all my friends are married or in relationships and I have nothing.

Therapist: Those are really upsetting thoughts to have. I am particularly interested in the thought about things being "awful" and "terrible." Can you tell me more about that?

Patient: Well, I think it's awful to be alone like this.

Therapist: So, when you think how it is awful, what kind of feeling goes with that?

Patient: I just feel terrible. I feel sad and hopeless, like there is nothing to live for.

Therapist: OK. So, this thought that it is awful makes you feel life isn't worth living and makes you feel sad and hopeless. As bad as it might feel, I am wondering whether you would feel differently if you weren't thinking it was awful and life is terrible. What if you thought that this is a really difficult time, but one that you might be able to manage with some help?

Patient: Are you saying that it's not bad?

Therapist: No, I am saying it is possible that it is bad, but when we think it's awful it might keep you from seeing some possibilities of getting better and feeling better. Let's take the idea that it is awful. Imagine if you were to take the current situation—a breakup in your relationship—and you gave it a rating of how bad it seems. What rating would you give from 0 to 100% where 100% was the worst thing anyone could ever imagine?

Patient: It seems like 99%.

Therapist: OK. Now let's draw a line here and put 0% and 100% and put "breakup" at 99%. Now what can you think about that is worse than 99%?

Patient: I guess losing my life—suffering in the process, a long painful illness.

Therapist: OK. So that is 100%. What would you put at 90% and 80%?

Patient: (*thinking for a moment*) It's hard to think that way. I tend to think in terms of extremes. I would say 90% would be losing a friend, 80% would be losing your job.

Therapist: How about 50%?

Patient: I don't know, losing some money, maybe. Getting the flu.

Therapist: How about 25%?

Patient: I'd have a hard time thinking of that. Let's see—having an argument with someone.

Therapist: Where would you put having a crippling illness for the next 20 years?

Patient: That would have to be 99%.

Therapist: So, it feels like the breakup is as bad as having a crippling illness for 20 years. Does that seem realistic?

Patient: I guess not.

Therapist: Even if you have this breakup, what are some pleasurable and meaningful things that you can still do, either now or in the future?

Patient: I don't know. I can still see my friends, go to work, exercise, enjoy the city, see my family. I can travel. Maybe in the future I will be able to find a better relationship. I guess a lot of things.

Therapist: So, when you place this at 99%—the same rating for a crippling 20-year illness—and 1% below dying slowly from a painful illness, does this seem realistic to you?

Patient: I guess not. Maybe I am overreacting.

Therapist: This is not to say that this isn't difficult or bad or that it feels awful. But it sounds like you see things in extremes—rather than shades of gray—and I am wondering if that adds to your feeling overwhelmed at times with these strong painful emotions.

Patient: You may have a point.

Homework

The patient can complete Form 9.10 (Place Events on a Continuum) and Form 9.11 (Placing Events in Perspective: What I Can Still Do).

Possible Problems

Many patients who are emotionally disregulated see events in all-or-nothing terms. Of course, this is the entire focus on the continuum technique: to be able to see things in shades of gray. Consequently, the patient may have difficulty identifying less noxious events. The therapist can assist by suggesting less "negative" events: "Where would you put getting the flu, losing $100, having an argument with a friend, wearing tight shoes?" Some patients may object that placing events along a continuum is invalidating. Again, anticipating this by prefacing the technique with identifying validation concerns can help avoid this difficulty.

Cross-Reference to Other Techniques

Behavioral activation techniques, such as activity scheduling, pleasure predicting, improving the moment, and other techniques that direct the patient toward positive change can help place the negative thought and emotion in perspective.

Forms

Form 9.10: Place Events on a Continuum

Form 9.11: Placing Events in Perspective: What I Can Still Do

TECHNIQUE: BUYING TIME

Description

Anxiety is often characterized by a sense of time urgency: the belief that something terrible is happening imminently or the belief that one has to have the answers to one's problems immediately (Ellis, 1962). If we view anxiety as an adaptive response to emergencies and threats that arose in the primitive environment of early man, then a sense of urgency would be an adaptive part of anxious experience. The ability to immediately escape or avoid or to detect danger would be a valued component of anxious responses to life-threatening events. Patients who have a sense of urgency to "feel better immediately" may find themselves abusing drugs and alcohol, bingeing or purging, acting out sexually, demanding immediate reassurance, or even performing self-mutilation (Riskind, 1997). Driven by a sense of urgency, anxious individuals seek the most effective immediate gratification for their needs, thereby contributing further to a sense of hopelessness (Leahy, 2005b).

Related to the sense of time urgency is the difficulty that people have in predicting their future mood and the effects of events (Klonsky, 2007). Thus, people often believe that they will have a durability of negative mood following negative life events and they often underestimate factors that may help them cope better. Part of the sense of urgency in overcoming a current mood is the overgeneralization of this mood to the future, discounting the meliorating effects of other positive life events.

The technique of buying time focuses the patient on the issue of time urgency and attempts to refocus to either delaying gratification, anticipating a sequence of positive changes, improving the moment, or decreasing the imminence or perception of rapid approach of danger. Using a variety of techniques to reduce urgency, the therapist assists the patient in tolerating current levels of stress with the possibility that events will change and emotions will dissipate with time.

Question to Pose/Intervention

"It seems that you are thinking that you need to feel better immediately given how bad you feel right now. It may be that your need to feel better immediately may actually make you more anxious, further spiraling you into a sense of emergency that things are getting worse. We can look at time differently to see if we can reduce this sense of urgency. There are a number of questions that we can consider. First, what do you see as the consequence of your sense of urgency and emergency? Second, if we take the current events and the way you feel, is it possible that you might feel better about these things in a few hours or a few days? Has that happened before? Third, what are some things that could happen in the next few hours or few days that could make you feel better? Perhaps there are some actions that you could plan and take to make a change for the future. Fourth, perhaps we can identify some alternative things for you to think about or do that could make you feel more calm. We can look at a list of pleasurable and relaxing activities that you could do now to improve the current moment. What if you did some of those things?"

Example

Therapist: I've noticed that you have a sense of urgency at times that you need to feel better immediately. And, then, at times you might drink more or binge eat or contact people for reassurance. Have you noticed this sense of urgency?

Patient: Yes. It seems to be happening on a regular basis. I just feel terrible and feel I can't stand it, so I need to do something.

Therapist: It's almost like you are panicking about feeling bad right now. What was it that was making you feel so bad last night?

Patient: I just thought I am going to be alone forever and I won't ever find someone.

Therapist: And what did you do?

Patient: I had a couple of glasses of wine and then began to binge and I felt spaced out.

Therapist: So, it seems that you were thinking that you really had to find someone right now or know you would have someone and then you acted out in these different ways. But I am wondering if we could look at this differently and figure out a way to turn off that sense of urgency that you are feeling.

Patient: That would be great. But it just feels so bad when it is happening.

Therapist: Well, that's why we need to focus on this. You can see that the consequences of feeling that there is an emergency have been costly for you. One thing to think about is how we can buy time—to get away from feeling bad right now and thinking of ways of feeling better in the future. For example, you are feeling bad about feeling lonely on Tuesday night, but I wonder how you are going to feel when you are at work on Wednesday morning. Do your feelings change?

Patient: They do. I felt better on Wednesday. I was with my friends at work and focusing on what I have to do.

Therapist: OK. So we can see that the feeling changes. And let's take this idea of being alone forever. This is a thought you have had before. But haven't you also had a series of relationships after those feelings of hopelessness?

Patient: Yeah. Last year I was feeling this way, and then I met Erik and it was OK for a while.

Therapist: So, your feelings don't last forever and things do change. It's important to keep in mind that you can feel differently when events change. But you might not know that on Tuesday night. So, one thing you can do is "stretch time" and recognize that events change, feelings change, and you change. I was wondering why you thought you needed to know for sure on Tuesday night what your life would be like in the future. It's almost as if you are saying that if you don't know for sure then it will be terrible.

Patient: I often think that way. I have this sense that I need to know for sure. But then I don't and so I think it's going to be terrible.

Therapist: There are a lot of things we don't know for sure that turn out to be OK. So this may be a bias in the way you think. I remember you telling me last month that you thought you were going to get fired and it seemed like a real urgency and then your boss told you that you were doing a good job. A sense of urgency is a common feeling for you.

Patient: That's why I am always panicking.

Therapist: And I am also thinking about things that you could do in the present moment to improve the moment and feel better or feel differently on those lonely Tuesday nights. For example, what if you had a plan to make yourself feel calm. This could include taking a bubble bath, listening to music, exercising, watching a film, going on Facebook, or any number of things—sort of like a menu of what to do for now until something better comes along.

Patient: That might be a good idea.

Homework

The patient can be assigned the following: "Identify examples of a sense of urgency and list the triggers and what you do and feel right then. List the costs and benefits of feeling a sense of urgency. Are you equating a sense of urgency with a guaranteed bad outcome? Does this make sense? Have you been wrong in the past? Is your response to a sense of urgency more of the problem than actual events that occur? List the predictions that you are making that give rise to a sense of urgency and list reasons why events might change or turn out better. Ask yourself, 'How will I feel about this in a few hours, a day, a week, a month, a year?' Use Form 9.12, Overcoming Time Urgency, as a guide to help gain perspective. What could be some reasons why you might feel better or worse? What are some things that you can do to improve the moment and distract yourself from your sense of urgency?"

Possible Problems

Some patients feel so overwhelmed with the intensity of their emotions that they may have difficulty thinking through possible alternatives to time urgency. Stress reduction and mindful meditation techniques might be useful in reducing emotional intensity prior to considering cognitive techniques for coping with urgency.

Cross-Reference to Other Techniques

Acceptance, DBT techniques, and stress reduction techniques may help reduce time urgency.

Form

Form 9.12: Overcoming Time Urgency

CONCLUSIONS

In this chapter, we provide a number of useful techniques for helping patients manage their emotions by managing their thoughts. A more complete list, with thorough descriptions, can be found in Leahy's *Cognitive Therapy Techniques: A Practitioner's Guide* (Leahy, 2003a). Emotion regulation can be improved by changing the appraisal of the situation, thereby shortcutting the escalation of emotion. Indeed, by providing patients with a set of cognitive therapy techniques that can be used daily, and by anticipating the situations that may be most troubling, patients may find that they can inoculate themselves against the stress that elicits the emotions they struggle to regulate.

Although cognitive restructuring may not be viewed by some as a technique that is relevant to emotional regulation, we suggest that it may be a primary emotion regulation technique. Indeed, emotional dysregulation may be decreased if patients have access to more effective cognitive strategies of interpretation of events, including one's own emotion. Thus, patients who find themselves upset over being "rejected" may utilize a wide variety of cognitive restructuring techniques to cope with the event, including decatastrophizing, viewing the event in perspective, not taking it personally, and examining alternative interpretations. This restructuring may help decrease the emotional intensity, in some cases sufficiently so that other emotion regulation techniques may not be necessary. Alternatively, one can view cognitive restructuring as part of the therapeutic arsenal to be augmented with other techniques described in this book. Our approach, throughout this text, is to provide the clinician with a wide range of techniques and to allow the clinician the flexibility to choose what is optimal in a given situation.

CHAPTER TEN

Stress Reduction

The concept of "stress" has been at the center of emotion regulation research for almost half a century. Endocrinologist Hans Selye (1974, 1978) identified the general adaptation syndrome as a sequence of responses to stress. Stress was defined as the organism's response to a stressor (or stimulus impinging on it) that included physiological and cognitive components. According to Selye, the general adaptation syndrome comprises three phases: alarm, resistance, and exhaustion. During the alarm phase, the organism responds with either fight or flight (or in some cases "freezing"), activating the hypothalamic–pituitary–adrenocortical (HPA) axis, and the secretion of cortisol. This marks the mobilization of response to threat. During the resistance phase, the organism attempts to actively cope with the stress, mobilizing resources, energy, and behavior to actively solve the problems confronted. Finally, after continued mobilization of resources and coping, the organism begins a process of decompensation during the exhaustion phase, marked by misfiring of defensive and coping responses, digestive problems, fatigue, agitation, and irritability.

The experience of stress activates the sympathetic nervous system, leading to the release of norepinephrine, which stimulates organs, increases respiratory processes and heart rate, and increases the strength and energy available to muscles and prepares the organism for fight or flight. The sympathetic–adrenomedullary system also activates epinephrine and norepinephrine, redundantly affecting heart rate, perspiration, muscle strength, and other functioning (Aldwin, 2007; Gevirtz, 2007). The HPA axis is a slower system to be activated in response to stress. The HPA axis first activates the hypothalamus, which secretes corticotropin-releasing hormone, which in turn stimulates the pituitary, releasing adrenocorticotropic hormone, which activates the adrenal cortex and releases corticosteroids. Prolonged activation of the HPA suppresses the immune systems, exhausts the individual, and may result in greater vulnerability to illness. A considerable body of research supports the view that there are significant individual differences in response to stress, including vulnerability to problematic parenting, environmental stressors, and response to supportive environments (Belsky & Pluess, 2009).

Lazarus has expanded the stress model to incorporate cognitive appraisals underlying coping (Lazarus & Folkman, 1984). According to this model, there are primary and secondary appraisals for coping. Primary appraisal refers to the evaluation of the nature of the threat while secondary appraisal reflects assessment of one's ability to cope (Lazarus, 1999). For example, say someone had to lift a 50-pound object. She may recognize that the object to be lifted weighs 50 pounds, but she also recognizes that she is capable of lifting 100 pounds. In this instance, her resultant stress would be low. In contrast, if she assessed that she could lift only 45 pounds, she would experience greater stress.

Other models of stress propose that expectations, self-regulating feedback loops, and other mechanisms and processes underpin the experience of stress. One view of emotion is that it helps the individual reestablish priorities (Simon, 1983). Expanding on this view, Carver and Scheier (2009) have advanced a cybernetic model of self-regulation that includes identification of the individual's purpose (goal, standard, reference value), a "comparator" function (which contrasts input with goals or purposes), and the output function (behavior and coping mechanisms) (Carver & Scheier, 1998). The cybernetic model emphasizes feedback loops that continually self-correct and help modulate the adaptation to stress. Emotion is linked to the expectations and comparisons that individuals make, such that corrections to increase effort are activated by discrepancies that one is failing to reach goals whereas decreases of effort result when one exceeds goals. This leads to the "counterintuitive" occurrence of "coasting"; that is, when the individual exceeds goals and is feeling pleasure, there is a decrease of effort. Thus, expectations help define the experience of stress and the responses activated to cope.

An integral part of emotion regulation is the capacity to tolerate and reduce stress. The emotional schema model proposes that beliefs about the controllability of emotion, danger, impairment, and duration of emotion can further exacerbate emotional dysregulation. Reducing stress by utilizing a variety of behavioral techniques can positively impact this process, indicating to the individual that emotion can be controlled; it is temporary, not dangerous, and not impairing. Stress can be cognitively generated by anticipating negative experiences and interpreting current experiences in a threatening or negative way. Stress may also be the result of external demands, problems, and relationship conflicts. Physiological conditions, such as lack of sleep or illness, and environmental conditions, such as noise or crowds, can cause stress. Regardless of the source, stress affects the body, activating the fight-or-flight response. With activation of the sympathetic nervous system, an individual experiences increases in the rate of respiration, muscle tension, heart rate, and blood pressure. Blood flow to the extremities is decreased.

The competing process within the body to the stress response is the relaxation response. The relaxation response activates the parasympathetic nervous system, effectively putting the breaks on the physiological changes that accompany the fight-or-fight response. The relaxation response can be activated through relaxation exercises.

Another key component of stress is time management and one's orientation toward time. Riskind has proposed that time perception is a factor in the perception of threat and the ability to cope (Riskind, 1997; Riskind, Black, & Shahar, 2009). According to his "looming vulnerability model," anxious individuals perceive a threatening stimulus as rapidly approaching, reducing the ability to adapt their behavior, problem solve, or simply "get out of the way." Anxiety can be reduced by reassessing the velocity of the "impending" stressor, identifying all the events that would have to ensue before "impact," and considering alternative coping strategies that might mitigate the effect of the threatening stimulus. In addition, imagery that allows the "slowing down" of the movement of the threatening stimulus also reduces anxiety or stress.

A sense of time urgency can severely impact stress. For example, overscheduling, having difficulty prioritizing tasks, difficulty "breaking away" from one task to take on another, multitasking, and viewing time as rushing in can significantly affect stress. Patients who feel overwhelmed often view tasks that they need to address as vague, uncontrollable, and even dangerous, resulting in a sense of both urgency and helplessness. Moreover, demands for "answers right now" lead to a continual sense of apprehension, panic, and emergency. In order to address these time urgency issues and the sense of feeling overwhelmed, we indicate how patients can reevaluate their sense of time pressure and reduce stress by realistic time management.

TECHNIQUE: PROGRESSIVE MUSCLE RELAXATION

Description

Just as the body has a stress response, there is also the capacity for a relaxation response. One of the fundamental relaxation skills is progressive muscle relaxation, developed by Edmund Jacobsen over 60 years ago (E. Jacobson, 1942). Psychological stress is accompanied by increased physical tension. However, many people are not aware of body tension. By first cultivating an awareness of this tension and then learning to relax the muscles in the body, patients can decrease stress. In progressive muscle relaxation, patients tense and release each of the major muscle groups in sequence in the body from head to toe: forehead, eyes, mouth, jaw, neck, shoulders, back, chest, biceps, forearms, hands, abdomen, quadriceps, calves, and feet. Each of the muscles is tensed for 4 to 8 seconds, with patients bringing their full awareness to the tension. Then the muscle group is released, and patients focus their full awareness on the sensation of relaxation. By contrasting the states of tension and relaxation, patients are cultivating an awareness of both. This exercise should be practiced for 10 to 15 minutes twice a day.

Question to Pose/Intervention

"One way to decrease stress is relaxation. But relaxation is a skill that needs to be cultivated with practice. One of the fundamental relaxation techniques is progressive muscle relaxation. Stress affects the body by causing increased muscle tension. Often we are not aware of this tension. By letting go of muscle tension, we can decrease stress and trigger the body's relaxation response. One way to do this is to tense each major muscle group of the body from head to toe, one muscle group at a time. As you tense each major muscle group, bring your full awareness to the tension in that part of the body. Then release the tension and bring your full awareness to the absence of tension and whatever other pleasurable sensations you feel."

Example

Therapist: How has your mood been this week?

Patient: Stressed.

Therapist: What are you doing to manage your stress?

Patient: My doctor prescribed medication for me, but it makes me too tired to focus at work.

Therapist: Another way to cope with stress is by practicing relaxation. Stress affects the body physically, causing increased muscle tension. By relaxing this tension, we can decrease stress.

Patient: Actually, now that you mention it, my neck and shoulders are stiff.

Therapist: Most us hold our tension from the shoulders and above. I'd like to teach you a relaxation technique called progressive muscle relaxation. We'll progressively tense and then release each of the major muscle groups in the body from head to toe. Hold the tension for 5 seconds and release the tension for 5 seconds. As you tense each muscle group, I'd like you to bring your full awareness to the tension. After you release the tension, I'd like you to bring your full awareness to the sensations you are experiencing in that muscle group. When you tense your muscle, silently say to yourself, "Tense," and when you release the tension, silently say, "Relax." (*Instructs the patient in going through each muscle group.*)

Homework

The therapist should instruct patients to practice the exercise twice daily for 10 to 15 minutes, using Form 10.1 (Instructions for Progressive Muscle Relaxation) as a guide. Instructions for the exercise can be reviewed.

Possible Problems

Some patients report that they may feel some cramping in a muscle, and they should be told that tensing can be done gently rather than intensely. Others may attempt to go through the exercise rapidly, without allowing relaxation to be experienced in the moment. They may be told to prolong the period of tensing and relaxing and to focus on their sensations. Common sensations include feeling of tightness alternating with feeling of letting go, relaxation, warmth, tingling, and tightness. Patients may report attempting the technique when stressed but finding it ineffective. In this case, the therapist should emphasize that relaxation is a skill that requires practice. Once the skill is developed through practice in situations of relatively little stress, it can be used more effectively in situations of heightened stress.

Cross-Reference to Other Techniques

Related techniques include mindfulness practice, diaphragmatic breathing, and self-soothing.

Form

Form 10.1: Instructions for Progressive Muscle Relaxation

TECHNIQUE: DIAPHRAGMATIC BREATHING

Description

When the body is experiencing stress, respiration is shallow and rapid. Breathing occurs from the chest rather than the abdomen. When breathing is rapid and shallow, more oxygen is "blown off" and the concentration of oxygen in the blood (and brain) is reduced, resulting in more attempts to gain oxygen through deep and intense breathing. This may result in hyperventilation syndrome and greater increases of anxiety. Some patients mistakenly believe that they need to take "deep breaths," which only exacerbates the hyperventilation cycle, often resulting in dizziness, feelings of panic, a sense that one is smothering, and heightened anxious arousal.

Shallow, rapid breathing stimulates the sympathetic nervous system, which is activated when we are anxious. With each inhalation, the chest and ribs expand. By contrast, slow breathing from the belly or diaphragm activates the parasympathetic nervous system, which brings about a relaxation response. With each inhalation, the diaphragm expands and the chest remains relatively still.

Question to Pose/Intervention

"How we breathe affects how we feel. When we are stressed or anxious, we breathe shallowly and rapidly from the chest. This type of breathing stimulates the body's sympathetic nervous system, the body's fight-or-flight system. If we are relaxed and begin to breathe this way, we can induce some of the physical sensations of anxiety. When we are relaxed, we breathe slowly and deeply from the diaphragm. This type of breathing activates the parasympathetic nervous system, which puts the brakes on the body's fight-or-flight system. In other words, diaphragmatic breathing activates the body's relaxation response. However, this type of breathing is a skill. The more often you practice breathing this way, the more effectively you will be able to use it to calm yourself down."

Example

Therapist: Are you feelings anxious?

Patient: Yes. How did you know?

Therapist: You're breathing quickly and from the chest. That type of breathing is associated with anxiety.

Patient: I didn't realize there were different types of breathing.

Therapist: Yes, there's relaxed breathing and anxious breathing. How you breathe affects how you feel.

Patient: What's relaxed breathing?

Therapist: When we're relaxed, we breathe slowly and deeply from the belly or diaphragm. Watch. As I inhale, my abdomen expands, and it flattens as I exhale. My chest isn't moving. When we breathe this way, we're triggering the body's relaxation response.

Patient: I am not sure I completely understand.

Therapist: I'd like you to lie down and place this book on your chest. (*Patient lies down.*) Now I would like you to breathe the way you usually breathe. (*Patient breathes.*) I noticed that you are breathing and that the book on your chest is rising and falling. This is because you are breathing from your chest and not from your abdomen. Now place the book on your stomach and imagine that you are taking in each breath in the shape of a candy cane; each breath comes in from your nose and gently goes out through your abdomen. See if the book will rise from your abdomen. Give it a try, and I'll give you feedback.

Homework

The patient can practice diaphragmatic breathing every day for at least 10 minutes, using Form 10.2 (Instructions for Diaphragmatic Breathing) as a guide.

Possible Problems

Patients may continue to breathe from the chest rather than the abdomen. For this reason, it is recommended that the therapist observe them practice this technique in the therapy session before assigning it for homework. Some patients report feeling more anxious when using this technique and some may begin to hyperventilate. This is not an unusual or dangerous response, and the proper breathing technique should be practiced in the session until it is mastered sufficiently to be practiced at home. Patients may also be hyperventilating as a general rule, and their hyperventilation may be increased if they take deep breaths or if they yawn. For example, one patient noticed that she would hold her breath when she was anxious and needed to remind herself to "continue breathing."

Cross-Reference to Other Techniques

Related techniques include progressive muscle relaxation, self-soothing, mindfulness, and positive imagery.

Form

Form 10.2: Instructions for Diaphragmatic Breathing

TECHNIQUE: SELF-SOOTHING

Description

The capacity to self-soothe is an important emotional regulation skill. It involves using the five senses (taste, touch, hearing, smell, and vision) to help make intense negative emotions tolerable. For example, the stress an individual experiences while working to meet a deadline might be eased by listening to classical music and drinking a cup of herbal tea.

Many clients with emotion regulation difficulties have not learned to soothe themselves when experiencing intense negative emotions, particularly if their expression of negative emotions as children was dismissed or punished by caregivers. Lacking these skills, clients may rely on others to soothe them or seek to escape emotional distress in dysfunctional ways. Alternatively, some clients may be reluctant to self-soothe because they believe that they are not worthy of kindness and nurturance, or they believe that others should soothe them. In Dialectical Behavior Therapy (DBT; Linehan, 1993b), clients are taught how to self-soothe as part of distress tolerance skills training. The skills are taught with the stated objective of making unbearable pain bearable, rather than removing the pain completely.

Question to Pose/Intervention

"Intense negative emotions are inevitable in life. Rather than try to avoid them at all costs, it's important to develop skills to make them bearable. One way to make distress tolerable is by practicing self-soothing. This involves using your five senses to take the edge off of emotional pain. In other words, when you self-soothe, you bring your awareness to your sense of taste, touch, smell, hearing, and vision. We do for ourselves what we might do for a friend who is upset. For example, I might self-soothe by sitting in a comfortable chair by the fireplace while listening to calming music and petting my cat.

Example

Therapist: It sounds like a stressful week. You've been working 12 hours every day.

Patient: Well, I have no choice. We're on a deadline and I have to get it done.

Therapist: What skills can you use to decrease your stress?

Patient: Nothing. I don't have time to go to the gym or hang out with friends.

Therapist: One skill that might be useful is self-soothing while you're working. Use your senses to take the edge off—vision, hearing, smell, touch, and taste. It won't get rid of the stress, but it might ease it a bit.

Patient: Well, I'm in the office. I can't burn incense. What do you propose?

Therapist: There are unobtrusive ways to self-soothe. You could keep scented lotion in your desk and listen to music. What do you think? Would you be willing to try?

Patient: It's worth a shot. I could also buy some flowers and put them on my desk.

Homework

The client can review the list of suggested self-soothing activities and practice them.

Possible Problems

The client may report that self-soothing did not work. In this instance, the therapist should clarify what the patient means by "work." It is not uncommon for clients to practice the skill with the expectation of eliminating distress, rather than easing it. The therapist should emphasize that the goal of self-soothing is to make emotional pain tolerable, not to eliminate pain.

Cross-Reference to Other Techniques

Related techniques include activity scheduling, time management, progressive muscle relaxation, and diaphragmatic breathing.

Form

Form 10.3: Self-Soothing

TECHNIQUE: ACTIVITY SCHEDULING
AND PLEASURE PREDICTING

Description

Behavioral activation has long been a component of behavioral treatments for depression and anxiety (Martell et al., 2010; Rehm, 1981) with considerable support for its independent efficacy (Cuijpers, van Straten, & Warmerdam, 2007; Sturmey, 2009). From a behavioral perspective, stress can be viewed as the inability to produce positive consequences, the reduction of the rewarding value of consequences, the increase of aversive experiences, or the noncontingency of behavior and consequences. Put more simply, this means that depression (e.g., anxiety, stress) may result from difficulty obtaining rewarding experiences, the lack of skills to obtain these rewards, an increase of unpleasant experiences, and the perception or actuality that one cannot affect outcome. From this perspective, decreasing stress would entail the following:

1. Identifying possible rewarding behaviors.
2. Increasing the value of rewards (e.g., by increasing their frequency, intensity, or salience).
3. Reducing negative experiences.
4. Increasing the perception of controllability of outcomes (contingency).

Many of these goals may be attained by using activity scheduling and pleasure predicting. In the previous section, we identified the use of behavioral activation in self-soothing, focusing on the present moment. In this section, we focus on behavioral activation over the course of a week, month, or year. This is based on the view that much of stress can be a consequence of the lack of future time perspective that identifies positive activities that are controllable in the future. Indeed, one might claim that the way out may be forward.

Question to Pose/Intervention

"Sometimes when we are stressed we feel there is very little to look forward to. We can focus on how bad we feel right now and fail to appreciate that there are positive activities on the horizon. Another part of our stress is that we do not plan activities, and things just happen to us. One way to deal with this might be to plan activities for the next day, week, or month so that you have some positive goals to look forward to. I am going to ask you to plan some activities for the coming week, and schedule them at specific times. When you think of these activities, I am going to ask you to consider how much pleasure you think you will get and how much of a sense of mastery you will have. We can think of 'mastery' as the sense that you are accomplishing something. I will also ask you to keep track of what you actually do and how much pleasure and mastery you actually experience."

Example

Therapist: One way of handling your stress and anxiety is to have things to look forward to. For example, think about the next day. What could you look forward to?

Patient: I don't think that way. I just get wrapped up in how I feel right now.

Therapist: Yes, and that may be the problem that we can solve. For example, what if you had a couple of positive things to look forward to today, tomorrow, and this week? Each day—something positive. And then you thought about those positives every day? What would that be like?

Patient: A lot different from the way I am. I guess I might feel more optimistic.

Therapist: If you plan some positives and carry them out—actually do them—you might feel more optimistic, more in control of your life, and less wrapped up in the feelings at the present. You would be able to make things happen for yourself. The more positives that you plan and carry out, the less stress and anxiety you will experience.

Patient: It sounds like a good idea. But how do I know it will work?

Therapist: You can only know if you do it for a while and see what happens.

Homework

The patient is asked to complete Form 10.4, Weekly Activity Scheduling: Pleasure Predicting and Actual Outcome. In reviewing the homework, the therapist and the patient can examine where the patient under- or overpredicted pleasure or mastery. Activities with higher pleasure ratings can then be incorporated in ongoing reward menus and assigned more frequently. Low pleasure and mastery activities can be eliminated or decreased in frequency for future planned activities.

Possible Problems

Some patients have difficulty identifying positive activities in the future because their present mood of depression or anxiety leads them to believe that nothing will be pleasurable. The therapist can indicate the following: "When you are feeling down, it is likely that you will think that nothing could make you feel better. There are a couple of ways of looking at this. First, you can simply do these activities and find out if your predictions are accurate. Sometimes people find that things turn out better than expected, which can be encouraging. Second, it may be that these activities may not be as pleasurable as they once were. You can think of this in terms of practicing the activity until it becomes pleasurable. It's like exercise: It may take a while to see the results." Another common problem with activity scheduling is that patients may have negative dysfunctional thoughts while engaging in the activity. For example, one patient kept thinking, "What a loser I am that I have to do this kind of thing to feel better." Identifying negative thoughts, or even ruminations, about activities can be helpful in reducing the aversive consequences of pleasure predicting. Again, we find it helpful to use the analogy of physical exercise: "If you wanted to get back into shape, would you think you were a loser because you had to exercise a bit more?" Doing pleasurable activities can be reframed as "self-care," "assertion of your rights to have pleasure," and "taking control of your life."

Cross-Reference to Other Techniques

Other relevant techniques include self-soothing, reward menu, and time management.

Form

Form 10.4: Weekly Activity Scheduling: Pleasure Predicting and Actual Outcome

TECHNIQUE: TIME MANAGEMENT

Description

Much of the stress that one experiences can be the result of feeling no control over time and activity. Patients who are stressed often complain that they do not have the time to get things done or that there is no time for pleasurable activities. In most cases, the patients are taking a reactive role, simply responding to the stimuli in front of them. For example, the patient goes to work and simply gets caught up in the first activity that he thinks about. Time is not planned or controlled, and nothing is prioritized. Often the patient will choose to engage in relatively lower priority activities because they are easier or more pleasant. Time management helps the patient establish priorities, identify off-task behavior, engage in self-monitoring and self-control, assign adequate time for travel and tasks, plan ahead, and provide time for self-reward.

Question to Pose/Intervention

"You seem to feel overwhelmed throughout the day, and you can't seem to get done the important things that you need to do. Perhaps we can examine how you can manage your time a little better. The first thing to figure out is what is of most importance, medium importance, and least importance. We have to first set these priorities. Then we need to identify what you are doing that is least important, that is, 'off task' from the activities of highest importance. Finally, we need to assign the appropriate amount of time for each activity, allowing for some rewarding or stress-free time in between."

Example

Therapist: It sounds like you are wasting a lot of time at work and feeling that you aren't getting things done. Let's do some time management on this.

Patient: OK. I do need to get a better handle on my time.

Therapist: Right. Let's start by making a list of the most important activities to do.

Patient: OK. I need to answer the e-mails on these accounts and work on the project.

Therapist: Those sound like essential work on your job. Now, how are you going off task and goofing off?

Patient: Well, I'm searching the web and looking at different news sites and I'm even shopping around for prices on various things—in fact, things I don't buy. And I send e-mails and text messages to my friends.

Therapist: Well, those things could be fun, but they are going to take time away from work. How much time do you think you are spending off task, goofing off like this?

Patient: Probably 3 hours each day.

Therapist: So that might be 15 hours per week—over 700 hours a year, probably. How do things feel at the end of the day when you goof off like this?

Patient: Pretty lousy. Like I am not getting things done.

Therapist: OK. So let's keep track of the off-task behaviors that we mentioned. Perhaps you could make a note of them and bring that in next week. Now, how about the highest priority activities? Could you do those first? This way you will get the most important things done and then you could even assign yourself some goof-off time as a reward for getting the most important things done.

Note: In addition to identifying high-, medium-, and low-priority activities and assigning them, the therapist can ask the patient if he is giving himself enough time to get things done or to travel to and from work. Some patients complain of continually feeling rushed, simply because they overschedule activities. Other patients have difficulty deciding to "finish" an activity, sometimes finding it hard to let it go. Assigning enough time for travel and tasks and limiting the amount of time on a task can assist in better time management.

Homework

Using Forms 10.5, 10.6, 10.7, and 10.8, patients can complete a list of high-, medium-, and low-priority tasks, examine their activity schedule to see how they are actually spending their time, and identify and eliminate off-task behaviors. In addition patients can identify fun activities from the reward menu, which can be used as reinforcers for engaging in higher priority behaviors. For example, surfing the Internet for 10 minutes can be a reinforcer for completing 1 hour of work.

Possible Problems

Some patients find that they get so absorbed in off-task behaviors that they have a difficult time breaking free. The therapist can examine the pros and cons (short term and long term) for these activities, engage in role plays to help patients challenge their thoughts about these activities, and use alarm systems (either a watch, timer, or computer-based time alarm) to alert them to on-task and off-task behaviors. Other patients procrastinate on higher priority tasks. Anti-procrastination training can be helpful. The therapist and patient identify the pros and cons of doing the higher priority behavior, examine beliefs about how unpleasant and difficult the higher priority behavior will be, develop self-contracts for doing them, and experiment with doing on-task behaviors for short periods of time.

Cross-Reference to Other Techniques

Other relevant techniques include pleasure predicting and activity scheduling.

Forms

Form 10.5: List of Priorities

Form 10.6: Self-Monitoring Off-Task Behaviors

Form 10.7: Planning Ahead

Form 10.8: Anti-Procrastination

TECHNIQUE: RELAXING AND POSITIVE IMAGERY

Description

One way to decrease stress and negative emotions is to focus one's awareness on positive and relaxing images. Often it is not possible to physically leave a situation that evokes distress. However, with the use of relaxing and positive imagery, it is possible to mentally escape situations that evoke distress. The use of the imagination can affect us emotionally and physically. By imagining oneself in a relaxed and positive situation, actual relaxation may be experienced. To be effective, the scene should be visualized in as much detail as possible with as many senses incorporated as possible. For example, in imagining a beach scene, it is important to imagine the warmth of the sun, the hot sand, the sound of the waves and seagulls, the smell of the ocean and suntan lotion. The individual should imagine him- or herself relaxing in this scene. It may be a place that actually exists or is completely fabricated. It is important to practice visualization at times of relatively little stress so that it can be used effectively in times of great distress. As with the other distress tolerance skills discussed in this chapter, visualization skills become stronger with repeated practice.

Question to Pose/Intervention

"It's not always possible to leave a distressing situation. However, by using visualization, it's possible to mentally leave the situation. In your imagination, you can create a perfectly relaxing and safe scene. Make it as vivid as you can by bringing all your sense into play. For example, when I'm distressed I might imagine that I am in a tree house at night. I can see the stars through the branches. I hear the crickets chirping and leaves rustling in the breeze. I imagine myself sitting there feeling completely relaxed. By bringing my awareness to this scene, and experiencing it in my imagination, I decrease my distress."

Example

In this example, the therapist is helping the patient with a fear of enclosed spaces cope with an upcoming CT scan.

Therapist: You sound pretty stressed about the upcoming CT scan. I thought we could spend some time mapping out some coping strategies you could use during the test.

Patient: There's not a lot I can do. I'm not supposed to move so I can't use progressive muscle relaxation. I don't think I can use deep breathing either.

Therapist: When it's not possible to leave a distressing situation physically, you can leave it with the use of your imagination. During the test, you could create a relaxing and comfortable place and imagine yourself in it. What is a relaxing and safe place for you?

Patient: I always feel relaxed at the beach.

Therapist: OK great. Close your eyes. Try to imagine the beach scene in as much detail as possible. Bring it to life by using as many of your senses as you can. What do you see, feel, hear, smell, and taste?

Patient: I feel the sand under my feet and the sun on my face. I hear the waves and children laughing. I smell suntan lotion.

Therapist: OK great. Stay with that image and bring your awareness to how relaxed you feel.

Patient: I'm actually starting to feel a little relaxed.

Therapist: Focus on the relaxed feelings. If you have difficulty relaxing, tell yourself, "I'm letting go of tension." Remember the details: the sights, the smells, the sounds. You can return here as many times as you like. Keep in mind that the use of visualization to relax is a skill. It's important to practice it regularly so that you can use it more effectively in times of distress. When is the scan?

Patient: Next Friday.

Therapist: That gives you plenty of time to practice. The easiest place to practice is lying in bed. You can practice in the evening before sleep and in the morning before getting out of bed.

Homework

For homework, patients can practice imagining a relaxing scene and bringing their awareness to the experience of it, using Form 10.9 as a guide.

Possible Problems

It may be difficult for patients who are distressed to sustain their focus on the imagined scene. For these individuals, the exercise can be modified so that the visualization is guided. The therapist can ask patients to write a detailed description of the relaxing scene and the imagined experience of being there. Then this description can be read by either the patients or their therapist and recorded for them to use a guided visualization exercise. Some patients experience dysphoria when imagining positive scenes. Common thoughts are "I used to enjoy that and now I don't" or "I am only imagining things, not experiencing them." Again, the therapist can emphasize that practicing a wide variety of self-help skills can increase the likelihood of actually engaging in positive activities, including some that are imagined in the visualization.

Imagination and visualization may be construed as the first step in developing plans and carrying out solutions.

Cross-Reference to Other Techniques

Related techniques include focusing on the breath, reward menu, and activity scheduling.

Form

Form 10.9: Instructions for Using Positive Imagery

TECHNIQUE: THE ALEXANDER LIE-DOWN
RELAXATION TECHNIQUE

Description

The Alexander technique (AT) is a method of letting go of unnecessary tension in the body and mind by finding unhelpful habits of motion and attention and applying directed awareness and selective relaxation to change these habits. Traditional training in AT involves a patient meeting with an AT teacher, who presents a series of simple exercises, involving body awareness, economy of motion, and more efficient movement in everyday tasks. Although this is an educational rather than a medical discipline, AT has some demonstrated effectiveness in reducing the experience of stress and stress-related medical symptoms (Jones, 1997; Little et al., 2008).

Historically, AT has been used by performers, such as actors and musicians, and work in AT is included in the curriculum of some major music education institutions, such as the Juilliard School in New York and the Royal College of Music in London. AT's emphasis on contacting the present moment and using awareness to reduce stress has led to some of its techniques and principles being adopted by experiential psychotherapies, such as Gestalt therapy (Tengwall, 1981). Although AT shares certain conceptual similarities with meditation and mindfulness training, it is not directly linked to any spiritual philosophy or specific theory of cognition. It is a focused series of techniques that can be used to help promote relaxation and stress management and may contribute to greater relaxation and more efficient posture and movement when engaging in other mindfulness and relaxation-based techniques.

The exercise presented here is a variation of a fundamental AT self-help practice known as the Alexander lie-down technique. The practice is a deceptively simple, 20-minute relaxation exercise that, in some ways, resembles a yogic or meditative practice. Proponents of the AT lie-down technique report that regular practice of this deep relaxation method can result in a higher energy level, lower experienced stress, and more efficient movement and functioning in daily activities (American Society for the Alexander Technique, 2006). This brief exercise involves less thought, conceptual material, and even physical effort than many of the techniques thus far presented. It is particularly appropriate for patients who experience physical tension or chronic pain as part of their symptom presentation.

Question to Pose/Intervention

"Do you give yourself the opportunity to relax deeply in any way during your daily life? Have you experienced lowered energy or a physical experience of feeling drained as a result of stress or being overwhelmed? Would you be willing to engage in a brief relaxation exercise for about 20 minutes a day for the next week or so as a part of our work together? The Alexander lie-down technique is a simple relaxation exercise that involves you doing nothing, as much as you can, for about 20 minutes. This practice involves lying down in a simple, relaxing posture that is designed to use gravity, and the natural balance of your body, to facilitate deep rest and restoration for your body and mind. It can be learned in a few minutes and can be practiced, as you find it useful, for years."

Example

Patient: This has been an overwhelming week at home, with all of the work I need to do on the computer to manage our family business. I find that I just can't relax these days.

Therapist: It does sound like you have a lot of work and little time to deal with it all. You've said that you can't relax. What do you do to relax?

Patient: Well, I usually exercise, read, or talk with a friend. Sometimes, lately, I've even tried to do some of the meditation exercises that we've looked at, but none of that really leads me to relax.

Therapist: It sounds like you are trying very hard, not just in your family business and in your relationships, but in trying to do the right thing to help you relax.

Patient: I have, really.

Therapist: As we have discussed, exercise, reading, socializing, and even meditation, all might contribute to some relaxation, but they all can sometimes be rather activating and involve a fair amount of effort.

Patient: I know what you mean.

Therapist: I would like to take some time in our session today to introduce a form of relaxation that is very simple, and that really involves doing nothing, as much as you can, but inviting a deep sense of rest and physical relaxation. Would that be OK?

Patient: Sure. That actually sounds nice, if it could help.

Therapist: (*Uses the instructions given in Form 10.10 for the lie-down technique.*)

Homework

The Alexander lie-down technique (Form 10.10) can be practiced 20 minutes per day as a homework exercise. It can also be practiced in shorter intervals, particularly as a response to stress during long periods of work.

Possible Problems

There are several aspects of the AT lie-down technique that might make some patients either physically or mentally uncomfortable. If the exercise involves any pain or serious discomfort, patients should feel free to discontinue it at any time and inform their therapist. There is no special reason to assume that this would be the case, but as the exercise does involve getting up and down from the floor and lying in a particular position, it is important to make certain that the patients use their own sensitivity to practice in a way that works for them. Also, demonstrating this exercise can be unusual in many office spaces, because it does involve lying down on a blanket. Sufficient physical space is needed for this, obviously. More than just the physical space, lying on the floor in a state of deep rest may be something that patients are very unaccustomed to doing in a therapist's office. For some patients, the therapist might choose to briefly yet patiently demonstrate the posture and technique involved and suggest that patients begin the exercise for themselves as homework.

Like other relaxation exercises, the Alexander lie-down technique might not directly lead to relaxation. If patients report that the exercise is "not working," the therapist should remind patients that developing skill in applied relaxation takes time and practice. The therapist may use CT techniques to identify and challenge the automatic thoughts that accompany this apparent lack of results. More often, patients may fall asleep during the Alexander lie-down technique. This problem can be addressed by having patients practicing the lie-down with their eyes open, until they become sufficiently fluent in the application of the technique to enter into a state of restfulness without falling asleep.

Cross-Reference to Other Techniques

The Alexander lie-down technique may help patients to develop facility in selective attention, relaxation, and stable posture that is involved in sitting meditation practices such as the mindfulness of the breath or making space exercise. Because it involves deep rest and relaxation, it is a worthwhile complementary practice for patients who are practicing progressive muscle relaxation. Patients who have mastered the Alexander lie-down technique and the 3-minute breathing space or 3-minute coping breathing space may blend these two practices together for a brief, relaxing dose of mindfulness and stress reduction at regular intervals during periods of sustained stress.

Form

Form 10.10: Instructions for the Alexander Lie-Down Technique

TECHNIQUE: INTENSIFY POSITIVE EXPERIENCES BY BEING MINDFUL OF THEM

Description

Positive emotional experiences are needed to buffer the impact of negative ones. Yet, for many patients with emotion regulation difficulties, positive experiences seem fleeting or insignificant. Factors that can detract from positive emotional experiences include worry, thoughts about when the experience will end, and the belief that one is unworthy of positive experiences. In order for patients to derive the full benefit of positive emotional experiences, it is important that they are mindful of them. In other words, patients need to bring their full awareness to positive experiences as they are happening and let distracting thoughts go.

Question to Pose/Intervention

"In order to get the maximal benefit of positive experiences, it is important to be mindful of them as they are happening or bring full awareness to them. Often we are physically present for positive events but mentally elsewhere. As a result, we don't enjoy them as much. For example, you might attend yoga class but spend the entire class worrying about a problem. As a result, your ability to enjoy it is decreased. By shifting your awareness from your thoughts back to the class, your experience becomes more enjoyable."

Example

The therapist is reviewing the patient's pleasant activity log that was completed for homework.

Therapist: It doesn't look like you enjoyed any of these activities very much. Do you think there was anything interfering with your ability to enjoy them?

Patient: I'm not sure what you mean.

Therapist: Well, sometimes we do things for enjoyment. Although we're physically present for these activities, mentally we are not. In other words, our thoughts take us out of the situation.

Patient: That's true. I spent most of the week worried about the exam that I have next week. I couldn't really focus on any of the things I did.

Therapist: So it sounds like worry thoughts interfered with your enjoyment of these activities. To get the maximal benefit from positive experiences, it's important to focus your awareness on them. It's important to practice letting go of the thoughts, like worries, that decrease our enjoyment.

Patient: How can I do that?

Therapist: By shifting your awareness from your thoughts to what's happening in the moment. So, for example, if you are at a tennis match, focus on the players and the sound of the tennis ball. As the focus of your awareness drifts to worry thoughts, bring it back.

Homework

For homework, patients can practice bringing their awareness to pleasurable activities.

Possible Problems

Patients may be frustrated by the difficulty of sustaining awareness on positive events. The therapist should emphasize that the ability to focus awareness on present experience is a skill that requires practice. Additionally, the therapist should normalize the tendency of the mind to wander. Mindful breathing can be included in the homework as a method of increasing awareness of the present moment. In addition, some patients discount the positive experiences as trivial. The therapist can ask patients what life would be like if they could never again experience any of these everyday, "trivial" experiences.

Cross-Reference to Other Techniques

Related techniques include mindfulness, compassionate imagery, and reward menu.

Forms

None

TECHNIQUE: COPING WITH CRAVINGS AND URGES: URGE SURFING

Description

Cravings, urges, and desires that are not immediately satisfied are form of distress. Because it may be counter to an individual's interest to act on cravings, urges, and desires, it is important to develop the skill of tolerating them. Acting on urges and cravings reinforces or strengthens them by removing discomfort and bringing short-term pleasure. For example, an unfulfilled craving for cocaine is uncomfortable. If an individual acts on the craving by using cocaine, he or she escapes distress and experiences a short-term elevation in mood, both of which reinforce the cravings for cocaine. Repeatedly acting on urges and desires may strengthen the commonly held belief that they are irresistible.

Urge surfing is a mindfulness-based technique for relapse prevention, a treatment for addictions designed to help the patient overcome urges to use drugs and alcohol (Daley & Marlatt, 2006). However, this technique can also be used effectively to manage other urges, including urges to binge, self-injury, and act on one's emotion. Urge surfing is premised on the idea that urges are time-limited phenomena. Without the opportunity to act on them, urges are typically not long lasting. Just as emotions reach their peak intensity and then ebb, so do cravings, urges, and desires. Trying to suppress an urge or struggling against an urge only intensifies it. In other words, "fighting the urge only feeds it." When practicing urge surfing, the patient takes a mindful stance toward the urge and observes it in a detached, nonjudgmental way. Rather than struggle with the urge, the patient observes it rise and fall. He or she experiences the urge as a wave, riding it until it subsides.

Question to Pose/Intervention

"Urges and cravings can be distressing when we cannot or should not satisfy them. For example, if I'm on a diet, it's not in my interest to satisfy my craving for chocolate cake. Rather, I need to tolerate the craving. Sometimes cravings feel irresistible. But they are not. The fact is that cravings and urges will pass as a function of time. Like waves, they reach their peak intensity and then ebb. If we think of them that way, we can just surf or ride the wave of the urge into shore. When you're having an urge, bring it into your awareness and observe it nonjudgmentally. Don't push it away or try to block it. "

Example

In this example, the therapist teaches urge surfing to a patient with binge-eating disorder.

Therapist: You say you have difficulty overcoming your urges to binge.

Patient: Yes, they're irresistible.

Therapist: Did you act on every urge you had this week?

Patient: No. That's true, I didn't.

Therapist: But your thought is that they're irresistible. That's a common belief—that urges are irresistible. Acting on them repeatedly can strengthen that belief. They may seem irresistible if they creep up on us and we act on them without awareness. The key is bringing them into awareness, becoming more mindful of them so we can choose how to respond to them.

Patient: OK. But, what should I do if I have one?

Therapist: One option is to simply ride it out or urge surf. How long do you think an urge to binge lasts?

Patient: I don't really know. It seems to last indefinitely, but I guess that's impossible.

Therapist: Have you ever had an urge to binge when you couldn't act on it? How long did it last?

Patient: I had one this week during a conference call. After the call ended, the urge was gone. It must have been 20 minutes.

Therapist: It's important to be aware that urges are time limited. They're like waves, reaching a peak intensity and then ebbing. Rather than being hit by the wave, imagine yourself surfing it. Don't fight it or resist it. Let go of tension in your body and breathe. Just ride it out.

Homework

For homework, the patient can practice surfing his or her urges to engage in particular dysfunctional behavior. To increase the likelihood of success and develop a sense of mastery, the patient can be instructed to begin his or her practice with lower intensity urges and then progress to more intense urges.

Possible Problems

The patient may lack sufficient awareness of his or her urges to practice this technique. In other words, the patient may be acting on his or her urges impulsively before he or she is aware of them. In this instance, the therapist should ask the patient to monitor urges in an effort to cultivate greater awareness of them. The patient should monitor the frequency, intensity, and duration of urges. Through monitoring, the patient will obtain valuable information about what is triggering the urges and in what contexts they are most intense. With this knowledge, the patient can practice urge surfing in a graded fashion, beginning with the least intense urges. Alternatively, the patient can practice surfing urges that would not be problematic to act on as a way to gain mastery of the technique. For example, the patient can practice surfing urges to speak, dance, or satisfy one's curiosity.

Cross-Reference to Other Techniques

Related techniques include experiencing emotion as a wave, observing and describing emotions, and mindfulness.

Forms

None

CONCLUSIONS

Stress management has a long history in psychology, dating back to the 19th century in a variety of self-help formats. In this chapter, we have highlighted a variety of stress management techniques that might be helpful in regulating emotion and in reducing the likelihood of stressful events in the future. Time management, planning activities, building reward menus, and soothing oneself in the present moment are all techniques that can counteract current stress and reduce the impact of events in the future. In addition to the techniques described here, stress management can also include dietary guidelines, regular exercise, massage, the use of dance and creative outlets for expression and stress reduction, emotional journaling, and assertion. Moreover, many patients may experience stress as a result of angry and hostile reactions to events. All of the foregoing can be included in a more comprehensive treatment of stress.

CHAPTER ELEVEN

Conclusions

We have reviewed nine "strategies" of emotion regulation in this book. What do they have in common, and how would they be integrated into a comprehensive approach? In this final chapter, we try to demonstrate how an integrative emotional schema approach can provide a flexible, comprehensive strategy of emotion regulation for a common clinical issue: coping with a breakup of an intimate relationship.

We began with a consideration of integrative theories of emotion, such as that proposed by Gross's distinction between antecedent and response coping and Barlow's unified theory. The various chapters in this book address different coping strategies—some focusing on antecedent coping (such as cognitive restructuring), others focusing on response strategies (such as mindfulness, acceptance, and stress reduction). We have proposed that an overarching model of emotional schemas can incorporate the important distinctions that Gross has advanced as well as the implications of a unified theory of emotion as described by Barlow. In particular, EST proposes that the evolutionary adaptation and universality of emotion is a fundamental component of all emotions, but that emotions are also an object of cognition and, therefore, can be socially constructed so that beliefs about durability, lack of control, legitimacy, and other dimensions can further impact the up- or down-regulation of emotion. EST helps in identifying the patient's theory of emotions and theory and strategies of emotional control. These beliefs about emotion can then be modified using the many techniques described in this book.

Perhaps the clearest way of summing up this argument is to examine what beliefs and strategies one can utilize when confronting a breakup of a relationship. A comprehensive model is shown in Figure 11.1. Consider two individuals—Andy, who is adaptive, and Carl, who is confused—who have independently been informed that their "significant other" has broken up with them. Adaptive Andy recognizes that he has a range of emotions: sadness, anger, anxiety, confusion, and even a little relief. He also believes that having a lot of different emotions is not self-contradictory but rather reflects the complexity of human relationships. He normalizes his emotions, expresses them tactfully with his friend, Frank, and believes that he doesn't need to have everything clear and simple. Thus, he doesn't ruminate. He realizes it is a stressful time, so he practices some relaxation, goes to a yoga class, schedules pleasurable activities, and accepts the imperfect validation that his friend occasionally offers. Andy does not ruminate about the relationship because he does not think it will help, and he is able to tolerate his mixed and confused feelings, partly because he views them as temporary and partly because having mixed

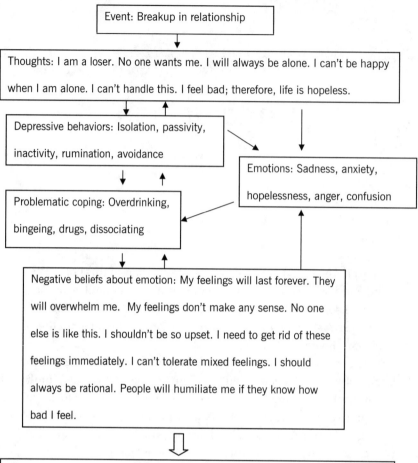

FIGURE 11.1. Emotional schema conceptualization.

feelings makes sense to him. He sometimes has an urge to drink more than usual, but he is able to ride the wave and let the urge come and go. He stands back, on occasion, observes himself and others, and doesn't have a sense of urgency to "make things happen." He feels sad but also directs compassionate supportive statements toward himself, reminding him that he is the kind of person that he wants to be and that he is deserving of love and support. And he is willing to give that love and support to himself. He thinks about long-term goals and values: hoping to find a better relationship in the future, valuing the fact that he appreciates commitment and love, and recognizing that he may have to be unhappy for a while. He can let the feeling come and go because he knows that he has to go through it to get past it. Andy is truly adaptive and has the wisdom to use the techniques described in this book.

However, Confused Carl is not as fortunate. He has many of the negative emotional schemas that we have outlined. He believes he should only feel one way and cannot understand or accept his mixed feelings. He ruminates while isolating himself and remains inactive. He needs an answer, clarity, and certainty and demands fairness in life. He feels ashamed of his emotional vulnerability and soothes himself by having a drink—and then another. When his sadness comes over him, he believes he must get rid of it immediately, so he eats junk food and spends hours perusing pornography. He is afraid to cry, but finally does, further activating his belief that he is pathetic and weak. He hates himself and believes that showing compassion and love toward himself is a sign of further weakness. He cannot accept his emotion and dwells on how bad he feels. When he sees his friend Tom, he spills out his complaints about the breakup and becomes increasingly angry that Tom "doesn't get it." He tells Tom, "It's easy for you." As Tom tries to empathize, Carl complains further, "Don't patronize me!" Because Carl has difficulty sleeping, he tries to drink himself to sleep at night and wakes in the morning with a hangover, which he treats with a wake-up drink followed by endless cups of espresso during the day. He has stopped working out and says that he has to wait to feel better before he goes out and sees friends or returns to the gym to get back into shape. Carl believes that his emotions are in charge and he has given up trying.

As these two stories illustrate, patients can require assistance on many levels and at many stages of emotion dysregulation. Adaptive Andy is already using the adaptive emotional schemas, already accepting his emotions, receiving imperfect validation, activating himself to engage in positive behavior, using compassionate mind toward himself, clarifying and affirming his goals and values, and committing himself to living a purposeful life. Adaptive Andy is taking all the steps to legitimize his emotions, act in spite of his feelings, and support himself. He is not likely to be our patient. He won't need us.

Confused Carl, on the other hand, needs our help. He needs to examine his pejorative theory of his emotion. Confused Carl has many of the negative beliefs about emotion that we have outlined. He fears his emotions, feels ashamed, believes he is weak and inferior because of his feelings, thinks his feelings do not make sense, and cannot accept or tolerate the mixed feelings that come over him. He believes he has to suppress—eliminate—painful feelings, and he turns to maladaptive coping, such as drinking, isolation, blaming, and ruminating. He is a good candidate for what this book is all about.

So, how do we help Confused Carl? He needs to direct compassionate mind toward himself to help him legitimize his emotional needs and soothe his painful feelings. He needs to realize that he can act opposite the way he feels, he can build a supportive network by being more skilled in seeking validation and supporting the people who support him. He can learn to be mindful and accepting of his emotions and of himself by taking a nonjudgmental stand toward the way he feels and learn how to make the best of a temporarily bad situation. He can learn to tolerate the ambiguity, unfairness, and apparent self-contradiction of feelings while clarifying a set of values that will make his life more purposeful and more worth enduring.

To help patients like Carl, we can develop integrative strategies using the emotional schema conceptualization, that is, by recognizing the difficulties that they are experiencing regarding their emotions. Using a case conceptualization based on emotional schemas, the clinician and the patient can collaborate to develop a treatment plan for coping based on both antecedent and response-based strategies, as outlined in Figures 11.1 and 11.2. Our clinical experience is that there is no one set of interventions that works for every patient, and the clinician can enhance the effectiveness of therapy through flexibility of approach without requiring a strong allegiance to one model.

This book was a collaborative effort by three clinicians who see patients on a regular basis. We recognize, as the readers of this book also know, that every patient is a unique experience, every patient has a unique world of emotions. Helping patients identify their beliefs about their emotions—and encouraging them to recognize alternatives to feeling overwhelmed or to feeling a need to numb themselves against their emotions—can help patients live with their feelings without being afraid of themselves. Patients come to therapy because of the way they feel—or because they would like to have other feelings. We hope that the ideas, strategies, and examples in this book will pave the way for that journey.

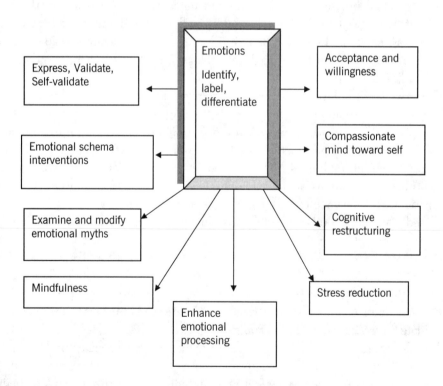

FIGURE 11.2. Emotion regulation interventions.

Reproducible Forms

Leahy Emotional Schemas Scale

Directions: We are interested in how you deal with your feelings or emotions—for example, how you deal with feelings of anger, sadness, and anxiety or with sexual feelings. We all differ in how we deal with these feelings, so there are no right or wrong answers. Please read each sentence carefully and rate it, using the following scale, as to how you've dealt with your feelings during the past month. Write the number of your response next to the sentence.

Scale:

1 = very untrue of me
2 = somewhat untrue of me
3 = slightly untrue of me
4 = slightly true of me
5 = somewhat true of me
6 = very true of me

1. When I feel down, I try to think about a different way to view things. ____

2. When I have a feeling that bothers me, I try to think of why it is not important. ____

3. I often think that I respond with feelings that others would not have. ____

4. Some feelings are wrong to have. ____

5. There are things about myself that I just don't understand. ____

6. I believe that it is important to let myself cry in order to get my feelings "out." ____

7. If I let myself have some of these feelings, I fear I will lose control. ____

8. Others understand and accept my feelings. ____

9. You can't allow yourself to have certain kinds of feelings—like feelings about sex or violence. ____

10. My feelings don't make sense to me. ____

11. If other people changed, I would feel a lot better. ____

12. I think I have feelings that I am not really aware of. ____

13. I sometimes fear that if I allowed myself to have a strong feeling, it would not go away. ____

14. I feel ashamed of my feelings. ____

15. Things that bother other people don't bother me. ____

16. No one really cares about my feelings. ____

17. It is important for me to be reasonable and practical rather than sensitive and open to my feelings. ____

18. I can't stand it when I have contradictory feelings—like liking and disliking the same person. ____

(cont.)

19. I am much more sensitive than other people. ____

20. I try to get rid of an unpleasant feeling immediately. ____

21. When I feel down, I try to think of the more important things in life—what I value. ____

22. When I feel down or sad, I question my values. ____

23. I feel that I can express my feelings openly. ____

24. I often say to myself, "What's wrong with me?" ____

25. I think of myself as a shallow person. ____

26. I want people to believe that I am different from the way I truly feel. ____

27. I worry that I won't be able to control my feelings. ____

28. You have to guard against having certain feelings. ____

29. Strong feelings only last a short period of time. ____

30. You can't rely on your feelings to tell you what is good for you. ____

31. I shouldn't have some of the feelings I have. ____

32. I often feel numb emotionally, like I have no feelings. ____

33. I think that my feelings are strange or weird. ____

34. Other people cause me to have unpleasant feelings. ____

35. When I have conflicting feelings about someone, I get upset or confused. ____

36. When I have a feeling that bothers me, I try to think of something else to think about or do. ____

37. When I feel down, I sit by myself and think a lot about how bad I feel. ____

38. I like being absolutely definite about the way I feel about *someone else*. ____

39. Everyone has feelings like mine. ____

40. I accept my feelings. ____

41. I think that I have the same feelings other people have. ____

42. I aspire to higher values. ____

43. I think that my feelings now have *nothing* to do with how I was brought up. ____

44. I worry that if I have certain feelings, I might go crazy. ____

45. My feelings seem to come from out of nowhere. ____

46. I think it is important to be rational and logical in almost everything. ____

47. I like being absolutely definite about the way I feel about *myself*. ____

48. I focus a lot on my feelings or my physical sensations. ____

49. I don't want anyone to know about some of my feelings. ____

50. I don't want to admit to having certain feelings, but I know that I have them. ____

Fourteen Dimensions
of the Leahy Emotional Schemas Scale

The following dimensions describe various interpretations and coping strategies for emotions based on the Leahy Emotional Schemas Scale. Items marked by parentheses are reverse scored. Note: Items 22 and 43 do not fall within specified dimensions.

Validation

Item 8	Others understand and accept my feelings.
(Item 16)	No one really cares about my feelings.
(Item 49)	I don't want anyone to know about some of my feelings.

Comprehensibility

(Item 5)	There are things about myself that I just don't understand.
(Item 10)	My feelings don't make sense to me.
(Item 33)	I think that my feelings are strange or weird.
(Item 45)	My feelings seem to come from out of nowhere.

Guilt

Item 4	Some feelings are wrong to have.
Item 14	I feel ashamed of my feelings.
Item 26	I want people to believe that I am different from the way I truly feel.
Item 31	I shouldn't have some of the feelings I have.

Simplistic View of Emotion

Item 18	I can't stand it when I have contradictory feelings—like liking and disliking the same person.
Item 35	When I have conflicting feelings about someone, I get upset or confused.
Item 38	I like being absolutely definite about the way I feel about *someone else*.
Item 47	I like being absolutely definite about the way I feel about *myself*.

Higher Values

Item 21	When I feel down, I try to think of the more important things in life—what I value.
(Item 25)	I think of myself as a shallow person.
Item 42	I aspire to higher values.

Control

(Item 7)	If I let myself have some of these feelings, I fear I will lose control.
(Item 27)	I worry that I won't be able to control my feelings.
(Item 44)	I worry that if I have certain feelings, I might go crazy.

(cont.)

Numbness

Item 15   Things that bother other people don't bother me.

Item 32   I often feel numb emotionally, like I have no feelings.

Need to Be Rational

Item 17   It is important for me to be reasonable and practical rather than sensitive and open to my feelings.

Item 46   I think it is important to be rational and logical in almost everything.

Item 30   You can't rely on your feelings to tell you what is good for you.

Duration

Item 13   I sometimes fear that if I allowed myself to have a strong feeling, it would not go away.

(Item 29)   Strong feelings only last a short period of time.

Consensus

(Item 3)   I often think that I respond with feelings that others would not have.

(Item 19)   I am much more sensitive than other people.

Item 39   Everyone has feelings like mine.

Item 41   I think that I have the same feelings other people have.

Acceptance of Feelings

(Item 2)   When I have a feeling that bothers me, I try to think of why it is not important.

(Item 12)   I think I have feelings that I am not really aware of.

(Item 20)   I try to get rid of an unpleasant feeling immediately.

Item 40   I accept my feelings.

(Item 50)   I don't want to admit to having certain feelings, but I know that I have them.

(Item 9)   You can't allow yourself to have certain kinds of feelings—like feelings about sex or violence.

(Item 28)   You have to guard against having certain feelings.

Rumination

(Item 1)   When I feel down, I try to think about a different way to view things.

(Item 36)   When I have a feeling that bothers me, I try to think of something else to think about or do.

Item 37   When I feel down, I sit by myself and think a lot about how bad I feel.

Item 24   I often say to myself, "What's wrong with me?"

Item 48   I focus a lot on my feelings or my physical sensations.

Expression

Item 6   I believe that it is important to let myself cry in order to get my feelings "out."

Item 23   I feel that I can express my feelings openly.

Blame

Item 11   If other people changed, I would feel a lot better.

Item 34   Other people cause me to have unpleasant feelings.

Emotion Log

Directions: For each emotion in the left column, put a check in the box for the days on which you notice that you have these emotions. You can add other emotions that are not listed in the left column.

Emotion	Monday	Tuesday	Wednesday	Thursday	Friday	Saturday	Sunday
Happy							
Interested							
Excited							
Caring							
Affection							
Love							
Loved							
Compassion							
Grateful							
Proud							
Confident							
Hurt							
Sad							
Regret							
Irritated							
Angry							
Resentful							
Disgust							
Contempt							
Ashamed							
Guilty							
Envious							
Jealous							
Anxious							
Afraid							
Other							

From Greenberg (2002). Copyright 2002 by the American Psychological Association. Reprinted by permission.

Possible Emotions Someone Could Have
in This Situation

Directions: In the left column, list all of the different emotions that you are having in this situation, including unpleasant, neutral, and pleasant emotions. For example, you might be feeling sad, lonely, angry, anxious, confused, indifferent, relieved, challenged, curious, happy, or other emotions. In the right column, list the specific thoughts that are associated with these emotions. For example, for the emotion of anger, you might be thinking, "They don't respect me." In the bottom left column, list other possible emotions you could have and the thought that would go with those emotions. For example, you might be feeling "angry," but another possible emotion could be "anxiety." What thoughts go with "anxiety"?

Emotions I Am Experiencing	Thoughts
Other Emotions I Could Have	Thoughts

Costs and Benefits of Thinking
My Emotions Are Abnormal

Directions: In the left column, list any emotions that you consider abnormal, unusual, or about which you might feel ashamed or guilty. Then in the next two columns list the costs and benefits of believing that these emotions are abnormal. What would change and how would you feel about your emotions if you thought that they were not abnormal? Would your life be better or worse? For example, you might think that the costs of being angry are that you are unhappy and that you have more conflicts with people, but you might also think that the benefits are that you are standing up for yourself.

Emotions I consider abnormal	Costs	Benefits

Survey of Other People
Who Have These Emotions

Directions: List whatever emotions are troubling you in the left column and in the right column list people you know or characters in stories, poems, movies, or songs that depict these emotions. What do you make of the fact that a lot of different people have these feelings?

Emotions that I have	People who have these feelings

Activity Schedule, Emotions, and Thoughts

Directions: Our emotions often change depending on what we are doing and thinking. Keep track of your hourly activities, noting the emotions and the intensity or degree of emotion and then your thoughts and the degree to which you believe these thoughts. For example, you might rate the intensity of your anger at 90% when you think, "He is trying to ridicule me" and you might believe this thought 80%. If you believed the thought, "He is trying to ridicule me" at 20%, you might have a lot less anger. Is there any relationship among activities, thoughts, and emotions? Are emotions temporary—do they increase and decrease with intensity? What leads your emotions to decrease in intensity?

Time	Activity	Emotion (0–100%)	Thoughts (degree of belief 0–100%)
A.M. 7			
8			
9			
10			
11			
12 noon			
P.M. 1			
2			
3			
4			
5			
6			
7			
8			
9			
10			
11			
12 midnight			

Costs and Benefits of Believing
That Emotions Are Temporary

Directions: What are the costs and benefits of believing that your emotions are temporary? What would change if you believed that an unpleasant feeling you had was only temporary?

Costs	Benefits

What would change if you believed that your emotions are temporary?

How to Accept Difficult Feelings

Directions: Examples of how to accept feelings include the following: "Don't fight the feeling; allow it to happen. Stand back and observe it. Imagine that the feeling is floating along and you are floating along next to it. Watch it go up and down, come and go, moment to moment." See if you can set a limit on feeling the way you feel—for example, 10 minutes—and then move on to something else. You can also distract yourself with other activities, do pleasurable things, or practice mindful awareness—stepping back, simply observing that you feel the way you feel, and letting it go.

Question to ask yourself	Examples
• What is the feeling that is hard to accept?	
• What does it mean to you if you accepted that you had this feeling?	
• What are the advantages and disadvantages of accepting the feeling?	
• Set a time limit to focus on the feeling.	
• Shift attention to other activities and things around you.	
• Are there productive, rewarding, or pleasurable things to do?	
• Practice mindful awareness.	

Examples of Mixed Feelings

Directions: We may have a lot of different feelings about the same person, place, or thing. For example, we might have mixed feelings about our parents, partners, friends, experiences, places we visit, and things that we do. It's important to realize that mixed feelings are normal and may illustrate the ability to have a richer and more complex experience. In the following form, list some people, places, things, or experiences about which you have mixed feelings and then list those feelings.

People, places, experiences, and things about which I have mixed feelings	The variety of feelings that I have

Advantages and Disadvantages
of Accepting Mixed Feelings

Directions: You may have mixed feelings about having mixed feelings! That's also normal. Please list the advantages and disadvantages to you of accepting that you have mixed feelings.

Advantages	Disadvantages

Looking for Positive Emotions

Directions: There are many positive emotions that you may have experienced and continue to experience. It is important to integrate these emotions in your everyday life. Look at the list of these 10 positive emotions and then in the right column list examples of these emotions in the past or currently. Try to keep track of these on a daily basis.

Positive emotions	Memories and examples of these emotions
Joy	
Gratitude	
Serenity	
Interest	
Hope	
Pride	
Amusement	
Inspiration	
Awe	
Love	

Emotional Goal Inventory

Directions: Sometimes we get stuck in an emotion like sadness, anger, anxiety, or fear, and we just don't know how to get out of it. One technique that you can use to become "unstuck" is to identify a different emotion that you would like to experience and develop a story or plan of how you can experience that emotion.

Emotion that I want to aim for:
Describe some thoughts, behaviors, and experiences that can help you experience more of this emotion:
How can you plan to aim for these other emotions?

Additional Meanings in Life

Directions: Think about the many things in your life that may give you meaning and purpose. We have listed some suggestions in the left column, but you can add as many categories or experiences of meaning and purpose that you want. In the middle column, rate how important each item is to you, from 0 (not at all important) to 5 (essential). In the right column, list some things that you can do—actions, thoughts, meditation, or anything—to help you pursue what is meaningful. The goal is to clarify what matters and to direct you toward the purposes in your life.

What gives me meaning and purpose in my life?	How important is this to me?	Examples of things that I can do to pursue this
Friendship		
Love for others		
Being a good parent, son or daughter, or partner		
Belonging to a community		
Helping others		
Competence in my work		
Advancing my career		
Being a team player		
Living a healthy lifestyle		
Getting exercise and being active		
Appreciating my surroundings and my life		
Gratitude		
Experiencing beauty		

(cont.)

What gives me meaning and purpose in my life?	How important is this to me?	Examples of things that I can do to pursue this
Feeling connected to something larger than myself		
Justice		
Learning and growing		
Adventure and trying new things		
Expressing myself		
Making good decisions		
Working hard and getting things done		
Curiosity and openness		
Humor and fun		
Improving my finances		
Connecting with tradition		
Spirituality		
Learning new things and new skills		
Being in contact with nature		
Meditation and prayer		

Possible Emotions That I Can Also Have

Directions: In the left column we have listed a number of positive emotions that you could aim for. Check the items that you might want to aim for and write some ideas about what you would have to think or do to experience that emotion. For example, you might feel angry about something that has happened (perhaps a friend treated you badly), but you could imagine feeling love for someone else or curious about a different activity. Think about how your emotions can change or be flexible depending on where you put your focus or attention.

Type of emotion	What could I think or do that would lead to this emotion?
Happy	
Interested	
Excited	
Caring	
Affection	
Forgiving	
Accepting	
Love	
Loved	
Compassion	
Grateful	
Proud	
Confident	
Other	

Relationship to Higher Values

Directions: Sometimes we feel sad, anxious, or angry because we are missing something that is important to us. Let's say you feel sad about a relationship breakup. Write your response to each of the following items.

Questions to ask yourself about your values	Your response
Doesn't this mean that you have a higher value that's important to you—for example, a value of closeness and intimacy? What is this value and what does the value mean to you?	
Doesn't this value say something good about you?	
If you aspire to higher values, doesn't this mean that you will have to be disappointed at times?	
Would you want to be a cynic who values nothing? What would your life be like?	
Are there some worthwhile and meaningful experiences that you have because you have this value?	
Are there other people who share your higher values?	
What advice would you give them if they were going through what you are going through?	

VIA Survey of Character Strengths

Go to the website *www.viacharacter.org* and click on "Survey" to complete the The VIA Survey of Character. This is a 240-item questionnaire that has been developed to identify various character strengths that you have. On the website you can get a free summary of your responses. This survey takes about 30–40 minutes to complete. Bring the results of this survey to your next session with your therapist.

Examples of When I Feel
or Don't Feel Validated

Directions: Sometimes we feel that other people understand us, validate the way we feel, and give us support. Write some specific examples of this in the left column. In the right column, write examples of when you didn't feel validated.

I felt validated (cared for, supported) when ...	I didn't feel validated (cared for, supported) when ...

Problematic Ways of Getting People
to Respond to Me

Directions: Sometimes we don't feel people understand us, and we respond in ways that might be viewed by others as problematic. Try to be honest with yourself and indicate whether you have ever used any of the following behaviors. Give specific examples. Now think about the consequences of using these strategies in response to invalidation. Is this behavior going to help you? Perhaps there are alternatives that you might consider.

Problematic behavior	Examples
Complain over and over	
Raise my voice	
Yell or scream	
Criticize the other person for not understanding	
Pouting	
Throwing things	
Make it sound like something terrible is happening to me	
Threaten to harm myself	
Threaten to leave	
Repeat myself over and over	
Other	

My Beliefs about Validation

Directions: When we believe that someone is not hearing our feelings, we tend to have a string or series of thoughts. Take your first thought about what it means to you if someone doesn't validate you. Now ask yourself, "If that were true, it would bother me because it would mean ... what?" Keep repeating this response for each thought until you can't think of anything else it could mean. Let's say that you begin with the thought, "She doesn't hear what I am saying," and then you have a string of other thoughts like, "It means she doesn't care" and "No one cares." What will this make you feel? Are there different ways of thinking about "She doesn't hear what I am saying?" Could there be another way of looking at the beliefs in the list below—for example, "Maybe people are imperfect" or "Maybe I can try to clarify what I am feeling?"

Beliefs about validation	Degree of belief (0–100%)
I want other people to agree with me.	
If people offer me advice, they are neglecting my feelings.	
Unless you've gone through what I have gone through, you can't really understand me.	
As long as people make an effort to understand me, I appreciate it.	
It's dangerous to trust people with your feelings. They might criticize you or make fun of you.	
Other examples	

Vertical Descent
for When I Do Not Feel Validated

Directions: When we believe that someone is not hearing our feelings, we tend to have a string or series of thoughts. Take your first thought about what it means to you if someone doesn't validate you. Now ask yourself, "If that were true, it would bother me because it would mean ... what?" Keep repeating this for each thought until you can't think of anything else it could mean. Look at your first thoughts in this diagram and ask yourself what the consequence is of interpreting someone's response in this way. For example, if you conclude that if someone doesn't hear you exactly the way you want to be heard, they don't care about you, then you are likely to feel really angry, alone, and even hopeless. But what if you had a different interpretation and thought, "Maybe no one is perfect" or "Maybe I can take some time to clarify what I am saying"?

When someone doesn't validate me, it bothers me because it makes me think ...

↓

↓

↓

↓

↓

What I Can Do When I Am Not Validated

Directions: Sometimes we don't feel that others understand how we feel—we feel invalidated. This can be upsetting. However, there may be a number of things that you can do to soothe your own feelings rather than rely on others. In the form below, list some examples of techniques you could try as alternatives for when you feel invalidated.

Alternatives to validation	Examples
I can accept that others are imperfect.	
I can recognize that there are a lot of ways that people have supported me.	
I can focus on solving some of my problems.	
I can find ways to soothe myself in the present moment.	
I can distract myself with other activities and goals.	
I can challenge the idea that being invalidated is awful.	
Other	

Adaptive Things to Say or Do
When I Feel Invalidated

Directions: Sometimes when people don't understand us we can be more effective if we say or do certain things. Some suggestions for adaptive things to do or say are presented in the list below. Add to this list any additional things that you've said or done that has helped you get validation and provide examples.

Some useful things to say or do when I don't feel understood or validated	Examples
I don't think I am making myself clear. Here is what I am trying to say.	
I really appreciate your making an effort to understand me, but I think you might not understand right now what I am going through.	
Can you rephrase for me what you hear me saying so that I can find out if I am making myself clear?	
I would feel understood better if you could say or do the following . . .	
Thanks for taking the time to listen and care.	
I know I may be going on a bit long right now, but I do appreciate your making an effort.	
Your support means a lot to me.	
Other examples	

Examples of Minimizing My Needs

Directions: Sometimes we act as if our needs and our feelings are not really important. We might feel undeserving of having our needs met, apologize for our needs, or even space out when our emotions are discussed. In the left column of the form below, identify ways that you might be minimizing your needs and in the right column give some examples. Now think about the consequence of invalidating your own needs. Would you minimize the needs or suffering of a friend? Why not? Would it sound invalidating, cruel, or dismissive? What alternative, compassionate, and validating things would you say to a friend? Is there some reason why you might not say these things to yourself rather than minimize your needs?

How I minimize my needs	Examples
It's a sign of weakness to feel you need others to support you and understand you.	
I am too needy.	
I don't like talking about my needs.	
I expect too much from life.	
I should just accept things the way they are because I will never get my needs met.	
I seem to choose people who treat me badly.	
Sometimes I try to act like a shallow person.	
I sometimes make fun of myself, as if I am a joke no one could take seriously.	
It's more important to make other people feel comfortable than to get my needs met.	
I don't really know what I need.	
I will often binge drink, overeat, use drugs, or do other things to numb myself emotionally.	
Other examples	

Compassionate Self-Validation

Directions: Think about the most compassionate, nurturant, loving, and kind person you can imagine. Now imagine that person talking with you, soothing you, telling you that your needs are important and that your pain is heard and felt. What would that person say? What would this compassionate voice sound like? How would you feel?

What my compassionate voice can tell me about my needs. What would it say or do?	How I would feel?

How to Be More Rewarding
and Get Support from Your Friends

Directions: In order to get your emotional needs met, it is important to make your relationships mutually rewarding. Think about ways in which you can reward your friends, help them understand you, strengthen your ties and bonds to one another, and expand your network of support. Eleven strategies are listed in the left column in the form below. In the right column, give some examples of how to incorporate these strategies in your daily life.

How to be more rewarding and get support from your friends	Examples
1. Are you acting like a downer?	
2. "I need my friends to understand Am I in a 'validation trap,' demanding validation?"	
3. Learn how to ask for help.	
4. When seeking validation, keep your listener in mind.	
5. Validate the validator.	
6. Talk about positives—things that you are doing that can help.	
7. If you describe a problem, describe a solution.	
8. Don't sound like your own worst enemy.	
9. Initiate positive contact with positive activities.	
10. Respect advice.	
11. Become part of a larger community.	

Emotion Myths

Directions: Some common myths about emotions are listed below. For each myth, formulate a challenge by stating why the myth is untrue.

1. There is a right way to feel in every situation.

   CHALLENGE: _____

2. Letting others know that I am feeling bad is a weakness.

   CHALLENGE: _____

3. Negative feelings are bad and destructive.

   CHALLENGE: _____

4. Being emotional means being out of control.

   CHALLENGE: _____

5. Emotions can just happen for no reason.

   CHALLENGE: _____

6. Some emotions are really stupid.

   CHALLENGE: _____

7. All painful emotions are a result of a bad attitude.

   CHALLENGE: _____

8. If others don't approve of my feelings, I obviously shouldn't feel the way I do.

   CHALLENGE: _____

9. Other people are the best judge of how I am feeling.

   CHALLENGE: _____

10. Painful emotions are not really important and should be ignored.

    CHALLENGE: _____

(cont.)

Please add your own beliefs or myths about emotion and challenge them here.

11. _____

    CHALLENGE: _____

12. _____

    CHALLENGE: _____

13. _____

    CHALLENGE: _____

14. _____

    CHALLENGE: _____

15. _____

    CHALLENGE: _____

Basic Facts about Emotions

- Humans are born with the capacity for basic emotions, including anger, joy, interest, surprise, fear, and disgust.

- Although humans are born with a biological readiness for shame and guilt, these emotions require more cognitive development and emerge later in life.

- Emotions are time limited and subside after reaching a peak intensity.

- Although emotions are of relatively brief duration, they are self-perpetuating.

- When an emotion persists for days, it becomes a mood. Unlike emotions, moods lack a clear prompting event. Moods may last for months, days, and years. Depression is a mood, but sadness is an emotion.

Adapted from Linehan (1993b). Copyright 1993 by The Guilford Press. Adapted by permission.

Model for Describing Emotions

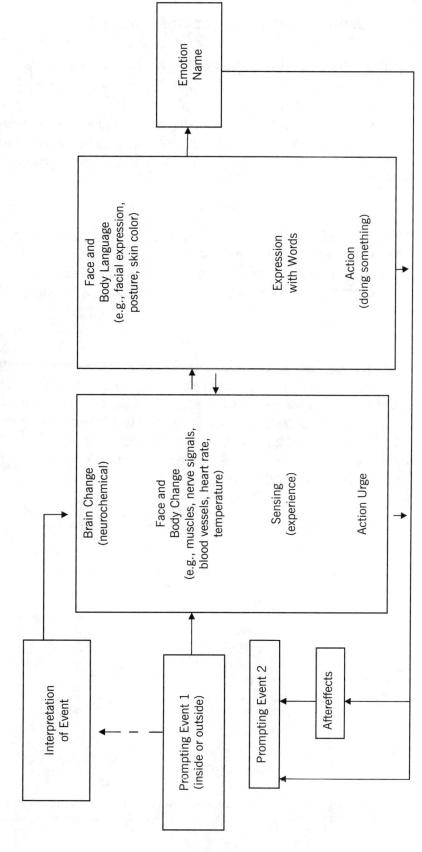

From Linehan (1993b). Copyright 1993 by The Guilford Press. Reprinted by permission.

Emotion Regulation in Psychotherapy: A Practitioner's Guide by Robert L. Leahy, Dennis Tirch, and Lisa Napolitano. Copyright 2011 by The Guilford Press. Permission to photocopy this form is granted to purchasers of this book for personal use only (see copyright page for details).

What Is the Function of Emotion?

COMMUNICATE/INFLUENCE OTHERS: The expression of emotion influences others whether we intend it or not. The expression of fear may communicate to others the presence of danger. The expression of sadness may evoke concern and empathy in others, and influence them to be caring. The expression of love may cause others to move closer to us. The expression of anger or disapproval may cause others to change their behavior.

MOTIVATE/PREPARE US TO TAKE ACTION: Emotions can motivate us and prepare us to take action. Intense fear can motivate us to flee danger or study for an upcoming exam, and love can motivate us to move closer to others. Emotions help us make decisions by letting us know.

COMMUNICATE TO THE SELF/SELF-VALIDATE: Emotions can provide us with valuable information about situations and people we anger. For example, our fear may indicate that the situation is dangerous, or our distrust may indicate that a person is untrustworthy. Although emotions provide us with valuable information, they should not be treated as facts. Emotions can be self-validating: we feel angry because we have good reason to, or we feel sad because something of value to us has been lost.

Adapted from Linehan (1993b). Copyright 1993 by The Guilford Press. Adapted by permission.

Observing and Describing Emotions

Select a current or recent emotion reaction and fill out as much of this sheet as you can. If you experienced more than one emotion, complete this form for each emotion.

EMOTION NAMES: _____

INTENSITY (0–100) _____

PROMPTING EVENT for my emotion: (who, what, when, where) What started the emotion?

INTERPRETATIONS (beliefs, assumptions, appraisals) of the situation?

BODY CHANGES and **SENSING:** What am I feeling in my body?

BODY LANGUAGE: What is my facial expression? Posture? Gestures?

(cont.)

ACTION URGES: What do I feel like doing? What do I want to say?

What **I SAID OR DID** in the situation: (Be Specific)

What **AFTEREFFECT** does the emotion have on me (my state of mind, other emotions, behavior, thoughts, memory, body, etc.)?

Function of Emotion
_____
_____
_____

Practicing a Nonjudgmental Stance
toward Emotions

Directions: Use this form to monitor the judgments you have about emotions and how these judgments affect you emotionally. See the following example.

Emotion that you judged	Judgments	Consequences of judgments
Sadness	It's weak. I'm a loser to feel this way.	Anger, shame

Experiencing Your Emotion as a Wave

Directions: The following are guidelines for experiencing your emotion as a wave. An emotion will reach its peak and intensity and then ebb.

- Experience your emotion as wave.

- Step back and simply notice it.

- Allow the emotion to rise, knowing that it will fall.

- Don't try to fight it or block it.

- Don't try to hold onto it.

- Breathe into it.

- Let go of the struggle.

- Relax.

- Ride the wave.

Emotion Induction Record

Directions: Use this form to record your emotion induction experience by answering the following questions.

What was used to induce the emotion? _____

_____

What emotion did you experience? _____

_____

Intensity of the emotion when you first experienced it (0–100%): _____

Peak intensity of emotion (0–100): _____

Time taken to reach peak intensity: _____

_____

Time taken to reach baseline: _____

_____

What I learned from this emotion induction: _____

_____

_____

_____

_____

_____

_____

_____

_____

_____

Experiment Record

Directions: Use this form to help you design an experiment to test your beliefs about emotions. Record your answers in the spaces provided.

What is the belief being tested? _____

_____

How strongly do you believe this? (0–100%) _____

How will this belief be tested? _____

_____

_____

What are you predicting will happen? _____

_____

_____

How confident are you in your prediction? (0–100%) _____

What was the actual outcome of the experiment? _____

_____

_____

Rerate the strength of your belief (0–100%) _____

Opposite Action

Directions: Opposite action is a technique you can use when you want to change your emotion or decrease its intensity. It's most effective when your emotion is not justified. To use this technique effectively it's important to first identify how the emotion you are experiencing is affecting you. In addition to acting opposite to the emotion's action urge, you also change the way the emotion is affecting your body, your thoughts, your facial expression, your body posture, what you do, and what you say. Please rate the emotion intensity before and after you use opposite action.

Emotion name: _____   **Intensity pre–post (0–100%):** _____

How does this emotion affect me physically (breathing, muscle tension, etc.)?

What is my action urge?

How does my emotion affect my facial expression, body posture, thinking, and behavior?

In light of the above information, this is what I will do to use opposite action:

Was the use of opposite action effective?

Daily Mindfulness Practice Record

Directions: Use this form each day to record your practice of mindfulness-based exercises. Remember to record each time you practice, whether you used a guided meditation audio file, and the duration of your practice period. Also, record when you practiced during the day or evening. Record any observations or questions that may have arisen during your practice. You can discuss these observations with your therapist during your next meeting.

Date	Daily practice	Observations, comments, and questions
Monday Date: _____	Did you practice? (Yes or No) Did you use an audio guide? (Yes or No)	
Tuesday Date: _____	Did you practice? (Yes or No) Did you use an audio guide? (Yes or No)	
Wednesday Date: _____	Did you practice? (Yes or No) Did you use an audio guide? (Yes or No)	
Thursday Date: _____	Did you practice? (Yes or No) Did you use an audio guide? (Yes or No)	
Friday Date: _____	Did you practice? (Yes or No) Did you use an audio guide? (Yes or No)	
Saturday Date: _____	Did you practice? (Yes or No) Did you use an audio guide? (Yes or No)	
Sunday Date: _____	Did you practice? (Yes or No) Did you use an audio guide? (Yes or No)	

Willingness Journal

Directions: Each day, rate your experience across three dimensions, using a 1–10 scale, with 10 being the most intense. The first dimension is the degree of willingness you experience throughout the day. The second dimension is the amount of distress that you experience while willingly engaging in valued behaviors. The third and final dimension is the degree of engagement you experience in your day.

Day	Monday	Tuesday	Wednesday	Thursday	Friday	Saturday	Sunday
Willingness	0–10 ____	0–10 ____	0–10 ____	0–10 ____	0–10 ____	0–10 ____	0–10 ____
Observations							
Distress	0–10 ____	0–10 ____	0–10 ____	0–10 ____	0–10 ____	0–10 ____	0–10 ____
Observations							
Engagement	0–10 ____	0–10 ____	0–10 ____	0–10 ____	0–10 ____	0–10 ____	0–10 ____
Observations							

Defusion Practices for Everyday Living

Directions: The following techniques are samples of different methods that you can use to help see thoughts and feelings for what they are, and not what *they say they are*. This week, use at least one of the defusion techniques each day. As the week progresses, jot down any observations that might arise about your experience, stepping outside of your thoughts and looking at them in these new ways. You may wish to employ these techniques when you feel caught up in your thoughts, find yourself either lost in ruminations about the past or consumed by worries about the future, or notice that you are stuck in the habit of making evaluations and judgments about yourself and others.

1. Breaking Identification with Thoughts

Your foot is a part of you, but it isn't all of you. When you have a dream, that dream unfolds in your mind, but it isn't "you." Similarly, our thinking, verbal minds are a part of who we are, but they aren't all of who we are. For this exercise, act as if your mind was something outside of yourself. For these purposes, we are almost thinking of our mind as something or someone separate from who we are. For example, "My mind is telling me that I need to stay inside today" or "Oh, my mind is doing it's old familiar pattern of regretting my last break-up."

2. Thanking the Mind

Take a moment to recognize that we humans evolved to possess a fascinatingly powerful problem-solving machine, which we call the mind. This problem-solving machine has been designed by evolution to be "always on," constantly seeking out possible threats and difficulties. It has also been designed to have a "better safe than sorry" mode of operating, so that it will interpret even ambiguous things in the environment as possibly negative. We carry this commentary in our minds about possible threats and problems.

When your mind is catching you up in worry and rumination, it really is just doing its job. So the next time you notice your mind offering up negative thoughts, step back from the thoughts, recognize them as a flow of mental events, and thank your mind for doing its job. For example, "Thanks, mind, for trying to warn me of the dangers of being rejected at this dinner party. I'm choosing to go anyway, but I know you are just doing your job, so thanks."

3. Taking Your Keys with You

Grab your key ring and match each challenging thought and feeling to one of the keys. As you go about your day, recognize that you are carrying these sometimes troubling mental events with you, just like you are carrying your keys. You need to carry your keys to function in your day, just like you need to carry these thoughts. Notice the thoughts, and your ability to carry them, whenever you notice the keys.

The techniques in this form are adapted from a number of acceptance and commitment therapy sources (such as Hayes, 2005; Hayes, Strosahl, & Wilson, 1999) and can also be found at *www.contextualpsychology.org.*

The Monsters on the Bus

Let's imagine that you find yourself in the role of a bus driver. You have your uniform, your shiny dashboard, your comfortable seat, and a powerful bus at your command. This bus that you are driving is very important. It represents your life. All of your experiences, all of your challenges and strengths, have brought you to this role, as the driver of your bus, your life. You have decided on a destination for this bus. It is a destination that you have chosen. This destination represents the valued directions that you are willing to pursue in your life. Getting to this destination is deeply significant to you. It matters that you get there. Every inch that you travel toward this valued aim means that you have, indeed, been taking your life in the right direction for you, in this moment. As you are driving, it is necessary that you keep to your course and follow the correct path toward your valued aim.

Like any bus driver, you are obliged to stop along the way and pick up passengers. The trouble with this particular journey is that some of these passengers are truly difficult to deal with. These passengers are actually monsters. Each one represents a difficult thought or feeling that you have had to contend with over the course of your life. Some monsters might be self-criticism. Others are feelings of panic and dread. Others represent frantic worries about what will come. Whatever has troubled you and distracted you from the rich possibilities of life is hopping on your bus in the shape of one of these monsters.

These monsters are unruly and they are rude. As you're driving, they are shouting insults at you and shooting spitballs. You can hear their calls as you drive. "You're a loser!" they shout. "Why don't you just give up? It's hopeless!" is heard ringing through the bus. One even shouts, "Stop the bus! This will never work!" You think about stopping the bus to scold and discipline these monsters. But if you did that, you would no longer be moving in the direction that matters to you. Perhaps you should pull over to the side of the road and throw these monsters off the bus. Again, this would mean you having to stop moving in the direction of your values. Maybe if you made a left turn and tried a different route the monsters would become quiet. But this too is a detour from living your life in a way that takes you toward realizing your freely chosen, valued aims.

All of a sudden you realize that while you have been preoccupied with devising strategies and arguments for dealing with the nagging monsters on the bus, you have already missed a couple of turns and have lost some time on your journey. You now understand that in order to get to where you want to go, and to continue moving in the direction that you have chosen in life, you need to continue driving and allow these monsters to continue their catcalls, teasing, and nagging all the while. You can make the choice to take your life in the right direction, while just making space for all of the noise that the monsters generate. You can't kick them off, and you can't make them stop. But you can make the choice to keep living your life in a way that is meaningful and rewarding to you, to keep driving the bus, even when the monsters yammer away as you go.

Adapted from Hayes, Strosahl, and Wilson (1999). Copyright 1999 by The Guilford Press. Adapted by permission.

"Stopping the War" Record

Directions: Use this form each day to record your practice of the "Stopping the War" exercise. Remember to record each time you practice. Record any observations or questions that may have arisen during your practice. You can discuss these observations with your therapist during your next meeting.

Date	Daily practice	Observations, comments, and questions
Monday Date: _____	Did you practice? (Yes or No)	
Tuesday Date: _____	Did you practice? (Yes or No)	
Wednesday Date: _____	Did you practice? (Yes or No)	
Thursday Date: _____	Did you practice? (Yes or No)	
Friday Date: _____	Did you practice? (Yes or No)	
Saturday Date: _____	Did you practice? (Yes or No)	
Sunday Date: _____	Did you practice? (Yes or No)	

Questions to Ask Yourself
after Completing Your First Week
of Engaging in the Lovingkindness Exercise

Directions: Complete this form and answer the following questions after you have engaged with the lovingkindness exercise for a week. It would be good to complete this, as best as you can, before meeting with your therapist and to bring it to the session to help inform your discussion of compassionate mind training. No matter how much, or how little, you have engaged in this practice, answer the following questions, as they can open up new perspectives and insights into your work with emotions.

1. How many days in the past week did you engage in the exercise?

2. For how long did you sit when you engaged in the exercise?

3. Did you use an audio guide, or did you engage in the exercise from memory?

4. What did you notice about your thoughts, feelings, and physical sensations as you engaged in this exercise?

5. How was this different from your typical way of being, thinking, and feeling?

(cont.)

6. How might this practice relate to, or even help you in dealing with, the current problems and difficult emotions that you have been facing?

7. Were there any obstacles or difficulties that presented themselves as you practiced this exercise?

8. How might you bring some of the quality of lovingkindness into your interactions with others?

9. How might you bring a quality of lovingkindness into your relationship with yourself?

Questions to Ask Yourself
after Completing Your First Week
of Imagining the Compassionate Self

Directions: Complete this form and answer the following questions after you have engaged with the compassionate self exercise for a week. It would be good to complete this, as best as you can, before meeting with your therapist and to bring it to the session to help inform your discussion of compassionate mind training. No matter how much, or how little, you have engaged in this practice, answer the following questions, as they can open up new perspectives and insights into your work with emotions.

1. How many days in the past week did you engage in the exercise?

2. When did you engage in the exercise?

3. Did you imagine your compassionate self while engaging in a meditation period, while moving through your daily activities, or both?

4. What did you notice about your thoughts, feelings, and physical sensations as you engaged in this exercise?

(cont.)

5. In what way, if any, did viewing the world from the perspective of your compassionate self affect you?

6. If you choose to share this information, how did your expressions or body language change when you were imagining your compassionate self?

7. Again, if you choose to answer this question, what were the qualities and attributes that you imagined in your compassionate self?

8. Were there any obstacles or difficulties that presented themselves as you practiced this exercise?

9. How might you use this image of a compassionate self to help you in the future?

Self-Compassionate Letter Writing

This exercise will involve your writing a letter to yourself from the perspective of a deeply compassionate, wise, and unconditionally accepting person. If you feel comfortable, you can imagine yourself as this loving, kind presence. This voice within you is an expression of your innate lovingkindness and intuitive wisdom.

In preparation, set aside some time when you can engage in this exercise in an unhurried fashion. Find a space that feels private and safe. Bring a pencil and some paper with you, and make sure that you have a surface to write on.

As you begin, take a minute or two to engage in mindful awareness of the flow of the breath. Feel your feet on the ground. Gently, allow your back to straighten and feel yourself rooted to the earth. As much as you can, let go of judgments, analyses, and even descriptions, and bring bare attention to the flow of breath in and out of the body.

After a few minutes of mindful breathing, allow your attention to rest on the flow of your thoughts as you breathe in. Letting go of the attention to the breath, bring your current life situation to mind. What conflicts, problems, or self-criticisms come to mind? What is your mind beginning to tell you? What emotions arise within you?

As you breathe out, let go of these thoughts and feelings. On the next available in-breath, direct your attention to an image of yourself as a compassionate and wise being. In your compassionate mind, you possess wisdom and emotional strength. You are unconditionally accepting of all that you are, in this moment, and are completely noncondemning. Your compassionate self radiates emotional warmth. For a moment, recognize the calmness and wisdom that you possess. Take a moment to feel the physical sensations that company the arising of a compassionate mind. Recognize the strength and healing quality of a vast and deep kindness. Recognize that this lovingkindness, this powerful compassion exists within you as an abundant reservoir of strength.

As you begin, remember the simple act of self-validation. There are many good reasons for the distress you are currently experiencing. Your brain and mind have evolved and emerged through millions of years of life progressing on this planet. You were not designed to deal with the particular pressures and complexities of our current social environment. Your learning history has presented you with strong challenges and situations that have caused you pain. Can you open yourself to a compassionate understanding that your struggle is a natural part of life, and that it is not your fault?

In the next few minutes, allow yourself to compose a compassionate letter that gives a voice to your compassionate self. Allow yourself to compose a letter that will fill at least the remainder of this page. When you next meet with your therapist, if you feel willing, bring this letter to the session. Together, you and your therapist can read and reflect on the words and feelings that you have allowed yourself to express here.

(cont.)

MY SELF-COMPASSIONATE LETTER:

Questions to Ask Yourself
to Enhance Your Emotional Awareness

1. What just happened that activated your emotional response?

2. Using the five senses, what can you notice in your environment around you?

3. Turning your awareness inward, what physical sensations do you notice in your body in this moment?

4. Where in your body are you experiencing sensations that you relate to your emotions just now?

5. If you were to give a label, or the name of a feeling, to your emotion, what would it be?

6. What thoughts are going through your mind that you associate with this emotion?

(cont.)

7. What needs or wants do you associate with this emotional state?

8. What urges toward action arrive with this emotion?

9. Is this a clearly defined emotion, or are you experiencing a mix of emotions? If so, what are the labels for the emotions you are feeling?

10. Does this emotion feel like a response to something directly in your environment or history (a "primary emotion"), or is it a response to another emotion (a "secondary emotion")? If it is an emotion about another emotion, what is the primary emotion you are responding to?

11. Does this feel like an emotion that you want to move towards or an emotion that you want to move away from?

12. How can you best make space for this emotion and take care of yourself in this moment?

Emotionally Intelligent Thought Record
(Long Form)

Directions: Over the course of the next week, use this series of questions to help yourself practice a growing awareness of your thoughts, emotions, physical sensations, and possible responses. You can use this work sheet when you notice something affecting the way you are feeling during times of stress or even when you suddenly notice that your emotions have shifted in a negative direction. You can use this work sheet in real time to tune into what is going on in the present moment. Sometimes, though, this won't be possible. This is not a problem. You can still use this work sheet after some time has passed, by looking back on your memories of an event and asking yourself these questions as if things were happening in this moment. As you use this record, be aware, as much as you can, of the present-moment-focused "bare attention" that you have been developing through training in mindful awareness. If any questions or observations arise as you practice, write them down so that you might share them with your therapist during your next meeting.

---

1. Situation

What is going on around you, in your environment, right now? Where are you?

Who is with you? What are you doing? What are you noticing in the environment that is affecting you?

(cont.)

2. Physical Sensations

Sometimes our response to something in our environment can be felt in the body, like "butterflies in the stomach," for example. Bringing our attention, as best as we can, to these sensations can be helpful. Developing awareness and sensitivity to these experiences can take practice, so if you don't notice anything in particular, just allow yourself that experience, while maybe taking a moment or two to give your attention some time to observe whatever may be present. In this situation, what physical sensations do you notice yourself experiencing in your body? Where in your body do you feel such sensations? What are the qualities of such sensations?

3. Emotions

Labeling our emotions using "feeling words" can be helpful. Taking a moment to truly make space for and allow this emotional experience, what feeling word would best describe and "label" this emotion that you are feeling in this moment? How intensely would you say you are feeling this emotion? If you were to rate this emotion on a scale of 0–100, with 100 being the most intense feeling you could have and 0 being no presence of this feeling at all, what would that rating be?

(cont.)

4. Thoughts

What thoughts are going through your mind in this situation? Ask yourself, "What is going through my mind right now? What is my mind telling me?" What is "popping into your head" in this situation? What does this situation say about you? What does this situation suggest about your future? As best as you can, notice the flow of thoughts that unfold in your mind in this situation. What are some of the thoughts that are arriving?

5. "Learning to Stay"

We human beings have learned to try to get rid of, or get away from, things that seem threatening or unpleasant. This makes solid sense when you think about it. As you and your therapist have discussed, attempts to suppress or eliminate distressing thoughts and feeling sometimes makes them that much stronger. So, for a moment, take this opportunity to learn to stay with your experience, just as it is. Following the flow of your breath in this moment, as much as you can, make space for whatever unfolds before your mind. In the following space, write down any observations you may have about this simple act of gently making space for your experience, moment by moment.

(cont.)

6. Responding "Inside"

Now that you have noticed, and allowed yourself to more fully experience, the sensations, emotions, and thoughts that have shown up in this situation, how might you best respond in this moment? Adopting a mindful, "emotionally intelligent" attitude, you can recognize that these thoughts and feelings are events in the mind, and not reality itself. Working with your therapist, you can learn many ways to respond to distressing thoughts and feelings. Here are a few questions to ask yourself to practice this week:

- "What are the costs and benefits to me of believing these thoughts?"
- "How might I act if I really believed this?"
- "How might I act if I didn't believe this?"
- "What might I say to a friend who was facing this situation?"
- "What needs are involved in this event, and how can I best take care of myself now?"
- "Can I mindfully observe these events in my mind, choose a course of action, and act in a way that will serve my aims?"

In the following space, write your responses and observations.

(cont.)

7. **Responding "Outside"**

Ask yourself the following questions:

- "How can I best pursue my own aims and values in this situation?"
- "Is there a problem here that I need to solve in order to live my life in a meaningful and valued way?"
- "How can I interact with others in this situation in an effective way that suits my aims and values?"
- "Does this situation call for a behavioral response? Does any action need to be taken?"
- "Is doing nothing an option?"
- "How can I take care of myself best in this situation?"

In the space below, record any responses or observations that involve ways in which you can use this situation as a step in a life that feels rewarding and in tune with your personal values.

FORM 8.3

Emotionally Intelligent Thought Record
(Short Form)

---

1. Situation

What is going on around you, in your environment, right now? Where are you? Who is with you? What are you doing?

---

2. Physical Sensations

In this situation, what physical sensations do you notice yourself experiencing in your body? Where in your body do you feel such sensations?

(cont.)

---

3. Emotions

Using one word, describe and "label" this emotion that you are feeling in this moment. How intensely would you say you are feeling this emotion on a scale of 0–100?

---

4. Thoughts

What thoughts are going through your mind in this situation?

---

5. "Learning To Stay"

For a moment, take this opportunity to learn to stay with your experience, just as it is. Follow the flow of your breath. In the space that follows, write down any observations you may make about this.

(cont.)

6. Responding "Inside"

How might you best respond to your thoughts and emotions in this moment?

What would a self-compassionate, rational, and balanced response be?

7. Responding "Outside"

In this situation, are there any actions in the world that you need to take to pursue your valued directions? If so, what would these actions be?

Distinguishing Thoughts from Feelings

Directions: When you are feeling upset, you are probably having upsetting thoughts. Let's say you are feeling sad. You might be thinking, "Nothing will ever get better." Or let's say you feel angry. Your thought might be, "He's treating me with disrespect." In the left column, describe the situation (what was going on), in the center column describe your feelings (e.g., sad, angry, anxious), and in the right column describe your thoughts.

Situation	Feelings	Thoughts
Describe what was going on, what led up to it, what the context was.	Identify your feelings or emotions (*examples*: sad, helpless, anxious, afraid, numb, hopeless, angry, jealous, empty, happy, relieved, curious).	What were you thinking?

Categories of Automatic Thoughts

1. **Mind reading:** You assume that you know what people think without having sufficient evidence of their thoughts. "He thinks I'm a loser."
2. **Fortune telling:** You predict the future negatively: Things will get worse, or there is danger ahead. "I'll fail that exam," or "I won't get the job."
3. **Catastrophizing:** You believe that what has happened or will happen will be so awful and unbearable that you won't be able to stand it. "It would be terrible if I failed."
4. **Labeling:** You assign global negative traits to yourself and others. "I'm undesirable" or "He's a rotten person."
5. **Discounting positives:** You claim that the positive things you or others do are trivial. "That's what wives are supposed to do—so it doesn't count when she's nice to me," or "Those successes were easy, so they don't matter."
6. **Negative filtering:** You focus almost exclusively on the negatives and seldom notice the positives. "Look at all of the people who don't like me."
7. **Overgeneralizing:** You perceive a global pattern of negatives on the basis of a single incident. "This generally happens to me. I seem to fail at a lot of things."
8. **Dichotomous thinking:** You view events or people in all-or-nothing terms. "I get rejected by everyone" or "It was a complete waste of time."
9. **Shoulds:** You interpret events in terms of how things should be, rather than simply focusing on what is. "I should do well. If I don't, then I'm a failure."
10. **Personalizing:** You attribute a disproportionate amount of the blame to yourself for negative events, and you fail to see that certain events are also caused by others. "The marriage ended because I failed."
11. **Blaming:** You focus on the other person as the *source of* your negative feelings, and you refuse to take responsibility for changing yourself. "She's to blame for the way I feel now" or "My parents caused all my problems."
12. **Unfair comparisons:** You interpret events in terms of standards that are unrealistic—for example, you focus primarily on others who do better than you and find yourself inferior in the comparison. "She's more successful than I am" or "Others did better than I did on the test."
13. **Regret orientation:** You focus on the idea that you could have done better in the past, rather on what you can do better now. "I could have had a better job if I had tried," or "I shouldn't have said that."
14. **What if?:** You keep asking a series of questions about "what if" something happens, and you fail to be satisfied with any of the answers. "Yeah, but what if I get anxious?" or "What if I can't catch my breath?"
15. **Emotional reasoning:** You let your feelings guide your interpretation of reality. "I feel depressed; therefore, my marriage is not working out."
16. **Inability to disconfirm:** You reject any evidence or arguments that might contradict your negative thoughts. For example, when you have the thought "I'm unlovable," you reject as *irrelevant* any evidence that people like you. Consequently, your thought cannot be refuted. "That's not the real issue. There are deeper problems. There are other factors."
17. **Judgment focus:** You view yourself, others, and events in terms of evaluations as good–bad or superior–inferior, rather than simply describing, accepting, or understanding. You are continually measuring yourself and others according to arbitrary standards, and finding that you and others fall short. You are focused on the judgments of others as well as your own judgments of yourself. "I didn't perform well in college," or "If I take up tennis, I won't do well," or "Look how successful she is. I'm not successful."

From Leahy and Holland (2000). Copyright 2000 by Robert L. Leahy and Stephen J. Holland. Reprinted by permission.

Four-Column Thought Form

Directions: Each of us has a particular style of thinking. On this form, please note the situation (e.g., sitting at home alone, talking with someone, doing your work) that is associated with a negative feeling (e.g., sad, angry, anxious). Then note the specific thoughts that you are having that are associated with this feeling in this situation. Using the checklist of automatic thought categories, note the specific category of your negative thought. After you have completed this form for a few days, make a list of the most common biases in your thinking and how this might affect the way that you feel.

Situation	Feeling	Automatic thought	Category of thought

Examining the Advantages
and Disadvantages of Thoughts

Negative thought	Advantages	Disadvantages
Weigh the advantages and disadvantages (divide 100 points between the two).	Advantages	Disadvantages
How would my life change if I believed this thought less?		

Note: Most negative thoughts may appear to have some advantages for you, even if they make you feel down. For example, self-criticism might seem to have advantages of motivating you, being realistic, or helping you figure out what to change.

Examining the Evidence for a Thought

Directions: We have many negative thoughts that we tend not to examine carefully. One way of testing the reality of your thought is to examine the evidence for and against this thought and to evaluate the quality of the evidence. For example, you might be using your emotions as evidence ("I feel bad; therefore, I am bad"), but is this the highest quality of evidence? Would you be able to convince someone else with this evidence? How would other people view the evidence? Weigh the evidence for and against your thought by dividing 100 points and then indicate what you would conclude after looking at all the evidence.

Negative thought:				
Evidence favoring thought	Quality of evidence (0–10)	Evidence against thought	Quality of evidence (0–10)
What do you think about the quality of the evidence for and against your thought?			
Weigh the evidence for and against your thought (divide 100 points)		Costs = Benefits =	
Conclusions			

Defense Attorney Form

Directions: Imagine that your negative thoughts about yourself, experience, and the future were the voice of a prosecutor at a trial. Write down all these "charges" in the left column. Now imagine that you are an attorney hired to defend yourself against these charges. You will want to use all the evidence to support your client (you). You will challenge the validity of the evidence, call witnesses to defend you, and present evidence to support yourself. Write out your defense against these charges.

The "prosecution's charges"	Your defense

What Would the Jury Think?

Directions: Imagine that you took one of your negative thoughts and put it on trial. Go through the questions in the left column and give your responses. Would this thought stand up to scrutiny?

Questions that the jury might consider	Your response
Has the prosecutor proved that the defendant is guilty of terrible things?	
Are there any problems with the evidence presented by the prosecutor?	
What is the strongest point that the prosecutor made? What do you make of this?	
What is the strongest point that the defense attorney made? What do you make of this?	
Is the prosecutor really fair? Why or why not?	
What do you think fair-minded people would think if they saw this trial?	

Advice I Would Give My Best Friend

Directions: You may be going through a hard time right now, and so you might think of the advice you would give a friend with the same problem. What would you suggest or tell your friend? Is this different from the way you are talking to yourself? Why is that?

Problem I am having or negative thoughts	Advice I would give a friend
Why would I give a friend advice I don't give myself?	

Why It's Hard for Me to Take Good Advice

Directions: It's often easier to give advice than to advise yourself. Go through each of the columns and try to examine why it's hard to take your own good advice.

The good advice that's hard for me to take	Why it's hard for me to take my good advice	Why I should take my good advice

Place Events on a Continuum

Directions: Take the current event that is upsetting you and rate it for how bad it feels, with 0 corresponding to the absence of anything negative and 100 corresponding to the worst thing imaginable that could happen to anyone. Now think of events that correspond to each of the 10-point ratings in the following scale. What would be 80, 70, 40, 20, etc? Describe why the current event is rated so high for you and why these other events are not as "terrible." Is it possible that you might be viewing what is happening now as worse than it really could turn out to be?

0	10	20	30	40	50	60	70	80	90	100

Emotion Regulation in Psychotherapy: A Practitioner's Guide by Robert L. Leahy, Dennis Tirch, and Lisa Napolitano. Copyright 2011 by The Guilford Press. Permission to photocopy this form is granted to purchasers of this book for personal use only (see copyright page for details).

Placing Events in Perspective:
What I Can Still Do

Directions: Sometimes when bad things happen to us, we fail to recognize that there are still things we can do to make our lives pleasurable and meaningful. Take the current event that is upsetting you. What can you still do, either now or sometime in the future, that could be positive for you? You might also make a list of things you can no longer do since this negative event occurred. But what does this list show you? If you can still do a lot of pleasurable and meaningful things, then does the negative event seem less terrible to you?

Even though this happened, I can still do the following, either now or in the future:

Overcoming Time Urgency

Directions: We often have a hard time seeing things in the perspective of time. Go through each of the following questions on the left and give your best response on the right. How do things look different with a different perspective of urgency or time?

Current negative mood or thoughts	Your response
What do you see as the consequence of your sense of urgency and emergency?	
Is it possible that you might feel better about these things in a few hours or a few days? Has that happened before?	
What are some things that could happen in the next few hours or few days that could make you feel better?	
How can you distract yourself from your current mood and do things that are more pleasurable?	
Why is this *not* a real emergency?	
Can you focus on making the present moment better?	

Instructions for Progressive Muscle Relaxation

Directions: Sitting comfortably in chair or lying down, practice tensing and relaxing each of the major muscle groups listed next. As you tense each muscle group, hold the tension for 4 to 8 seconds. Bring your full awareness to the tension. Then release the tension in that muscle, bringing your full awareness to the sensation of relaxation. Remember that relaxation is a skill that requires practice.

Major muscle groups

1. Left foot
2. Right foot
3. Left calf
4. Right calf
5. Left quadriceps
6. Right quadriceps
7. Abdomen
8. Buttocks
9. Left hand and forearm

10. Right hand and forearm
11. Left bicep
12. Right bicep
13. Shoulders
14. Chest
15. Back
16. Neck
17. Mouth
18. Face

Instructions for Diaphragmatic Breathing

What Is It?

Diaphragmatic breathing is also called belly breathing. It's how we breathe when we're relaxed. Breathing this way when we are stressed helps us to feel more relaxed. By contrast, when we are stressed, we breathe rapidly and from the chest.

Diaphragmatic breathing is a skill that requires practice. It is recommended that you build up this skill through daily practice when you are relatively calm. This will enable you to use diaphragmatic breathing more effectively when you are distressed.

How Do I Practice?

It's easiest to practice diaphragmatic breathing lying down or sitting. To make sure you are breathing correctly, you may want to place one hand on your chest and the other on your abdomen.

To begin, inhale normally through your nose. As you inhale, think of sending the air into the belly or diaphragm, bypassing the chest. Feel the abdomen expand.

Exhale through your mouth, making a *shhh* sound. As you exhale, feel the abdomen flatten. Draw out the exhalation before taking your next breath.

It should feel comfortable. There is no need to pause between the inhalation and exhalation.

Continue breathing this way for at least 5 minutes.

Self-Soothing

Self-soothing is using the senses to make distress more tolerable. Bring your awareness to your sense of taste, touch, smell, hearing, and vision to take the edge off emotional pain.

Vision

Bring your awareness to things you see like beautiful paintings, photos of people you love, flowers, a candle flame, children playing, animals, scenes of nature, patterns, architecture, and vibrant colors; look at birds in flight, watch a sunset, look up at night to see the stars, watch people dancing.

Taste

Have a cup of tea, eat a special meal, savor the taste of chocolate or other food you don't ordinarily indulge in, splurge on fresh-squeezed orange juice, chew a piece of gum.

Sound

Listen to sounds of nature, like birds singing or leaves rustling; play calming music; listen to the sound of laughter; listen to children playing; listen to the voice of someone you love.

Touch

Wear silky, soft fabrics, snuggle under the covers of your bed, brush your hair, rub lotion on your hands, take a hot bath.

Smell

Light incense or a scented candle, wear your favorite perfume, use scented soap and shampoo, light a wood fire on a cold day, bake a pie and savor the aroma.

Adapted from Linehan (1993b). Copyright 1993 by The Guilford Press. Adapted by permission.

Weekly Activity Scheduling:
Pleasure Predicting and Actual Outcome

Directions: For each hour of the week fill in what you *plan to do* and how much pleasure (and effectiveness) you *think you will experience* using a scale of P0 (no pleasure) to P10 (most pleasure that you can imagine), with P5 indicating a moderate amount of pleasure. Note the amount of effectiveness—or feeling of competence—and rate your experience from E0 to E10. For example, if you predict that you will derive a pleasure rating of 6 and an effectiveness rating of 4 if you exercise at 8 A.M. on Monday, then write "exercise, P6 and E4" in the box for Monday at 8 A.M. Then write out what you actually experienced in pleasure and effectiveness.

Hour	Monday	Tuesday	Wednesday	Thursday	Friday	Saturday	Sunday
A.M. 6							
7							
8							
9							
10							
11							
12 noon							
P.M. 1							
2							
3							
4							
5							
6							
7							
8							
9							
10							
11							
12 midnight							
1–6 A.M.							

List of Priorities

Directions: It's important to know what is important and what isn't. If you are like a lot of people, you are wasting valuable time on low-priority behaviors. This can include surfing the Internet, ruminating and worrying, watching television, or engaging in other activities that may not be that relevant to your important goals. The first thing to do is identify what is of importance. Using the following table, list activities that are of highest, medium, and lowest priority.

Highest priority	Medium priority	Lowest priority

Self-Monitoring Off-Task Behaviors

Directions: Keep track of any low-priority, off-task, or goof-off behaviors that are not part of your plan to manage your time more effectively. Write down where and when this occurs and how much time you are spending off task. Ask yourself if this is making you feel better or worse.

Monday	Tuesday	Wednesday	Thursday	Friday	Saturday	Sunday

Planning Ahead

Directions: You won't get things done unless you plan them. You can use the following activity schedule to assign the important activities that you need to get done—when you will do them and how much time you will spend. Also include some time for an activity that is rewarding for you so that you will have something to look forward to.

Monday	Tuesday	Wednesday	Thursday	Friday	Saturday	Sunday

Anti-Procrastination

Directions: Ask yourself the questions from the left-hand column and fill in your responses in the right-hand column.

Questions to ask yourself	Your response
What is the task I really need to get done?	
What are the costs and benefits for me in doing this?	Costs: Benefits:
How will I feel after I get this done?	
Am I exaggerating how difficult or unpleasant this will be?	
What can I reward myself with if I get it done?	
Schedule a time and palce for this task.	
What was the actual outcome?	

Instructions for Using Positive Imagery

Directions: Often it is not possible to physically leave a distressing situation. With the use of relaxing and positive imagery, it's possible to mentally escape the situation. By imagining oneself in a relaxed and positive situation, actual relaxation may be experienced. Keep in mind that the use of visualization to relax is a skill. It's important to practice it regularly so that you can use it more effectively in times of distress.

How?

- Visualize a safe and relaxing place. It could be the beach or the mountains. It can be a real place or a place you've never been.

- Visualize it in as much detail as possible, and incorporate as many senses as possible.

- What do you hear, smell, see, feel, and taste?

- Imagine yourself relaxing in this scene.

- If you have difficulty relaxing, tell yourself, "I'm letting go of tension."

- Remember the details—the sights, the smells, the sounds.

- You can return here as many times as you like.

Instructions for the Alexander
Lie-Down Technique

1. Find a comfortable and quiet place, where you will be undisturbed for about 20 minutes. You will be lying on a mat or a blanket for about this amount of time. As a result, try to find a floor space that is quite clean and at is a comfortable temperature. Unfold the mat to create an area that will be sufficient to cover the ground beneath your body if you were lying on your back. Bring three or four paperback books with you and place them at the top of the mat. These books will support the back of your head, like a pillow, when you are lying down.

2. Take a seat on the mat with your legs straight out in front of you, with your gently erect spine balanced comfortably on your sit bones. As you follow these instructions, allow yourself to engage in any movement slowly and softly, with an awareness of the flow of breath in and out of the body.

3. Bend your knees so that they are pointing at the ceiling, with your feet resting on the ground before you.

4. As you exhale, lean forward over your bent legs, feeling the top of your head as it extends forward. Your arms are simply hanging from your shoulders, in a relaxed fashion. Allow your spine to lengthen softly through this slow gesture.

5. Allow your spine to roll back as you move from this seated position, leaning forward, to take a position lying down on the mat. This can be done slowly and gently. If this feels uncomfortable or stressful to you at all, you can opt to use your hands as a support and walk your body with your hands down into a lying position.

6. Reach behind your head to adjust the books so that your head is supported in a comfortable fashion. This should be just high enough to fit beneath the curve in your neck. Again, this all can be done slowly and gently.

7. You are now lying on the floor with your head and neck gently supported. Your back is straight and lengthened. Your legs are together before you. Your knees are bent so that your legs stretching from the hips to the ankles form a triangle. All of the points of your body are supported.

8. Gently move your hands from lying at the sides of your body so that they are resting on your abdomen, feeling the flow of the breath in and out of the body.

9. For the next 20 minutes, your aim is to do nothing, as much as you can. Allow your eyes to close. Recognize that this is a time for conscious rest and relaxation. With each breath in, feel the presence of life in the body, drawing in attention and vitality. With each breath out, feel the release of tension and attention anywhere it may demonstrate itself in the body.

10. Allow yourself to gently follow the flow of the breath in and out of the body, breathing in and knowing that you are breathing in, breathing out and knowing that you are breathing out. Allow the breath to find its own rhythm and flow.

11. Notice the way your weight is supported by the mat. As you exhale, feel yourself sinking into the floor. As much as you can, allow yourself to breathe out and release any tension you feel in the body, breath by breath.

12. Throughout this period of rest, if you feel any discomfort anywhere in the body, allow yourself to make any necessary adjustments to your position to allow for greater comfort and relaxation.

13. Recognize the support that your body receives, as you feel the body lengthen and relax.

14. Remain in this position as you rest for about 20 minutes.

15. When you are ready, begin to leave the lie-down exercise by gently and slowly rocking from side to side. After a few moments, rock onto your left side and use your hands to gently walk the body up to a seated position.

16. When you rise from your seated position to a standing position, do this gradually, maintaining some of the rest and presence that you established during the lie-down exercise.

References

Ainsworth, M. S., Blehar, M. C., Waters, E., & Wall, S. (1978). *Patterns of attachment: A psychological study of the strange situation*. Mahwah, NJ: Erlbaum.

Aldao, A., Nolen-Hoeksema, S., & Schweizer, S. (2010). Emotion-regulation strategies across psychopathology: A meta-analytic review. *Clinical Psychology Review, 30*(2), 217–237.

Aldwin, C. M. (2007). *Stress, coping, and development: An integrative perspective* (2nd ed.). New York: Guilford Press.

Alloy, L. B., Abramson, L. Y., Safford, S. M., & Gibb, B. E. (2006). The Cognitive Vulnerability to Depression (CVD) Project: Current findings and future directions. In L. B. Alloy & J. H. Riskind (Eds.), *Cognitive vulnerability to emotional disorders* (pp. 33–61). Mahwah, NJ: Erlbaum.

Alloy, L. B., Reilly-Harrington, N., Fresco, D. M., Whitehouse, W. G., & Zechmeister, J. S. (1999). Cognitive styles and life events in subsyndromal unipolar and bipolar disorders: Stability and prospective prediction of depressive and hypomanic mood swings. *Journal of Cognitive Psychotherapy, 13*, 21–40.

American Psychiatric Association. (2000). *Diagnostic and statistical manual of mental disorders* (4th ed., text rev.). Washington, DC: Author.

American Society for the Alexander Technique. (2006). *Professional training in the Alexander Technique: A guide to AmSAT teacher training*. Retrieved March 17, 2010, from /www.alexandertech.org/training/TrainBroch.pdf.

Arntz, A., Bernstein, D., Oorschot, M., & Schobre, P. (2009). Theory of mind in borderline and cluster-C personality disorder. *Journal of Nervous and Mental Disease, 197*(11), 801–807.

Arntz, A., Rauner, M., & van den Hout, M. (1995). "If I feel anxious, there must be danger": Ex-consequentia reasoning in inferring danger in anxiety disorders. *Behaviour Research and Therapy, 33*(8), 917–925.

Baer, R. A. (2003). Mindfulness training as a clinical intervention: A conceptual and empirical review. *Clinical Psychology: Science and Practice, 10*(2), 125–143.

Bandura, A. (2003). Theoretical and empirical exploration of the similarities between emotional numbing in posttraumatic stress disorder and alexithymia. *Journal of Anxiety Disorders, 17*(3), 349–360.

Barkow, J. H., Cosmides, L., & Tooby, J. (Eds.). (1992). *The adapted mind: Evolutionary psychology and the generation of culture*. New York: Oxford University Press.

Barlow, D. H. (2002). *Anxiety and its disorders: The nature and treatment of anxiety and panic* (2nd ed.). New York: Guilford Press.

Barlow, D. H., Allen, L. B., & Choate, M. L. (2004). Toward a unified treatment for emotional disorders. *Behavior Therapy, 35*(2), 205–230.

Barlow, D. H., & Craske, M. G. (2006). *Mastery of your anxiety and panic: Patient workbook* (4th ed.). New York: Oxford University Press.

Baron-Cohen, S. (1991). The development of a theory of mind in autism: Deviance and delay? *Psychiatric Clinics of North America, 14*(1), 33–51.

Baron-Cohen, S., Scott, F. J., Allison, C., Williams, J., Bolton, P., Matthews, F. E., et al. (2009). Prevalence of autism-spectrum conditions: UK school-based population studies. *British Journal of Psychiatry, 194*(6), 500–509.

Batson, C. D., Shaw, L. L., & Oleson, K. C. (1992). Distinguishing affect, mood, and emotion: Toward functionally based conceptual distinctions. In M. S. Clark (Ed.), *Review of personality and social psychology* (pp. 294–326). Newbury Park, CA: Sage.

Beck, A. T. (1976). *Cognitive therapy and the emotional disorders.* New York: International Universities Press.

Beck, A. T. (1996). Beyond belief: A theory of modes, personality and psychopathology. In P. Salkovskis (Ed.), *Frontiers of cognitive therapy* (pp. 1–25). New York: Guilford Press.

Beck, A. T., Freeman, A., Davis, D., & Associates. (2004). *Cognitive therapy of personality disorders* (2nd ed.). New York: Guilford Press.

Beck, A. T., Rush, A. J., Shaw, B. F., & Emery, G. (1979). *Cognitive therapy of depression.* New York: Guilford Press.

Beck, J. S. (2011). *Cognitive therapy: Basics and beyond* (2nd ed.). New York: Guilford Press.

Belsky, J., & Pluess, M. (2009). Beyond diathesis stress: Differential susceptibility to environmental influences. *Psychological Bulletin, 135*(6), 885–908.

Bennett-Levy, J., Butler, G., Fennell, M., Hackmann, A., Mueller, M., & Westbrook, D. (Eds.). (2004). *Oxford guide to behavioural experiments in cognitive therapy.* Oxford, UK: Oxford University Press.

Berenbaum, H., & James, T. (1994). Correlates and retrospectively reported antecedents of alexithymia. *Psychosomatic Medicine, 56*(4), 353–359.

Bonanno, G. A., Keltner, D., Noll, J. G., Putnam, F. W., Trickett, P. K., LeJeune, J., et al. (2002). When the face reveals what words do not: Facial expressions of emotion, smiling, and the willingness to disclose childhood sexual abuse. *Journal of Personality and Social Psychology, 83*(1), 94–110.

Bond, F. W., & Bunce, D. (2000). Mediators of change in emotion-focused and problem-focused worksite stress management interventions. *Journal of Occupational Health Psychology, 5,* 156–163.

Borkovec, T. D., Alcaine, O. M., & Behar, E. (2004). Avoidance theory of worry and generalized anxiety disorder. In R. G. Heimberg, C. L. Turk, & D. S. Mennin (Eds.), *Generalized anxiety disorder: Advances in research and practice* (pp. 77–108). New York: Guilford Press.

Bower, G. H. (1981). Mood and memory. *American Psychologist, 36*(2), 129–148.

Bower, G. H., & Forgas, J. P. (2000). Affect, memory, and social cognition. In E. Eich, J. F. Kihlstrom, G. H. Bower, J. P. Forgas, & P. M. Niedenthal (Eds.), *Cognition and emotion* (pp. 87–168). New York: Oxford University Press.

Bowlby, J. (1968). *Attachment and loss: Vol. I. Attachment.* London: Hogarth.

Bowlby, J. (1973). *Attachment and loss: Vol. II. Separation.* London: Hogarth.

Brown, K. W., & Ryan, R. M. (2003). The benefits of being present: Mindfulness and its role in psychological well-being. *Journal of Personality and Social Psychology, 84,* 822–848.

Buckholdt, K. E., Parra, G. R., & Jobe-Shields, L. (2009). Emotion regulation as a mediator of the relation between emotion socialization and deliberate self-harm. *American Journal of Orthopsychiatry, 79*(4), 482–490.

Butler, A., Chapman, J. M., Forman, E. M., & Beck, A. T. (2006). The empirical status of cognitive-behavioral therapy: A review of meta-analyses. *Clinical Psychology Review, 26*(1), 17–31.

Butler, E. A., Egloff, B., Wilhelm, F. H., Smith, N. C., Erickson, E. A., & Gross, J. J. (2003). The social consequences of expressive suppression. *Emotion, 3*(1), 48–67.

Campbell-Sills, L., Barlow, D. H., Brown, T. A., & Hofmann, S. G. (2006). Acceptability and suppression of negative emotion in anxiety and mood disorders. *Emotion, 6*(4), 587–595.

Carver, C. S., & Scheier, M. (1998). *On the self-regulation of behavior.* Cambridge, UK: Cambridge University Press.

Carver, C. S., & Scheier, M. F. (2009). Action, affect, and two-mode models of functioning. In E. Morsella, J. A. Bargh, & P. M. Gollwitzer (Eds.), *Oxford handbook of human action. Social cognition and social neuroscience* (pp. 298–327). New York: Oxford University Press.

Caspi, A., Moffitt, T. E., Morgan, J., Rutter, M., Taylor, A., Arseneault, L., et al. (2004). Maternal expressed emotion predicts children's antisocial behavior problems: Using monozygotic-twin differences to identify environmental effects on behavioral development. *Developmental Psychology, 40*(2), 149–161.

Cassidy, J. (1995). Attachment and generalized anxiety disorder. In D. Cicchetti & S. L. Toth (Eds.), *Rochester symposium on developmental psychopathology: Vol. 6. Emotion, cognition, and representation* (pp. 343–370). Rochester, NY: University of Rochester Press.

Chapman, A. L., Rosenthal, M. Z., & Leung, D. W. (2009). Emotion suppression in borderline personality disorder: An experience sampling study. *Journal of Personality Disorders, 23*(1), 29–47.

Ciarrochi, J. V., & Bailey, A. (2009). *A CBT practitioner's guide to ACT: How to bridge the gap between cognitive behavioral therapy and acceptance and commitment therapy.* New York: New Harbinger.

Ciarrochi, J. V., Forgas, J., & Mayer, J. (2006). *Emotional intelligence in everyday life: A scientific inquiry* (2nd ed.). New York: Psychology Press/Taylor & Francis.

Ciarrochi, J. V., & Mayer, J. D. (2007). The key ingredients of emotional intelligence interventions: Similarities and differences. In J. V. Ciarrochi & J. D. Mayer (Eds.), *Applying emotional intelligence: A practitioner's guide* (pp. 144–156). New York: Psychology Press.

Clark, D. A. (2002). Unwanted mental intrusions in clinical disorders: An introduction. *Journal of Cognitive Psychotherapy, 16*(2), 123–126.

Clark, D. A., & Beck, A. T. (2009). *Cognitive therapy of anxiety disorders: Science and practice.* New York: Guilford Press.

Clark, D. A., Beck, A. T., & Alford, B. A. (1999). *Scientific foundations of cognitive theory and therapy of depression.* New York: Wiley.

Clark, D. M. (1986). A cognitive approach to panic. *Behaviour Research and Therapy, 24*(4), 461–470.

Clarkin, J., Yeomans, F. E., & Kernberg, O. F. (2006). *Psychotherapy for borderline personality: Focusing on object relations* Washington, DC: American Psychiatric Press.

Cloitre, M., Cohen, L. R., & Koenen, K. C. (2006). *Treating survivors of childhood abuse: Psychotherapy for the interrupted life.* New York: Guilford Press.

Cohn, M. A., & Fredrickson, B. L. (2009). Positive emotions. In S. J. Lopez & C. R. Snyder (Eds.), *Oxford handbook of positive psychology* (2nd ed., pp. 13–24). New York: Oxford University Press.

Corcoran, R., Rowse, G., Moore, R., Blackwood, N., Kinderman, P., Howard, R., et al. (2008). A transdiagnostic investigation of 'theory of mind' and 'jumping to conclusions' in patients with persecutory delusions. *Psychological Medicine, 38*(11), 1577–1583.

Cribb, G., Moulds, M. L., & Carter, S. (2006). Rumination and experiential avoidance in depression. *Behaviour Change, 23*(3), 165–176.

Cuijpers, P., van Straten, A., & Warmerdam, L. (2007). Behavioral activation treatments of depression: A meta-analysis. *Clinical Psychology Review, 27*(3), 318–326.

Culhane, S. E., & Watson, P. J. (2003). Alexithymia, irrational beliefs, and the rational-emotive explanation of emotional disturbance. *Journal of Rational-Emotive and Cognitive Behavior Therapy, 21*(1), 57–72.

Dalgleish, T., Yiend, J., Schweizer, S., & Dunn, B. D. (2009). Ironic effects of emotion suppression when recounting distressing memories. *Emotion, 9*(5), 744–749.

Damasio, A. (2005). *Descartes' error: Emotion, reason, and the human brain.* New York: Penguin.

Darwin, C. (1965). *The expression of the emotions in man and animals.* Chicago: University of Chicago Press. (Original work published 1872)

Davidson, R. J. (2000). Affective style, psychopathology, and resilience: Brain mechanisms and plasticity. *American Psychologist, 55,* 1196–1214.

Davidson, R. J., Fox, A., & Kalin, N. H. (2007). Neural bases of emotion regulation in nonhuman primates and humans. In J. J. Gross (Ed.), *Handbook of emotion regulation* (pp. 47–68). New York: Guilford Press.

Depue, R., & Morrone-Strupinsky, J. V. (2005). A neurobehavioral model of affiliative bonding: Implications for conceptualizing a human trait of affiliation. *Behavioral and Brain Sciences, 28*(3), 313–395.

DeRubeis, R. J., & Feeley, M. (1990). Determinants of change in cognitive therapy for depression. *Cognitive Therapy and Research, 14*(5), 469–482.

DeWaal, F. (2009). *The age of empathy: Nature's lessons for a kinder society.* New York: Harmony.

DiGiuseppe, R., & Tafrate, R. C. (2007). *Understanding anger disorders.* New York: Oxford University Press.

Dugas, M. J., Buhr, K., & Ladouceur, R. (2004). The role of intolerance of uncertainty in etiology and maintenance. In R. G. Heimberg, C. L. Turk, & D. S. Mennin (Eds.), *Generalized anxiety disorder: Advances in research and practice* (pp. 143–163). New York: Guilford Press.

Dugas, M. J., & Robichaud, M. (2007). *Cognitive-behavioral treatment for generalized anxiety disorder: From science to practice.* New York: Routledge.

Dunn, B. D., Billotti, D., Murphy, V., & Dalgleish, T. (2009). The consequences of effortful emotion regulation when processing distressing material: A comparison of suppression and acceptance. *Behaviour Research and Therapy, 47*(9), 761–773.

Eibl-Eibesfeldt, I. (1975). *Ethology, the biology of behavior* (2d ed.). New York: Holt, Rinehart & Winston.

Eisenberg, N., & Fabes, R. A. (1994). Mothers' reactions to children's negative emotions: Relations to children's temperament and anger behavior. *Merrill-Palmer Quarterly, 40*(1), 138–156.

Eisenberg, N., Gershoff, E. T., Fabes, R. A., Shepard, S. A., Cumberland, A. J., Losoya, S. H., et al. (2001). Mother's emotional expressivity and children's behavior problems and social competence: Mediation through children's regulation. *Developmental Psychology, 37*(4), 475–490.

Eisenberg, N., Liew, J., & Pidada, S. U. (2001). The relations of parental emotional expressivity with quality of Indonesian children's social functioning. *Emotion, 1*(2), 116–136.

Eizaguirre, A. E., Saenz de Cabezon, A. O., Alda, I. O. d., Olariaga, L. J., & Juaniz, M. (2004). Alexithymia and its relationships with anxiety and depression in eating disorders. *Personality and Individual Differences, 36*(2), 321–331.

Ekman, P. (1993). Facial expression and emotion. *American Psychologist, 48*, 384–392.

Ekman, P., & Davidson, R. J. (1994). *The nature of emotion: Fundamental questions.* New York: Oxford University Press.

Eliot, R., Watson, J. C., Goldman, R. N., & Greenberg, L. S. (2003). *Learning emotion focused therapy.* Washington, DC: American Psychological Association.

Ellis, A. (1962). *Reason and emotion in psychotherapy.* Secaucus, NJ: Citadel Press.

Ellis, A., & MacLaren, C. (1998). *Rational emotive behavior therapy: A therapist's guide.* San Luis Obispo, CA: Impact.

Fairburn, C. G., Cooper, Z., Doll, H. A., O'Connor, M. E., Bohn, K., Hawker, D. M., et al. (2009). Transdiagnostic cognitive-behavioral therapy for patients with eating disorders: A two-site trial with 60-week follow-up. *American Journal of Psychiatry, 166*(3), 311–319.

Fairburn, C. G., Cooper, Z., & Shafran, R. (2003). Cognitive behaviour therapy for eating disorders: A "transdiagnostic" theory and treatment. *Behavior Research and Therapy, 41*(5), 509–528.

Farb, N. A. S., Segal, Z., Mayberg, V., Bean, H. J., McKeon, D., & Fatima, Z. (2007). Attending to the present: Mindfulness meditation reveals distinct neural modes of self-reference. *Social Cognitive and Affective Neuroscience, 2*(4), 313–322.

Flavell, J. H. (2004). Theory-of-mind development: Retrospect and prospect. *Merrill-Palmer Quarterly, 50*(3), 274–290.

Foa, E. B., & Kozak, M. J. (1986). Emotional processing of fear: Exposure to corrective information. *Psychological Bulletin, 99*, 20–35.

Folkman, S., & Lazarus, R. S. (1988). Coping as a mediator of emotion. *Journal of Personality and Social Psychology, 54*(3), 466–475.

Fonagy, P. (2000). Attachment and borderline personality disorder. *Journal of the American Psychoanalytic Association, 48*(4), 1129–1146; discussion, 1175–1187.

Fonagy, P. (2002). *Affect regulation, mentalization, and the development of the self.* New York: Other Press.

Fonagy, P., & Target, M. (1996). Playing with reality: I. Theory of mind and the normal development of psychic reality. *International Journal of Psychoanalysis, 77*(Pt. 2), 217–233.

Fonagy, P., & Target, M. (2007). The rooting of the mind in the body: New links between attachment theory and psychoanalytic thought. *Journal of the American Psychoanalytic Association, 55*(2), 411–456.

Forgas, J. P. (1995). Mood and judgment: The affect infusion model (AIM). *Psychological Bulletin, 117*(1), 39–66.

Forgas, J. P. (2000). Feeling is believing? The role of processing strategies in mediating affective influences on beliefs. In N. H. Frijda, A. S. R. Manstead, & S. Bem (Eds.), *Emotions and belief: How feelings influence thoughts* (pp. 108–143). New York: Cambridge University Press.

Forgas, J. P., & Bower, G. H. (1987). Mood effects on person-perception judgments. *Journal Of Personality and Social Psychology, 53*(1), 53–60.

Forgas, J. P., & Locke, J. (2005). Affective influences on causal inferences: The effects of mood on attributions for positive and negative interpersonal episodes. *Cognition and Emotion, 19*(7), 1071–1081.

Forman, E. M., Herbert, J. D., Moitra, E., Yeomans, P. D., & Geller, P. A. (2007). A randomized controlled effectiveness trial of acceptance and commitment therapy and cognitive therapy for anxiety and depression. *Behavior Modification, 31*(6), 772–799.

Fox, N. A. (1995). Of the way we were: Adult memories about attachment experiences and their role in determining infant–parent relationships: A commentary on van IJzendoorn (1995). *Psychological Bulletin, 117*(3), 404–410.

Fraley, R. C. (2002). Attachment stability from infancy to adulthood: Meta-analysis and dynamic modeling of developmental mechanisms. *Personality and Social Psychology Review, 6*(2), 123–151.

Fraley, R. C., Fazzari, D. A., Bonanno, G. A., & Dekel, S. (2006). Attachment and psychological adaptation in high exposure survivors of the September 11th attack on the World Trade Center. *Personality and Social Psychology Bulletin, 32*(4), 538–551.

Fredrickson, B. L., & Branigan, C. (2005). Positive emotions broaden the scope of attention and thought-action repertoires. *Cognition and Emotion, 19*(3), 313–332.

Fredrickson, B. L., & Losada, M. F. (2005). Positive affect and the complex dynamics of human flourishing. *American Psychologist, 60*(7), 678–686.

Freeston, M. H., Ladouceur, R., Gagnon, F., Thibodeau, N., Rheaume, J., Letarte, H., et al. (1997). Cognitive-behavioral treatment of obsessive thoughts: A controlled study. *Journal of Consulting and Clinical Psychology, 65*, 405–413.

Germer, C. K., Seigel, R. D., & Fulton, P. R. (Eds.). (2005). *Mindfulness and psychotherapy.* New York: Guilford Press.

Gevirtz, R. N. (2007). Psychophysiological perspectives on stress-related and anxiety disorders. In P. M. Lehrer, R. L. Woolfolk, & W. E. Sime (Eds.), *Principles and practice of stress management* (3rd ed., pp. 209–226). New York: Guilford Press.

Gigerenzer, G. (2007). *Gut feelings: The intelligence of the unconscious.* New York: Viking.

Gigerenzer, G., Hoffrage, U., & Goldstein, D. G. (2008). Fast and frugal heuristics are plausible models of cognition: Reply to Dougherty, Franco-Watkins, and Thomas (2008). *Psychological Review, 115*(1), 230–239.

Gilbert, P. (2007). Evolved minds and compassion in the therapeutic relationship. In P. Gilbert & R. L. Leahy (Eds.), *The therapeutic relationship in the cognitive behavioral psychotherapies* (pp. 106–142). New York: Routledge.

Gilbert, P. (2009). *The compassionate mind.* London: Constable.

Gilbert, P. (2010). *Compassion focused therapy: Distinctive features.* London: Routledge.

Gilbert, P., & Irons, C. (2005). Focused therapies and compassionate mind training for shame and self-attacking. In P. Gilbert (Ed.), *Compassion: Conceptualisations, research and use in psychotherapy* (pp. 263–326). New York: Routledge.

Gilbert, P., & Leahy, R. L. (2007). *The therapeutic relationship in the cognitive behavioral psychotherapies.* New York: Routledge.

Gilbert, P., & Tirch, D. (2007). Emotional memory, mindfulness, and compassion. In F. Didonna (Ed.), *Clinical handbook of mindfulness* (pp. 99–110). New York: Springer.

Goleman, D. (1995). *Emotional intelligence.* New York: Bantam Books.

Gortner, E. M., Rude, S. S., & Pennebaker, J. W. (2006). Benefits of expressive writing in lowering rumination and depressive symptoms. *Behavior Therapist, 37*(3), 292–303.

Gottman, J. M. (1997). *The heart of parenting: How to raise an emotionally intelligent child.* New York: Simon & Schuster.

Gottman, J. M., Katz, L. F., & Hooven, C. (1996). Parental meta-emotion philosophy and the emotional life of families: Theoretical models and preliminary data. *Journal of Family Psychology, 10*(3), 243–268.

Gottman, J. M., Katz, L. F., & Hooven, C. (1997). *Meta-emotion: How families communicate emotionally.* Mahwah, NJ: Erlbaum.

Gratz, K., Rosenthal, M., Tull, M., Lejuez, C., & Gunderson, J. (2006). An experimental investigation of emotion dysregulation in borderline personality disorder. *Journal of Abnormal Psychology, 115*, 850–855.

Gray, J. A. (2004). *Consciousness: Creeping up on the hard problem.* Oxford, UK: Oxford University Press.

Greenberg, L. S. (2002). *Emotion-focused therapy: Coaching clients to work through their feelings.* Washington, DC: American Psychological Association.

Greenberg, L. S. (2007). Emotion in the therapeutic relationship in emotion-focused therapy. In P. L. Gilbert & R. L. Leahy (Ed.), *The therapeutic relationship in the cognitive behavioral psychotherapies* (pp. 43–62). New York: Routledge.

Greenberg, L. S., & Paivio, S. C. (1997). *Working with emotions in psychotherapy.* New York: Guilford Press.

Greenberg, L. S., & Safran, J. D. (1987). *Emotion in psychotherapy: Affect, cognition, and the process of change.* New York: Guilford Press.

Greenberg, L. S., & Safran, J. D. (1990). Emotional-change processes in psychotherapy. In R. Plutchik & H.

Kellerman (Eds.), *Emotion: Theory, research, and experience: Vol. 5. Emotion, psychopathology, and psychotherapy* (pp. 59–85). San Diego, CA: Academic Press.

Greenberg, L. S., & Watson, J. C. (2005). *Emotion-focused therapy for depression* (1st ed.). Washington, DC: American Psychological Association.

Grewal, D., Brackett, M., & Salovey, P. (2006). Emotional intelligence and the self-regulation of affect. In D. K. Snyder, J. Simpson, & J. N. Hughes (Eds.), *Emotion regulation in couples and families: Pathways to dysfunction and health* (pp. 37–55). Washington, DC: American Psychological Association.

Grilo, C. M., Walker, M. L., Becker, D. F., Edell, W. S., & McGlashan, T. H. (1997). Personality disorders in adolescents with major depression, substance use disorders, and coexisting major depression and substance use disorders. *Journal of Consulting and Clinical Psychology, 65*, 328–332.

Gross, J. J. (1998a). Antecedent- and response-focused emotion regulation: Divergent consequences for experience, expression, and physiology. *Journal of Personality and Social Psychology, 74*, 224–237.

Gross, J. J. (1998b). The emerging field of emotion regulation: An integrative review. *Review of General Psychology, 2*(3), 271–299.

Gross, J. J., & John, O. P. (2003). Individual differences in two emotion regulation processes: Implications for affect, relationships, and well-being. *Journal of Personality and Social Psychology, 85*(2), 348–362.

Gross, J. J., & Thompson, R. A. (2007). Emotion regulation: Conceptual foundations. In J. Gross (Ed.), *Handbook of emotion regulation* (pp. 3–24). New York: Guilford Press.

Guidano, V. F., & Liotti, G. (1983). *Cognitive processes and the emotional disorders.* New York: Guilford Press.

Gupta, S., Zachary Rosenthal, M., Mancini, A. D., Cheavens, J. S., & Lynch, T. R. (2008). Emotion regulation skills mediate the effects of shame on eating disorder symptoms in women. *Eating Disorders, 16*(5), 405–417.

Haidt, J. (2001). The emotional dog and its rational tail: A social intuitionist approach to moral judgment. *Psychological Review, 108*, 814–834.

Hanh, T. N. (1992). *Peace is every step: The path of mindfulness in everyday life.* New York: Bantam Books.

Harvey, A., Watkins, E., Mansell, W., & Shafran, R. (2004). *Cognitive behavioural processes across psychological disorders: A transdiagnostic approach to research and treatment.* Oxford, UK: Oxford University Press.

Hayes, S. C., Barnes-Holmes, D., & Roche, B. (Eds.). (2001). *Relational frame theory: A post-Skinnerian account of human language and cognition.* New York: Plenum Press.

Hayes, S. C., Luoma, J. B., Bond, F. W., Masuda, A., & Lillis, J. (2006). Acceptance and commitment therapy: Model, processes and outcomes. *Behaviour Research and Therapy, 44*(1), 1–25.

Hayes, S. C., & Smith, S. (2005). *Get out of your mind and into your life.* Oakland, CA: New Harbinger.

Hayes, S. C., & Strosahl, K. D. (Eds.). (2004). *A practical guide to acceptance and commitment therapy.* New York: Springer-Verlag.

Hayes, S. C., Strosahl, K. D., & Wilson, K. G. (1999). *Acceptance and commitment therapy: An experiential approach to behavior change.* New York: Guilford Press.

Hayes, S. C., Strosahl, K. D., Wilson, K. G., Bissett, R. T., Pistorello, J., Toarmino, D., et al. (2004). Measuring experiential avoidance: A preliminary test of a working model. *The Psychological Record, 54*, 553–578.

Hayes, S. C., Wilson, K. G., Gifford, E. V., Follette, V. M., & Strosahl, K. (1996). Experiential avoidance and behavioral disorders: A functional approach to diagnosis and treatment. *Journal of Consulting and Clinical Psychology, 64*, 1152–1168.

Hofmann, S., Sawyer, A., Witt, A., & Oh, D. (2010). The effect of mindfulness-based therapy on anxiety and depression: A meta-analytic review. *Journal of Consulting and Clinical Psychology, 78*(10), 169–183.

Hofmann, S. G., Schulz, S. M., Meuret, A. E., Suvak, M., & Moscovitch, D. A. (2006). Sudden gains during therapy of social phobia. *Journal of Consulting and Clinical Psychology, 74*(4), 687–697.

Holmes, E. A., & Hackmann, A. (Eds.). (2004). *Mental imagery and memory in psychopathology* (Special Edition: Memory, Vol. 12, No. 4). Hove, UK: Psychology Press.

Ingram, R. E., Miranda, J., & Segal, Z. V. (1998). *Cognitive vulnerability to depression.* New York: Guilford Press.

Isley, S. L., O'Neil, R., Clatfelter, D., & Parke, R. D. (1999). Parent and child expressed affect and children's social competence: Modeling direct and indirect pathways. *Developmental Psychology, 35*(2), 547–560.

Izard, C. E. (1971). *The face of emotion.* New York: Appleton-Century-Crofts.

Izard, C. E. (2007). Basic emotions, natural kinds, emotion schemas, and a new paradigm. *Perspectives on Psychological Science, 2*(3), 260–280.

Jacobson, E. (1942). *You must relax: A practical method of reducing the strains of modern living* (rev. ed.). Oxford, UK: Whittlesey House, McGraw-Hill.

Jacobson, N. S., & Margolin, G. (1979). *Marital therapy: Strategies based on social learning and behavior exchange principles.* New York: Brunner-Routledge.

Joiner, T. E., Jr., Brown, J. S., & Kistner, J. (Eds.). (2006). *The interpersonal, cognitive, and social nature of depression.* Mahwah, NJ: Erlbaum.

Joiner, T. E., Jr., Van Orden, K. A., Witte, T. K., & Rudd, M. D. (2009). *The interpersonal theory of suicide: Guidance for working with suicidal clients.* Washington, DC: American Psychological Association.

Jones, F. P. (1997). *Freedom to change: The development and science of the Alexander Technique.* London: Mouritz.

Kabat-Zinn, J. (1990). *Full catastrophe living: The program of the stress reduction clinic at the University of Massachusetts Medical Center.* New York: Delta.

Kabat-Zinn, J. (1994). *Wherever you go there you are.* New York: Hyperion.

Kabat-Zinn, J. (2009). Foreword. In F. Didonna (Ed.), *Clinical handbook of mindfulness* (pp. xxv–xxxiii). New York: Springer.

Kamalashila. (1992). *Meditation: The Buddhist way of tranquility and insight.* Birmingham, UK: Windhorse.

Keltner, D., Horberg, E. J., & Oveis, C. (2006). Emotions as moral intuitions. In J. P. Forgas (Ed.), *Affect in social thinking and behavior* (pp. 161–175). New York: Psychology Press.

Klonsky, E. D. (2007). The functions of deliberate self-injury: A review of the evidence. *Clinical Psychology Review, 27*(2), 226–239.

Kohut, H. (1977). *The restoration of the self.* New York: International Universities Press.

Kornfield, J. (1993). *A path with heart.* New York: Bantam.

Kring, A. M., & Sloan, D. M. (Eds.). (2010). *Emotion regulation and psychopathology: A transdiagnostic approach to etiology and treatment.* New York: Guilford Press.

Kunreuther, H., Slovic, P., Gowda, R., & Fox, J. C. (Eds.). (2002). *The affect heuristic: Implications for understanding and managing risk-induced stigma. Judgments, decisions, and public policy.* New York: Cambridge University Press.

Lazarus, R. S. (1982). Thoughts on the relations between emotion and cognition. *American Psychologist, 37*(9), 1019–1024.

Lazarus, R. S. (1991). Cognition and motivation in emotion. *American Psychologist, 46*(4), 352–367.

Lazarus, R. S. (1999). *Stress and emotion: A new synthesis.* New York: Springer.

Lazarus, R. S., & Folkman, S. (1984). *Stress, appraisal, and coping.* New York: Springer.

Leahy, R. L. (2001). *Overcoming resistance in cognitive therapy.* New York: Guilford Press.

Leahy, R. L. (2002). A model of emotional schemas. *Cognitive and Behavioral Practice, 9*(3), 177–190.

Leahy, R. L. (2003a). *Cognitive therapy techniques: A practitioner's guide.* New York: Guilford Press.

Leahy, R. L. (2003b). Emotional schemas and resistance. In R. L. Leahy (Ed.), *Roadblocks in cognitive-behavioral therapy: Transforming challenges into opportunities for change* (pp. 91–115). New York: Guilford Press.

Leahy, R. L. (2005a). A social-cognitive model of validation. In P. Gilbert (Ed.), *Compassion: Conceptualisations, research, and use in psychotherapy* (pp. 195–217). London: Routledge.

Leahy, R. L. (2005b). *The worry cure: Seven steps to stop worry from stopping you.* New York: Crown.

Leahy, R. L. (2007a). Emotion and psychotherapy. *Clinical Psychology: Science and Practice, 14*(4), 353–357.

Leahy, R. L. (2007b). Emotional schemas and resistance to change in anxiety disorders. *Cognitive and Behavioral Practice, 14*(1), 36–45.

Leahy, R. L. (2009). Resistance: An emotional schema therapy (EST) approach. In G. Simos (Ed.), *Cognitive behavior therapy: A guide for the practicing clinician* (Vol. 2, pp. 187–204). London: Routledge.

Leahy, R. L. (2010). *Beat the blues before they beat you: Depression free.* New York: Hay House.

Leahy, R. L., Beck, J., & Beck, A. T. (2005). Cognitive therapy for the personality disorders. In S. Strack (Ed.), *Handbook of personology and psychopathology* (pp. 442–461). Hoboken, NJ: Wiley.

Leahy, R. L., & Holland, S. J. (2000). *Treatment plans and interventions for depression and anxiety disorders.* New York: Guilford Press.

Leahy, R. L., & Kaplan, D. (2004, November). *Emotional schemas and relationship adjustment.* Paper presented at the meeting of the Association for Advancement of Behavior Therapy, New Orleans, LA.

Leahy, R. L., & Napolitano, L. A. (2005, November). *What are the emotional schema predictors of personality disorders?* Paper presented at the meeting of the Association for Behavioral and Cognitive Therapies, Washington, DC.

Leahy, R. L., & Napolitano, L. A. (2006). *Do metacognitive beliefs about worry differ across the personality disorders?* Paper presented at the meeting of the Anxiety Disorders Association of America, Miami, FL.

LeDoux, J. E. (1996). *The emotional brain: The mysterious underpinnings of emotional life.* New York: Simon & Schuster.

LeDoux, J. E. (2000). Emotion circuits in the brain. *Annual Review of Neuroscience, 23,* 155–184.

LeDoux, J. E. (2003). The emotional brain, fear, and the amygdala. *Cellular and Molecular Neurobiology, 23*(4–5), 727–738.

Linehan, M. M. (1993a). *Cognitive-behavioral treatment of borderline personality disorder.* New York: Guilford Press.

Linehan, M. M. (1993b). *Skills training manual for treating borderline personality disorder.* New York: Guilford Press.

Linehan, M. M., Bohus, M., & Lynch, T. R. (2007). Dialectical behavior therapy for pervasive emotion dysregulation: Theoretical and practical underpinnings. In J. Gross (Ed.), *Handbook of emotion regulation* (pp. 581–605). New York: Guilford Press.

Little, P., Lewith, G., Webley, F., Evans, M., Beattie, A., Middleton, K., et al. (2008). Randomised controlled trial of Alexander Technique lessons, exercise, and massage (ATEAM) for chronic and recurrent back pain. *British Medical Journal, 337,* 438–452.

Lundh, L.-G., Johnsson, A., Sundqvist, K., & Olsson, H. (2002). Alexithymia, memory of emotion, emotional awareness, and perfectionism. *Emotion, 2*(4), 361–379.

Luoma, J. B., Hayes, S. C., & Walser, R. (2007). *Learning ACT: An acceptance and commitment therapy skills-training manual for therapists.* Oakland, CA: New Harbinger.

Lutz, A., Brefczynski-Lewis, J., Johnstone, T., & Davidson, R. J. (2008). Regulation of the neural circuitry of emotion by compassion meditation: Effects of meditative expertise. *PLoS ONE, 3*(3), e1897.

Lynch, T. R., Chapman, A., Rosenthal, M. Z., Kuo, J. R., & Linehan, M. M. (2006). Mechanisms of change in dialectical behavior therapy: Theoretical and empirical observations. *Journal of Consulting and Clinical Psychology, 62*(4), 459–480.

Mahoney, M. J. (2003). *Constructive psychotherapy: A practical guide.* New York: Guilford Press.

Main, M., Kaplan, N., & Cassidy, J. (1985). Security in infancy, childhood, and adulthood: A move to the level of representation. In I. Bretherton & E. Waters (Eds.), Growing points of attachment theory and research. *Monographs of the Society for Research in Child Development, 50*(1–2, Serial No. 209), 66–104.

Marks, I. M. (1987). *Fears, phobias, and rituals: Panic, anxiety, and their disorders.* New York: Oxford University Press.

Martell, C. R., Addis, M. E., & Jacobson, N. S. (2001). *Depression in context: Strategies for guided action.* New York: Norton.

Martell, C. R., Dimidjian, S., & Herman-Dunn, R. (2010). *Behavioral activation for depression: A clinician's guide.* New York: Guilford Press.

Mathews, G., Zeidner, M., & Roberts, R. D. (2002). *Emotional intelligence: Science and myth.* Cambridge, MA: MIT Press.

Matthews, K. A., Woodall, K. L., Kenyon, K., & Jacob, T. (1996). Negative family environment as a predictor of boys' future status on measures of hostile attitudes, interview behavior, and anger expression. *Health Psychology, 15*(1), 30–37.

Mayer, J. D., & Salovey, P. (1997). What is emotional intelligence? In P. Salovey & D. J. Sluyter (Eds.), *Emotional development and emotional intelligence: Educational implications* (pp. 3–31). New York: Basic Books.

Mayer, J. D., Salovey, P., & Caruso, D. R. (2000). Models of emotional intelligence. In R. J. Sternberg (Ed.), *Handbook of human intelligence* (2nd ed., pp. 396–420). New York: Cambridge University Press.

Mayer, J. D., Salovey, P., & Caruso, D. R. (2004). Emotional intelligence: Theory, findings, and implications. *Psychological Inquiry, 15*(3), 197–215.

Mennin, D., Heimberg, R., Turk, C., & Fresco, D. (2002). Applying an emotion regulation framework to integrative approaches to generalized anxiety disorder. *Clinical Psychology: Science and Practice, 9,* 85–90.

Mennin, D. S., Turk, C. L., Heimberg, R. G., & Carmin, C. N. (2004). Regulation of emotion in generalized anxiety disorder. In M. A. Reinecke & D. A. Clark (Eds.), *Cognitive therapy over the lifespan: Evidence and practice* (pp. 60–89). New York: Guilford Press.

Miranda, J., Gross, J. J., Persons, J. B., & Hahn, J. (1998). Mood matters: Negative mood induction activates dysfunctional attitudes in women vulnerable to depression. *Cognitive Therapy and Research, 22*(4), 363–376.

Miranda, J., & Persons, J. B. (1988). Dysfunctional attitudes are mood-state dependent. *Journal of Abnormal Psychology, 97*(1), 76–79.

Mischel, W. (2001). Toward a cumulative science of persons: Past, present, and prospects. In W. T. O'Donohue, D. A. Henderson, S. C. Hayes, J. E. Fisher, & L. J. Hayes (Eds.), *A history of the behavioral therapies: Founders' personal histories* (pp. 233–251). Reno, NV: Context Press.

Mischel, W., & Shoda, Y. (2010). The situated person. In B. Mesquita, L. F. Barrett, & E. R. Smith (Eds.), *The mind in context* (pp. 149–173). New York: Guilford Press.

Monson, C. M., Price, J. L., Rodriguez, B. F., Ripley, M. P., & Warner, R. A. (2004). Emotional deficits in military-related PTSD: An investigation of content and process disturbances. *Journal of Traumatic Stress, 17*(3), 275–279.

Mowrer, O. H. (1939). A stimulus-response analysis of anxiety and its role as a reinforcing agent. *Psychological Review, 46,* 553–565.

Napolitano, L., & McKay, D. (2005). Dichotomous thinking in borderline personality disorder. *Cognitive Therapy and Research, 31*(6), 717–726.

Neff, K. D. (2003). Development and validation of a scale to measure self-compassion. *Self and Identity, 2,* 223–250.

Neff, K. D. (2009). Self-compassion. In M. R. Leary & R. H. Hoyle (Eds.), *Handbook of individual differences in social behavior* (pp. 561–573). New York: Guilford Press.

Neff, K. D., Kirkpatrick, K., & Rude, S. S. (2007). Self-compassion and its link to adaptive psychological functioning. *Journal of Research in Personality, 41,* 139–154.

Neff, K. D., Rude, S. S., & Kirkpatrick, K. (2007). An examination of self-compassion in relation to positive psychological functioning and personality traits. *Journal of Research in Personality, 41,* 908–916.

Nesse, R. M. (2000). Is depression an adaptation? *Archives of General Psychiatry, 57,* 14–20.

Nesse, R. M., & Ellsworth, P. C. (2009). Evolution, emotions, and emotional disorders. *American Psychologist, 64*(2), 129–139.

Nock, M. K. (2008). Actions speak louder than words: An elaborated theoretical model of the social functions of self-injury and other harmful behaviors. *Applied and Preventive Psychology, 12*(4), 159–168.

Nolen-Hoeksema, S. (2000). The role of rumination in depressive disorders and mixed anxiety/depressive symptoms. *Journal of Abnormal Psychology, 109,* 504–511.

Nolen-Hoeksema, S., Stice, E., Wade, E., & Bohon, C. (2007). Reciprocal relations between rumination and bulimic, substance abuse, and depressive symptoms in female adolescents. *Journal of Abnormal Psychology, 116*(1), 198–207.

Novaco, R. W. (1975). *Anger control: The development and evaluation of an experimental treatment.* Oxford, UK: Lexington.

Ochsner, K. N., & Feldman Barrett, L. (2001). A multiprocess perspective on the neuroscience of emotion. In T. J. Mayne & G. A. Bonnano (Eds.), *Emotion: Current issues and future directions* (pp. 38–81). New York: Guilford Press.

Ochsner, K. N., & Gross, J. J. (2005). The cognitive control of emotion. *Trends in Cognitive Sciences, 9*(5), 242–249.

Ochsner, K. N., & Gross, J. J. (2007). The neural architecture of emotion regulation. In J. J. Gross (Ed.), *Handbook of emotion regulation* (pp. 87–109). New York: Guilford Press.

Paxton, S. J., & Diggens, J. (1997). Avoidance coping, binge eating, and depression: An examination of the escape theory of binge eating. *International Journal of Eating Disorders, 22,* 83–87.

Pennebaker, J. W. (1997). Writing about emotional experiences as a therapeutic process. *Psychological Science, 8,* 162–166.

Pennebaker, J. W., & Francis, M. E. (1996). Cognitive, emotional, and language processes in disclosure. *Cognition and Emotion, 10,* 601–626.

Pennebaker, J. W., & Seagal, J. D. (1999). Forming a story: The health benefits of narrative. *Journal of Clinical Psychology, 55,* 1243–1254.

Phelps, E. A., & LeDoux, J. E. (2005). Contributions of the amygdala to emotion processing: From animal models to human behavior. *Neuron, 48*(2), 175–187.

Purdon, C., & Clark, D. A. (1999). Metacognition and obsessions. *Clinical Psychology and Psychotherapy, 6*(2), 102–110.

Quirk, G. J., & Gehlert, D. R. (2003). Inhibition of the amygdala: Key to pathological states? In P. Shinnick-Gallagher & A. Pitkanen (Eds.), *The amygdala in brain function: Basic and clinical approaches* (Vol. 985, pp. 263–272). New York: New York Academy of Sciences.

Rachman, S. J. (1997). A cognitive theory of obsessions. *Behaviour Research and Therapy, 35,* 793–802.

Rahula, W. (1958). *What the Buddha taught.* New York: Grove Press.

Rehm, L. P. (1981). *Behavior therapy for depression: Present status and future directions.* New York: Academic Press.

Rinpoche, M. Y. (2007). *The joy of living: Unlocking the secret and science of happiness.* New York: Harmony Books.

Riskind, J. H. (1997). Looming vulnerability to threat: A cognitive paradigm for anxiety. *Behaviour Research and Therapy, 35*(8), 685–702.

Riskind, J. H., Black, D., & Shahar, G. (2009). Cognitive vulnerability to anxiety in the stress generation process: Interaction between the looming cognitive style and anxiety sensitivity. *Journal of Anxiety Disorders, 24*(1), 124–128.

Robinson, P., & Strosahl, K. D. (2008). *The mindfulness and acceptance workbook for depression: Using acceptance and commitment therapy to move through depression and create a life worth living.* Oakland, CA: New Harbinger.

Roelofs, J., Rood, L., Meesters, C., Te Dorsthorst, V., Bogels, S., Alloy, L. B., et al. (2009). The influence of rumination and distraction on depressed and anxious mood: A prospective examination of the response styles theory in children and adolescents. *European Child and Adolescent Psychiatry, 18,* 635–642.

Roemer, E., & Orsillo, S. M. (2009). *Mindfulness- and acceptance-based behavior therapies in practice.* New York: Guilford Press.

Roemer, E., Salters, K., Raffa, S., & Orsillo, S. (2005). Fear and avoidance of internal experiences in GAD: Preliminary tests of a conceptual model. *Cognitive Therapy and Research, 29*(1), 71–88.

Rogers, C. (1965). *Client centered therapy: Its current practice, implications and theory.* Boston: Houghton-Mifflin.

Rothbaum, F., & Weisz, J. R. (1994). Parental caregiving and child externalizing behavior in nonclinical samples: A meta-analysis. *Psychological Bulletin, 116*(1), 55–74.

Safran, J. D., Muran, J. C., Samstag, L. W., & Stevens, C. (2002). Repairing alliance ruptures. In J. C. Norcross (Ed.), *Psychotherapy relationships that work* (pp. 23–254). New York: Oxford University Press.

Segal, Z. V., Williams, J. M. G., & Teasdale, J. D. (2002). *Mindfulness-based cognitive therapy for depression: A new approach to preventing relapse.* New York: Guilford Press.

Selman, R. L., Jaquette, D., & Lavin, D. R. (1977). Interpersonal awareness in children: Toward an integration of developmental and clinical child psychology. *American Journal of Orthopsychiatry, 47*(2), 264–274.

Selye, H. (1974). *Stress without distress.* New York: Dutton.

Selye, H. (1978). *The stress of life.* Oxford, UK: McGraw-Hill.

Siegel, D. (2007). *The mindful brain.* New York: Norton.

Siegel, R., Germer, C. K., & Olendzki, A. (2009). Mindfulness: What is it? Where did it come from? In F. Didonna (Ed.), *Clinical handbook of mindfulness* (pp. 17–35). New York: Springer.

Simon, H. A. (1983). *Reason in human affairs.* Stanford, CA: Stanford University Press.

Sloman, L., Gilbert, P., & Hasey, G. (2003). Evolved mechanisms in depression: The role and interaction of attachment and social rank in depression. *Journal of Affective Disorders, 74*(2), 107–121.

Smucker, M. R., & Dancu, C. V. (1999). *Cognitive-behavioral treatment for adult survivors of childhood trauma: Imagery rescripting and reprocessing.* Northvale, NJ: Jason Aronson.

Smyth, J. M., & Pennebaker, J. W. (2008). Exploring the boundary conditions of expressive writing: In search of the right recipe. *British Journal of Health Psychology, 13,* 1–7.

Sroufe, L., & Waters, E. (1977). Heart rate as a convergent measure in clinical and developmental research. *Merrill-Palmer Quarterly, 23*(1), 3–27.

Stewart, I., Barnes-Holmes, D., Hayes, S. C., & Lipkens, R. (2001). Relations among relations: Analogies, metaphors, and stories. In S. C. Hayes, D. Barnes-Holmes, & B. Roche (Eds.), *Relational frame theory: A post-Skinnerian account of human language and cognition* (pp. 73–86). New York: Plenum Press.

Stewart, S. H., Zvolensky, M. J., & Eifert, G. H. (2002). The relations of anxiety sensitivity, experiential avoidance, and alexithymic coping to young adults' motivations for drinking. *Behavior Modification, 26*(2), 274–296.

Stone, E. A., Lin, Y., Rosengarten, H., Kramer, H. K., & Quartermain, D. (2003). Emerging evidence for a central epinephrine-innervated alpha 1-adrenergic system that regulates behavioral activation and is impaired in depression. *Neuropsychopharmacology, 28*(8), 1387–1399.

Stuart, R. B. (1980). *Helping couples change: A social learning approach to marital therapy.* New York: Guilford Press.

Sturmey, P. (2009). Behavioral activation is an evidence-based treatment for depression. *Behavior Modification, 33*(6), 818–829.

Suveg, C., Sood, E., Barmish, A., Tiwari, S., Hudson, J. L., & Kendall, P. C. (2008). "I'd rather not talk about it": Emotion parenting in families of children with an anxiety disorder. *Journal of Family Psychology, 22*(6), 875–884.

Tamir, M., John, O. P., Srivastava, S., & Gross, J. J. (2007). Implicit theories of emotion: Affective and social outcomes across a major life transition. *Journal of Personality and Social Psychology, 92*(4), 731–744.

Tang, T. Z., & DeRubeis, R. J. (1999). Sudden gains and critical sessions in cognitive-behavioral therapy for depression. *Journal of Consulting and Clinical Psychology, 67*(6), 894–904.

Tang, T. Z., DeRubeis, R. J., Hollon, S. D., Amsterdam, J., & Shelton, R. (2007). Sudden gains in cognitive therapy of depression and depression relapse/recurrence. *Journal of Consulting and Clinical Psychology, 75*(3), 404–408.

Taylor, G. J. (1984). Alexithymia: Concept, measurement, and implications for treatment. *The American Journal of Psychiatry, 141,* 725–732.

Taylor, G. J., Bagby, R., & Parker, J. D. A. (1997). *Disorders of affect regulation: Alexithymia in medical and psychiatric illness.* New York: Cambridge University Press.

Tengwall, R. (1981). A note on the influence of F. M. Alexander on the development of Gestalt therapy. *Journal of the History of the Behavioral Sciences, 17*(1), 126–130.

Thera, S. (2003). *The way of mindfulness.* Kandy, Sri Lanka: Buddhist Publication Society.

Tirch, D., & Amodio, R. (2006). Beyond mindfulness and posttraumatic stress disorder. In M. G. T. Kwee, K. J. Gergen, & F. Koshikawa (Eds.), *Horizons in Buddhist psychology* (pp. 101–118). Taos, NM: Taos Institute.

Tirch, D. D., Leahy, R. L., & Silberstein, L. (2009, November). *Relationships among emotional schemas, psychological flexibility, dispositional mindfulness, and emotion regulation.* Paper presented at the meeting of the Association for Behavioral and Cognitive Therapies, New York.

Troy, M., & Sroufe, L. (1987). Victimization among preschoolers: Role of attachment relationship history. *Journal of the American Academy of Child and Adolescent Psychiatry, 26*(2), 166–172.

Turk, C., Heimberg, R. G., Luterek, J. A., Mennin, D. S., & Fresco, D. M. (2005). Delineating emotion regulation deficits in generalized anxiety disorder: A comparison with social anxiety disorder. *Cognitive Therapy and Research, 29,* 89–106.

Twemlow, S. W., Fonagy, P., Sacco, F. C., O'Toole, M. E., & Vernberg, E. (2002). Premeditated mass shootings in schools: Threat assessment. *Journal of the American Academy of Child and Adolescent Psychiatry, 41*(4), 475–477.

Urban, J., Carlson, E., Egeland, B., & Sroufe, L. (1991). Patterns of individual adaptation across childhood. *Development and Psychopathology, 3*(4), 445–460.

van IJzendoorn, M. (1995). Adult attachment representations, parental responsiveness, and infant attachment: A meta-analysis on the predictive validity of the Adult Attachment Interview. *Psychological Bulletin, 117*(3), 387–403.

Veen, G., & Arntz, A. (2000). Multidimensional dichotomous thinking characterizes borderline personality disorder. *Cognitive Therapy and Research, 24*(1), 23–45.

Völlm, B. A., Taylor, A. N. W., Richardson, P., Corcoran, R., Stirling, J., McKie, S., et al. (2006). Neuronal correlates of theory of mind and empathy: A functional magnetic resonance imaging study in a nonverbal task. *NeuroImaging, 29,* 90–98.

Wagner, A. W., & Linehan, M. M. (1998). Dissociation. In V. M. Follette, J. I. Ruzek, & F.R. Abueg (Eds.), *Cognitive-behavioral therapies for trauma.* New York: Guilford Press.

Wagner, A. W., & Linehan, M. M. (2006). Applications of dialectical behavior therapy to posttraumatic stress disorder and related problems. In V. M. Follette & J. I. Ruzek (Eds.), *Cognitive-behavioral therapies for trauma* (2nd ed., pp. 117–145). New York: Guilford Press.

Walser, R. D., & Hayes, S. C. (2006). Acceptance and commitment therapy in the treatment of posttraumatic stress disorder: Theoretical and applied issues. In V. M. Follette & J. I. Ruzek (Eds.), *Cognitive-behavioral therapies for trauma* (2nd ed., pp. 146–172). New York: Guilford Press.

Wang, S. (2005). A conceptual framework for integrating research related to the physiology of compassion and the wisdom of Buddhist teachings. In P. Gilbert (Ed.), *Compassion: Conceptualisations, research and use in psychotherapy* (pp. 75–120). New York: Routledge.

Wegner, D. M., Schneider, D. J., Carter, S., & White, T. (1987). Paradoxical effects of thought suppression. *Journal of Personality and Social Psychology, 53*, 5–13.

Wells, A. (2004). A cognitive model of GAD: Metacognitions and pathological worry. In R. G. Heimberg, C. L. Turk, & D. S. Mennin (Eds.), *Generalized anxiety disorder: Advances in research and practice* (pp. 164–186). New York: Guilford Press.

Wells, A. (2009). *Metacognitive therapy for anxiety and depression.* New York: Guilford Press.

Wenzlaff, R. M., & Wegner, D. M. (2000). Thought suppression. In S. T. Fiske (Ed.), *Annual review of psychology* (Vol. 51, pp. 59–91). Palo Alto, CA: Annual Reviews.

Wilson, D. S., & Wilson, E. O. (2007). Rethinking the theoretical foundation of sociobiology. *Quarterly Review of Biology, 82*(4), 327–348.

Wilson, K. G., & DuFrene, T. (2009). *Mindfulness for two: An acceptance and commitment therapy approach to mindfulness in psychotherapy.* Oakland, CA: New Harbinger.

Wolpe, J. (1958). *Psychotherapy by reciprocal inhibition.* Stanford, CA: Stanford University Press.

Yen, S., Zlotnick, C., & Costello, E. (2002). Affect regulation in women with borderline personality traits. *Journal of Nervous and Mental Diseases, 190*, 696.

Young, J. E. (1990). *Cognitive therapy for personality disorders: A schema-focused approach.* Sarasota, FL: Professional Resource Exchange.

Young, J. E., Klosko, J. S., & Weishaar, M. E. (2003). *Schema therapy: A practitioner's guide.* New York: Guilford Press.

Zajonc, R. B. (1980). Feeling and thinking: Preferences need no inferences. *American Psychologist, 35*, 151–175.

Zettle, R. D., & Hayes, S. C. (1987). A component and process analysis of cognitive therapy. *Psychological Reports, 61*, 939–953.

Zweig, R. D., & Leahy, R. L. (in press). Eating Disorders and Weight Management: Treatment Plans and Interventions. New York: Guilford Press.

Index

Note: Page numbers in *italics* indicate figures.